THE TRUTH

(Previous ~~Edition~~)

Many useful facts and opinions about the medical and social aspects of AIDS.
Nursing Times

Should be available to every GP for his own use and for lending to those concerned . . . well referenced yet written with a minimum of technical jargon.

The Physician

A wealth of research and published material from medical and popular sources in a detailed and extensively referenced book.
British Medical Journal

Useful and interesting book that patients will read and benefit from.
Journal of Royal College of General Practitioners

Excellent and thoroughly readable book.
Caring Professions Concern (CICP)

Probably the best single volume of the whole AIDS issue available today. I recommend it to pastors and those with care responsibility as well as others with more general interest.

Restoration

If *Which?* offers a best buy then *The Truth About AIDS* is my choice . . . the tone, suggestions and response seem to mirror exactly what Jesus would require of us all in the current crisis.

Third Way

Personal faith, questions and weaknesses are honestly shared by a Christian doctor who does not regard the finality of death as failure.
Life and Work

Dr Patrick Dixon MA MBBS read medical sciences at King's College Cambridge, completing medical training at Charing Cross Hospital, London. He specialised in the care of the dying and AIDS through work at St Joseph's Hospice in Hackney, and at University College Hospital as part of the Community Care Support Team, before starting an independent AIDS organisation. He is the founder of the leading national and international AIDS agency ACET (AIDS Care Education and Training) which has care and prevention programmes throughout the UK, as well as working in Uganda, Tanzania, Romania and Thailand. He is the leader of Bridge Church in West London, part of the Pioneer network of churches and a member of the Pioneer Team caring for churches, planting churches and training leaders. A public speaker and broadcaster, he is also author of AIDS and You *and* The Genetic Revolution.

The Truth About AIDS

DR PATRICK DIXON

KINGSWAY PUBLICATIONS
EASTBOURNE

ISBN 0 85476 495 X

Produced by Bookprint Creative Services
P.O. Box 827, BN21 3YJ, England for
KINGSWAY PUBLICATIONS LTD
Lottbridge Drove, Eastbourne, E. Sussex BN23 6NT
Printed in Finland

To all who feel rejected because of AIDS

Contents

Abbreviations

I hate jargon.

If you want a book full of technical terms then look elsewhere.

You will find a glossary at the back. It is not there to help you decipher this book, but to translate other things you may read or hear.

The term 'HIV' is used to describe a group of viruses which causes AIDS or related conditions in some or all of those infected. It is short for Human Immunodeficiency Virus.

'AIDS' is the only other abbreviation used often. It is short for Acquired Immune Deficiency Syndrome.

Many people who have developed AIDS, their families and their friends dislike the implied meanings of phrases such as 'AIDS sufferer', 'AIDS patient' and 'AIDS victim'. They prefer 'people who have developed AIDS'. I have tried to respect that, but to substitute five words for two throughout the book became cumbersome.

The message of this book is that AIDS is not just a medical condition. AIDS represents a lot of individual people who are experiencing a devastating tragedy.

Often I have used 'he' or 'his', although the person could equally well be a woman. Please do not infer from this that AIDS is a male gay disease. As you will see, nothing could be further from the truth.

Preface to Third Edition

The first edition of this book in November 1987 caused quite a stir. Packed with the latest facts and figures on AIDS, and backed by literally hundreds of scientific references and footnotes, it challenged what was being said.

Written originally to motivate churches to get involved in a practical, caring response, it found a much wider audience and has been revised and updated several times. Since then 19,000 new research papers have been published, governments have revised figures and forecasts, and major new problems have emerged. These are the reasons for a completely new edition, with over 300 new references.

Even in 1987 the African problem appeared vast, and Eastern Europe seemed likely to be hard hit. Both situations are more extensive than I feared then. Real progress on treatments and vaccines has been disappointingly slow despite press headlines. It is also depressing to see the lack of research being published on the effect of prevention programmes— only one in ten papers, and very few of these give us the answers we so urgently need on how to change behaviour most effectively. Western governments are revising down original forecasts for their own countries. At the same time there has been an abandonment of lower risk behaviour by some.

It is bizarre that now we are certain that at least 70% of all 15 million HIV infections worldwide have been heterosexually spread, some still say they do not accept significant heterosexual spread will happen in the West.

It is surprising that well-respected newspapers can still print stories suggesting that HIV is not the cause of AIDS, that there is no AIDS epidemic in Africa and that heterosexuals are only at risk from anal intercourse. It seems we have a long way to go in unravelling the confusion. There is therefore an urgent need for this new edition, which particularly addresses some of these recurring debates, and how we can respond.

Stigma, rejection, social isolation, ignorance and fear are unfortunately still hugely present in many countries. People with AIDS continue to fight illness and die in appalling conditions, and in many countries a mixture of politics, culture and other sensitivities still prevents effective high-impact education programmes.

As a direct result of this book, a major international AIDS initiative was launched in the UK in June 1988, called ACET (AIDS Care Education and Training). ACET (a Christian agency) has since grown to become the largest independent provider of practical care to those ill with HIV/AIDS at home in the UK, and is also the UK's largest provider of face-to-face AIDS lessons in schools. Over 600,000 pupils have received ACET's colour booklets on AIDS. ACET is also working overseas in partnership with churches, together with government and other non-governmental organisations such as UNICEF and the World Health Organisation. ACET has ongoing work in Uganda, Tanzania, Romania and Thailand. The need has never been more urgent for a practical, professionally-based response, backed by volunteers.

While every country is unique, basic principles of unconditional care and high-impact education remain the same. God calls us all, I believe, to accept all people and to extend his love to them regardless of whether or not we agree with what they do. My hope and prayer is that this new edition will further stimulate a massive, yet sensitive, worldwide response to AIDS.

May 1994

Acknowledgements

Thank you first to Kingsway Publications who initially suggested that I write this book, and in particular to Rachel Ashley-Pain for her excellent work on this and previous editions. She has devoted many hours to ensuring an accurate, readable and well-referenced text. Maintaining a technical book of this size in a rapidly changing field has been a big task.

Thank you to John Spencer FRCS who has been a continual source of wisdom and good counsel over the years and originally encouraged me when I was first thinking of becoming involved in the care of those who were very ill because of AIDS. He made many helpful suggestions to clarify parts of the first edition that were ambiguous or obscure.

This book would not have been possible without the enormous practical care, support and kindness from many in the group of churches I belong to (Bridge and Ealing).

I am indebted to Gerald Coates of Pioneer for his practical support, care, encouragement and shaping of priorities, together with other members of the Pioneer team. His emphasis on relationships, openness, honesty, integrity and community involvement has influenced my life and this book, and has led to the setting up of AIDS Care Education and Training (ACET) as a channel of practical help for those in need. I am part of another wonderful team of people at ACET whose influence now stretches to many nations through a network of practical care and prevention. This fourth edition draws on the wealth of six years of our national and international experience. I am particularly indebted to Maurice Adams, now Chief Executive, for his energetic advice, encouragement, support and expertise; to Jayne Clemence and Peter Glover for their innumerable comments and suggestions; and to the other team members, both past and present, who have all taught me so much about God's compassion and a Christian response. Caroline Akehurst of the Bureau of Hygiene and Tropical Diseases does a magnificent job with limited resources, producing various information services and bulletins on AIDS. Dr Caroline Collier was also helpful.

Dr George Rutherford, director of the AIDS unit in San Francisco, and his secretary Ann Schlegel, were of immense help during my visit there.

Bea Roman, then the director of development of the Shanti Project in San Francisco, contributed enormously to my understanding of the human toll of AIDS in the United States. The AIDS office of the Episcopal cathedral was also very helpful. Clive Calver, general director of the Evangelical Alliance, has been a great source of vision and support. Dr Rob George has been a helpful friend and encourager, and together with Roger Schofield has provided many helpful thoughts and insights into how the Christian community can respond to the challenge of AIDS. There are countless others I would like to thank but cannot name who have contributed stories and information—or just talked about what it is like to be dying of AIDS or to lose a good friend.

I owe a lot to St Christopher's Hospice and to all who have pioneered excellence in hospice care under Dame Cicely Saunders OBE. It was they who first fired my enthusiasm for the care of the dying. I spent four weeks there working on the wards as a nursing auxiliary when I was a medical student on one of their residential courses. It was a life-changing experience. Dr Hanratty, then medical director of St Joseph's Hospice in Hackney, has been a great influence on me and showed me the practical aspects of good pain control. It was he, along with the nursing Sisters, who convinced me that care of the dying would not become overwhelmingly depressing but was a most amazing privilege. I learned it is deeply satisfying as well as worthwhile.

I am also indebted to the Community Care Team at UCH, who taught me what it was to be a part of a truly multi-disciplinary team, with a real sense of belonging and mutual commitment.

Most of all a tribute is due to my wife, Sheila, as well as to our children, John, Caroline, Elizabeth and Paul. They have put up with a major disruption of family life while I have been doctoring, travelling, attending ACET, church and media commitments, or closeting myself away with pen, paper and computer printouts. Sheila is always encouraging and supportive, even when it has meant taking risks and sacrificing time together. Without her not a page of this book would have been written and none of it would have been checked or updated properly.

Thanks are due to Richard Ward for redrawing the graphs and maps.

A number of people have read parts of the manuscript at various stages and made innumerable comments and suggestions of which the majority have been incorporated into the book. However, the responsibility for the content is mine.

INTRODUCTION
Don't Tell People the Truth

Many people are scared of telling the truth about AIDS. They say it will cause panic. The trouble is, lack of trust in what is being said officially can cause near hysteria—as we have seen in reactions to infected surgeons or nurses recently.

My experience is that people respect you for being honest. No one believes you if you deliberately play down risks. You lose all credibility when you give the impression something is safe and someone dies after doing it. Common sense tells people that certain things must carry some risk.

It is stupid to say that if you follow guidelines you cannot become infected with the virus causing AIDS from looking after someone with the disease. Accidents happen. Guidelines may be hard to follow in all situations and they may have to be modified in the future in the light of experience. People know there are risks in nursing a person with AIDS, just as there are in being operated on by an infected surgeon. There must be. Anyone knows that. What is needed is to convince people that when you say these risks are very small you can really be trusted; that you are not giving people a false sense of security in order to persuade them to do something you know might be dangerous. When people really trust that you are telling the truth, the whole truth, and nothing but the truth—then they see what the risks really are and feel secure in knowing what they are dealing with. Knowing the truth allows them to make intelligent decisions about what to do.

15

I'm going to tell the truth as best I can.

There is a lot of extra information in the endnotes. These are in a shorthand that any librarian can understand. Sufficient information is given to turn to the exact pages of scientific publications. For reasons of space, authors' names and titles of papers have usually been omitted. Newspapers are from the UK unless stated. Use the Index and cross-references.

Not everything is referenced. Sometimes a figure or comment has been jotted down and used later although I cannot remember the source. Sometimes the source has been a personal interview. Where I want to protect the person's identity the reference is 'personal communication'. Many reference materials can be ordered from your local library or the librarian can advise you further. Student friends, doctors, or nurses will have access to much larger libraries.

This book is about people. Details of names, places, times and events have been altered where necessary to protect identity. If you think you are reading about someone or some place you know, you are probably mistaken. Some of the medical case reports in Chapter 3 are compiled from real events in a number of people's lives.

This book is written from the perspective of a doctor who is also a church leader.

Some Bible passages are written in the endnotes. These need to be read in context. Almost any argument can be constructed out of isolated Bible quotations. For three consecutive years recently I made it my business to read the Bible each year from start to finish—to catch its overall meaning and avoid 'verse grabbing' pitfalls. I encourage you to do the same.

Some parts of this book are sexually explicit and some may find this offensive. As a doctor I deal with real people in the real world who need accurate information and practical help. I regret giving offence, but my goal is to save lives and to help those affected.

I

The Extent of the Nightmare

It was 1981. In a Los Angeles doctor's office the men sitting in white coats were worried: within a few weeks they had diagnosed their fourth case of a condition so incredibly rare they had hardly expected to see it in their collective professional lifetime. They were baffled by the series of strange pneumonias that got worse despite normal antibiotics. All of the patients were men. All were young. All of them had died.

Three and a half thousand miles to the east, at a hospital in New York, several doctors were faced with a similar problem: strange tumours and lethal pneumonias in young men. What was going on?

The cases were all reported to the infectious disease centre. Could this be some sort of epidemic? Were the pneumonias and cancers caused by the same thing? What did the men have in common? Every day new reports of deaths came flooding in.[1] It was becoming clear that most, if not all, of the deceased were men who had had sex with other men. The disease quickly became labelled 'the gay plague'.

Dozens of strange infections were seen—with all the classic signs of weakened natural defences. The disease was called AIDS—Acquired Immune Deficiency Syndrome. It took some time to discover that the culprit was a tiny virus, called the Human Immunodeficiency Virus or HIV. It is now known that

17

someone can be infected with HIV for ten years or more before developing the illness called AIDS.

Just five years later, by November 1986, 15,345 people had already died, another 12,000 were dying, and a further 30,000 were feeling unwell.[2]

People were concerned that maybe up to a million people in the United States were also infected but were not yet ill.[3] At first the 'experts' predicted only one in ten of those infected would die, then two in ten, then three in ten, then nine out of ten.[4] Now many are saying that almost everyone with the infection will die.[5]

Most estimates from the early 1980s were exceeded. By April 1990 in the United States there were over 126,000 cases reported. (By the end of 1992 the number rose to 253,448 though with a broader case definition—171,480 had died.[6]) There were estimates of possibly 200–300,000 feeling unwell and maybe 700,000 infected, representing up to one in sixty of all men in the United States between the ages of twenty and fifty. In New York, AIDS is now the commonest cause of death for men and women aged twenty-five to fourty-four, with 100 AIDS deaths every week. One in every sixty-one babies is carrying HIV. By 1993 more people were dying of AIDS in the United States each year than died in the entire ten-year Vietnam War—compared to 6,000 deaths total in the UK.

The number of people already doomed in the United States makes the Vietnam tragedy look like a minor skirmish, with one new infection every thirteen minutes.[7] The coffins, if placed end to end, would stretch for 1,000 miles.[8] Yet all the time another similar but far more catastrophic disaster was silently destroying another continent, and no one had noticed.

The African experience

Some years after AIDS was first diagnosed in the United States, the first cases were recognised in Africa. Hindsight

AIDS cases, by year of diagnosis—United States, 1981–1990

(a) Total cases, cases among homosexual/bisexual men, and cases among women and heterosexual men reporting intravenous (IV)-drug use[9]

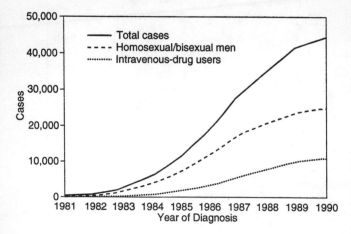

(b) Cases among persons reporting heterosexual contact with persons with, or at high risk of, HIV infection

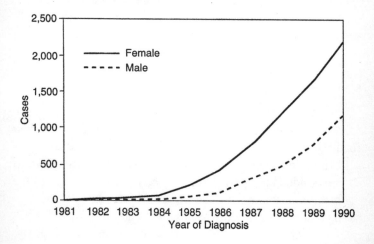

Southern Africa: estimated HIV prevalence among the sexually-active population.[10] *(See also Appendix F.)*

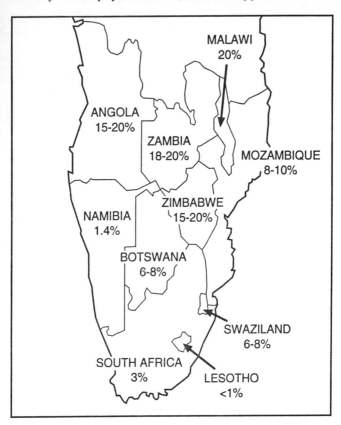

shows that for years thousands had been dying,[11] but their deaths were blamed on tuberculosis and other diseases.

In some towns and cities in Central Africa, up to a third of all young adults are now thought to be infected. A third of the truck drivers running the main north/south routes[12] and half the prostitutes in many towns are infected.[13] In some hospitals between eight and twenty-three pints of blood out of 100 are infected with HIV. One relief agency has talked unofficially about pulling out of Central Africa. 'What's the point in drilling more wells when most of the people will be dead in a few years?'[14] The World Health Organisation says 9 million were infected by early 1994.

Grandmothers are looking after their grandchildren because so many young men and women, the parents, have been wiped out by AIDS. Armies of troops in Central Africa are being depleted—not by rockets and machine guns, but by AIDS. Breadwinners for families and providers of the countries' wealth are missing. The educated élite living in the main towns and cities have often been worst hit. In the country, fields are uncultivated and cattle wander aimlessly.[15] One journalist visiting an African country recently, describes areas where whole families have been wiped out, plantations have gone back to bush and you can walk for miles without seeing anyone—a wasteland.[16] I have met someone who claims to have satellite photographs of a country in Central Africa taken two years apart, showing not deforestation, but reforestation as the amount of farming falls. It is an effect attributed to AIDS—the country is not at war. In 1991 I was told by a trusted colleague that he thought it would be hard to find a family in the African city where he lived who was not attending an AIDS funeral on average once a month. Deaths had soared among young adults in the previous three years. In Africa they call it the 'slim' disease. Some Africans believe if you sleep with only fat women you are safe. 'To be fat is to be healthy.'

Officials stand at the doors of some hospitals selecting the fit ones for treatment. Anyone who looks thin and weak is sent back into the bush—'Probably got AIDS; nothing we can do for him.' Many are sent away with perfectly treatable diseases such as tuberculosis.[17] You cannot tell the difference at the door. Years and years of careful preventive medicine is being undermined. How do you start educating about a disease which produces no illness for years, when nurses are still battling against ingrained habits just to get mothers to give their children a healthy diet?

The children's wards are full of dying children. Many are babies under one or two years old. Many are not dying of famine, but of AIDS. A terrible tragedy is that many caught the virus not while in their mothers' wombs, but from the use of unsterilised needles.[18] The problem is (as Thailand has found) that by the time a country identifies 10,000 cases it can have 500,000 infected. We must educate now.[19]

I visited Central Africa on an education project. The team I was with spoke to over 20,000 people about basic health protection. Education can be very effective.[20]

AIDS is *not* a gay plague; there are millions more women and children infected with HIV throughout the world than there are gay men. It gained this reputation in the United States because gay men were first to be diagnosed, yet seven out of ten of all infections worldwide so far, and nine out of ten last year, were heterosexually acquired.[21] Right now HIV is spreading through communities of drug addicts in the United States, to their husbands, wives, lovers, children, and out into the wider community. Sadly, too, many men, women and children have been infected from medical treatments— mainly from receiving blood or blood products prior to 1985. In other parts of the world there are 14 million people infected with HIV, of whom half a million are in Europe. Two million new infections will take place this year, half among women.[22]

The global pandemic

The World Health Organisation believes most of the 200 or so cases of new infection each day in Europe are occurring in the East.[23] In Romania, up to one in ten of all children in orphanages became infected before the revolution in 1990, and a similar percentage since.[24] The route appears to have been mainly infected needles rather than the widely reported microtransfusions used as a tonic.[25] Early unwillingness to

South and East Asia: estimated HIV prevalence among the sexually-active population.[26] *(See also Appendix F.)*

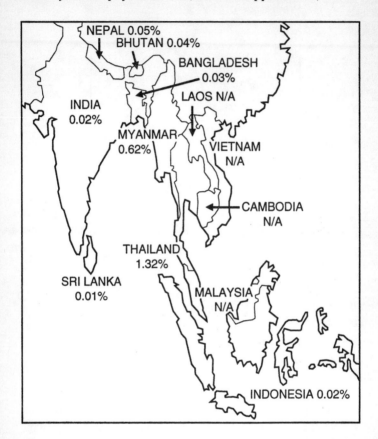

acknowledge the problem has been replaced by openness. District health campaigns have been targeted particularly at health care workers, but there is still a long way to go.

In Thailand, many experts have been predicting a serious AIDS epidemic for years because of the sex industry and international sex tourism. However, by the time the Thai government was prepared to acknowledge the situation, the

HIV in Thailand

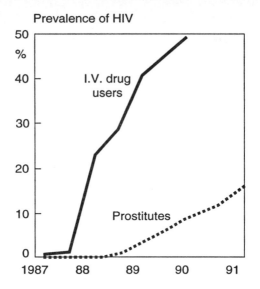

Prevalence of HIV

epidemic was well underway. In three years, half a million were infected—the great majority heterosexually.

The list goes on—Australia, New Zealand, Japan, India, Cambodia, the Philippines, Latin America, Russia, Albania. No country likes to admit that this embarrassing illness is causing difficulties. See pp 405–413 for every country.

In South East Asia, HIV is spreading so fast that it threatens to dwarf the African problem by the year 2000.[27] However, there is hope that if denial is replaced by openness, and if openness leads to intensive prevention, then the eventual size of the tragedy may be significantly reduced. South East Asia has the advantage of advanced warning—something Africa never had.

In India alone there may be more sexually-active people alive than adults in the whole of sub-Saharan Africa. What happens in the East is likely to have a massive impact on the world situation.[28] The Indian Health Organisation, an independent body from the government, has said there may be up to a million HIV-infected. In Bombay, some believe there may be over 100 new infections a day, partly related to prostitution—a third of prostitutes are infected.[29] While these estimates may be too high the World Health Organisation fears that HIV spread in India may now be even faster than in Thailand.

The global cost is growing too. By 1993 the World Health Organisation calculated the global social and economic costs of lost life were in excess of $5,000 million so far, excluding care and prevention programmes.[30] (See pp 276–281.)

The experience in the United Kingdom

The first reported case of AIDS in the United Kingdom was in 1981.[31] Today if you meet five gay men in a London bar, the chances are that one of them may be infected, although he may not know it. He may also have felt ill recently but put it down to some odd viral disease. He was right. He is beginning to experience the first symptoms of AIDS. All five may still be having sex with men (and maybe wives or other women too). In two years the numbers infected at a London clinic went up from four out of a hundred to a staggering twenty-one out of a hundred.[32] When you know that one in five of your possible partners could infect you, you start rethinking your behaviour. It is this terrible statistic that began to change gay lifestyles, not the government campaign that started two years later.[33] After all, if you knew that one in five of the people you went out with were positive, wouldn't it make you think again about 'safer sex' or sleeping with them at all?

By 1986 the numbers had risen from twenty-one to twenty-four out of a hundred. Infection levels are now relatively stable due to behaviour change, but with worrying signs of new risk-taking in some groups. For example, from 1981 to 1988 in England and Wales, the number of cases of

Projected and reported numbers of AIDS cases, England and Wales

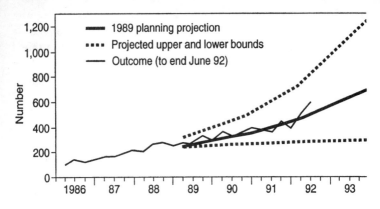

gonorrhoea in gay men fell (gonorrhoea levels are a good indication of risk-taking). In 1989, a 7.7% increase was seen. A worrying fivefold increase was seen in 1990 and 1991. Much of the increase seems to have been in younger men.[34] In one area of London, AIDS is now the commonest cause of death in men aged fifteen to forty-four.[35]

In Edinburgh, an estimated 1,500 people were infected in less than eighteen months through sharing contaminated needles. Because a drug habit is expensive, many female drug injectors turn to prostitution to obtain drugs. As a result, half of the prostitutes in Edinburgh are now infected with HIV. In London, one in sixty *heterosexual* men and women attending sex disease clinics are carrying HIV.[36]

UK forecasts revised down

By March 1994 there were 9,000 people with AIDS and 30,000 with HIV[37]—considerably less than the 50–80,000 forecast in the heady days of 1986 when it was feared that spread among gay men and drug users would continue at the same rate for the next few years.[38]

In fact, due to a remarkable reduction in risk-taking by gay men, and in needle sharing, infection rates have slowed down, with new infections almost balanced by deaths. However, no one should doubt the ever-present risk of further rapid spread if behaviour reverts to previous patterns. The spread among an estimated 100,000 drug injectors alone could be catastrophic in effect—and rapid.[39] Some have remained highly sceptical.

Although almost one in six AIDS cases and one in four of all HIV infections have been heterosexually acquired,[40] the great majority of such infections have arisen as a result of sexual activity in high-incidence countries. This has been a major component of the 1 in 500 twenty- to thirty-four-year-old women found to have HIV in London.

This highly-sensitive issue has been greatly underplayed by successive government ministers afraid of an anti-African backlash. However, hiding the truth was always a shortsighted strategy, especially since the facts were obvious to any journalist walking into an AIDS ward. For a long time, around six out of ten women with AIDS in London have been African, infected abroad. This is not a racist observation, just a tragic visible indicator of the devastation happening in many of the poorest nations. What is happening in London is of the utmost importance. It means that care agencies like ACET— which is alone involved in supporting up to a quarter of all those dying with AIDS in London—need to develop specialist cross-cultural expertise.

Denial of heterosexual risk

Many have tried to play down the heterosexual problem as a non-issue for white men and women.[41] This is remarkably shortsighted and inaccurate given that doctors and nurses are already caring for increasing numbers of white heterosexuals infected through heterosexual sex in the UK.[42]

Others then have suggested that heterosexuals only get HIV infection if they practise anal intercourse. This particular myth was exploded by a UK government study published in 1993 showing conclusively that HIV is spreading through non-traumatic vaginal sex.[43]

Some have still objected that almost every person infected heterosexually in countries like the UK has been infected through an 'at risk' partner—in other words, a partner who previously injected drugs or is bisexual or whatever. Although this is true, you would expect this in the early stages of an epidemic. Indeed, it was the situation among gay men in the UK during the early 1980s. Almost every case of infection was 'imported' and could be traced to sex with a gay man in the US.

It does not make any difference how your partner may have picked up the infection. The fact is that most people are unaware of a partner's previous risk exposure.

Having said all this, it is clear that heterosexual spread in the US or Europe is still far slower than in many developing countries. While viral variation could be the reason, with more virulent strains in some places (see Chapter 2) or some genetic susceptibility (see Chapter 5), the overwhelming evidence is that untreated sex diseases such as gonorrhoea and chancroid facilitate spread by damaging the protective surface of the genitalia.[44]

Some people have tried to make a link between hepatitis B and HIV, arguing that both are really blood-borne rather than sexually transmitted, except through anal intercourse. In fact the two viruses are totally different, with different mechanisms of infection, target cells and disease pictures. Hepatitis B, for example, is twenty times as infectious as HIV (see later chapters).

We can learn one thing from hepatitis B. In the 1970s the virus was thought not to transmit heterosexually—people made the same assumption about HIV ten years later. However, by 1989, new cases of heterosexual hepatitis B infection outnumbered cases due to homosexual intercourse by two to one, posing a global health hazard.[45] Fortunately, in contrast to HIV there is a vaccine available. Over the next decade we are likely to see widespread vaccination against this dangerous virus.[46]

The lesson is that the past does not always predict the future. The AIDS epidemic is in its very earliest stages. The infection rates in the UK are still so low in comparison to the rest of the world that it could be said that the UK epidemic has hardly begun. Most experts agree that in time—and we can argue about timescales—the great majority of HIV infection in the UK will be heterosexual, as is already the situation globally. The same is likely to be so in other developed nations. It is hard to come to any other conclusion when faced with the rapid spread of HIV in the two-thirds world and the massive growth in population movements, tourism and business travel.

In 1993 the UK Chief Medical Officer said that while it could take thirty years for the infection rate to reach 1% of the general population, by then half a million would be infected.[47]

Governments find AIDS figures hard to handle

In 1987 a senior official at the Department of Health said he expected only 30% of those infected with HIV to develop AIDS, while unofficially he thought everyone infected was going to die. I challenged this public statement in the first edition of this book. Now in released statements, officials admit that most of those infected are likely to die.

In the United Kingdom life insurance premiums have tripled for young men and doubled for young women because of AIDS.[48] This was an over-reaction, but premiums have not fallen.[49] Some people will say, 'Yes, but I'm not gay and I'm not an addict, so I'm not at risk.' A British study showed that 59% of gay men reported having sex with a woman.[50] See Chapter 4.

'Second generation' heterosexual transmission of HIV & AIDS—UK

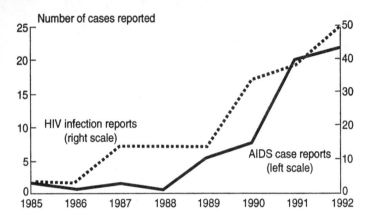

Women are becoming infected from sex with men with and without using condoms. Condoms reduce the risk enormously but not completely. Heterosexual spread of AIDS is now happening in South East Asia, as well as in many Western and Central American countries, not just in Africa.

Although, as we have seen, special reasons may be found why HIV has spread in Africa so widely, even outside Africa HIV behaves in many ways just like any other sexually-transmitted infection. And the behaviour of heterosexual men and women has been slow to change. During the height of the AIDS campaign, sexually-transmitted diseases rose by 30% in one London hospital among heterosexual men, and only one in ten were interested in using condoms.[51]

Doctors, nurses and dentists are becoming infected from patients they treat—usually following needlestick injuries—although the risk from such accidents is very low.[52] Children are becoming infected from being molested by their infected fathers.[53]   Transmission has also occurred during a bloody fight.[54] Organ transplants have infected people.[55] More than

Reports of HIV in heterosexuals—UK

'First generation' is heterosexual transmission from e.g. drug users. 'Second generation' is when the virus passes from one heterosexual to another with no other risk factors.

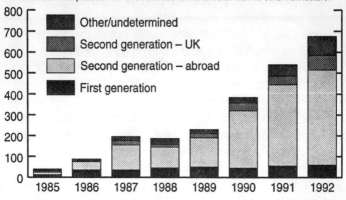

1,200 people in the United Kingdom—250 of whom were children—were infected from medical treatments before proper precautions were taken.

The majority of these children have haemophilia, a bleeding disorder treated using blood products. Until recently all of the blood was obtained from the United States. Although the British government had been warned that blood from the US could give people in the UK AIDS, they did not act immediately. By the end of March 1990, over thirty people had become infected with HIV from blood transfusions.[56] The United Kingdom became largely self-sufficient in blood products after a new laboratory costing £60 million (about $100 million) was opened on 29 April 1987.[57] Compensation has now been agreed in the UK and in a growing number of other nations.

In the United States, government and church estimates have been made that up to one third of all 57,000 Roman Catholic priests could be infected, and one high-ranking Anglican has said that he expects a similar proportion of United States Anglican clergy to be at risk also.

A US health official said, 'I and most of the public health directors I've talked to about this subject estimate that in our communities at least a third of Catholic priests under forty-five are homosexuals, and most are sexually active. They always engage in anonymous encounters, the highest risk sex of all, and when they want help they don't come to the clinics.'[58] Personal communication from a high-ranking church official in San Francisco gave the same figures. A number of priests in the United States have AIDS: some have been thrown out of the church; others have been hidden away.[59] Perhaps as a response to this situation, one Catholic Archdiocese in the US has begun insisting on HIV testing for aspiring priests and nuns—a move condemned in the press as outright discrimination, particularly as HIV infection may have arisen as a result of behaviour over ten years previously, prior to a change in faith and lifestyle.[60]

A survey of 1,500 United States Roman Catholic priests revealed that 20% are homosexually inclined and 10% are sexually active. However, surveys often underestimate due to the embarrassment of participants.

The highest-ranking cleric to die of AIDS so far is a Methodist bishop in Texas. No one knows how he became infected. In the United Kingdom *The Times* estimated that more than 100 Anglican clergy were already known to be positive by as early as 1987.[61] Several priests had already died from AIDS. An Anglican vicar quoted a doctor in saying that at least twenty clergy had full-blown AIDS. His own research suggested that 400 Anglican clergy belonged to the Gay Christian Movement.[62]

Some parts of the church in the United States and the United Kingdom are experiencing phenomenal growth as part of what some have called restoration and renewal. Thousands of young people across the country are becoming Christians each year. Often there are spectacular conversions resulting in radical changes in lifestyle.[63] Heroin addicts throw away their needles. Marriages are rebuilt. The results are often permanent—but so is the previous infection. AIDS could damage churches physically, emotionally, psychologically and spiritually—unless they are prepared.

At a conference for church leaders, I met a man who had been a drug addict before his conversion four or five years ago. He is now leading a church. This is happening all over the country. Some of these people will develop AIDS. The conference had representatives from sixty or so churches of a wide variety of denominations. Three different church leaders came to me saying they had long-standing members of their congregations who were infected with HIV or who were dying of AIDS. None of the three individuals was gay and none was from London or Edinburgh. Two were former drug addicts from the Midlands and one was a child on the south coast.

So what do we do? How can we prevent the disease? How can we cure it? How can we cope with it? The rest of this book addresses these four questions. But is AIDS really so different from any other disease, or is it just the mass hysteria and panic associated with it?

What is so special about AIDS?

At a recent major medical conference there was an argument: Is there anything special about AIDS or not?

AIDS is certainly unusual or unique in two respects. First, I do not know of any other illness today where people are beaten up, killed or denied basic medical care just because they happen to have a particular diagnosis.

Secondly, I do not know of any other illness which has so generated political debates, pressures, campaigning and aggressive activism.[64] Some companies are now saying it is hard to conduct normal medical research in the area of HIV or AIDS because the political pressures are so great that they threaten to overwhelm and interfere at every level.[65] Yet to a large extent those pressures are a result of the discrimination, prejudice and fear seen every day in many countries. It is true that some activism has been driven by members of the gay community in developed countries, rather than by drug users, heterosexuals or those with haemophilia, or those in the poorest nations—a fact which becomes very obvious at the larger international AIDS conferences.[66]

AIDS has also attracted the eccentric and the bizarre. I was recently sent literature from an organisation claiming that the US government made HIV as part of a deliberate plot to reduce the world population by 75% by 1996. The Mafia and the CIA are said to be deeply involved.[67] Equally bizarre are some of the 'cures' I am informed about, including eating earth and drinking vinegar, or high-cost preparations with no proven value.[68]

Yet in another sense there is nothing special about AIDS. It is just the latest in a long series of epidemics spread by sex.[69] Sleeping around has always carried risks to health. Now it can be lethal.

Sex diseases are common (STDs). Around 580,000 are treated with STDs in the UK each year,[70] with 12 million new cases annually in the US, two thirds in under-twenty-five-year-olds, a quarter in teenagers. Over 30 million in the US are estimated to have genital herpes. Some 56 million, or 20% of all US adults, are estimated to be carrying an STD at any time.[71] Many other nations show similar or higher rates. Worldwide there are an estimated 250 million new STD infections each year.[72] With ordinary STDs the damage is usually more obvious, immediate and less serious than with HIV. (World sexual activity: p 281; World STDs: p 319.)

More than 300 years ago a plague broke out in Europe and spread across the Western world. Vast numbers died. Early symptoms were mild, the second stage made people very ill, and half of those who developed the third stage died, many with brain damage. It was a terrible disease, and it was spread by sex. It was named 'syphilis'.

Syphilis only stopped being a major threat with the discovery of penicillin at the end of World War II. During the war, United States army recruits were warned that, after

Hitler, syphilis was Public Enemy Number One. A famous US Army war poster was of a prostitute walking with Hitler on one arm and the Japanese Emperor on the other. The caption read: 'VD (venereal disease) worst of the three.' Syphilis has not gone away; we are in the middle of a major heterosexual explosion of cases which often produce few or no symptoms and are untreated for a long period.

Gonorrhoea also became a curable sexual disease with penicillin—until the recent advent of penicillin-resistant strains which are now spreading rapidly across the globe and becoming harder and harder to treat. There is an unprecedented epidemic of genital herpes. Highly infectious, appallingly painful blisters prevent sex. (Fourteen thousand cases are reported every year in the United Kingdom and the numbers are rising.[73]) There is no cure and it can cause problems throughout a person's life. There is also a big increase in cancer of the neck of the womb (cervix), some of which is associated with a virus infection and is due to sleeping with multiple partners.

There is also the heart-rending problem of infertility. Have you ever wondered about the huge test-tube baby programme? As a medical student I remember attending the ward rounds of an obstetrics professor. He used to joke about a colleague who filled the ward with his infertile patients. He said he could tell which patients were his colleague's and not his own—his colleague's patients were the good-looking ones! The major part of his colleague's workload was people with badly damaged and scarred fallopian tubes—the thin delicate tubes which guide the egg from the ovary to the womb. The cause was an infection called pelvic inflammatory disease (PID), which can be caused by a tiny organism called chlamydia.[74] There is no treatment that can undo the damage of pelvic inflammatory disease. One in ten women develop it after being infected with chlamydia, gonorrhoea, or some other infections. It causes aches and pains that are chronically disabling, and it gradually causes the reproductive organs to stick together.

Then came a new disease—AIDS—that many people think has been around in Africa, the US and Europe for decades before recognition in the late 1980s.[75] Wherever it started, it spread slowly at first, undetected, and then explosively among men, women and young children. It was only detected as it hit the medical technology of the United States, was misdiagnosed as an American gay curiosity, and only traced to its probable roots some two or three years later.[76]

The difference between HIV-related diseases and other sexual epidemics is that HIV can infect you for years before you know it, and by the time you do it has spread to infect possibly hundreds of others. The other difference is that once you develop full-blown AIDS—which can take many years— you face almost certain death, unless you die of something else in the meantime. There is no cure and no vaccine, nor is either anywhere in sight. There are many misleading reports but no good results.

A rapidly-spreading, silent killer which is difficult to detect, infectious and lethal causes panic. Radiation disasters are similar: you cannot hear, see, feel, or touch the enemy, nor feel the damage it is doing until too late—sometimes not for years. No wonder the Chernobyl disaster caused such terrible pandemonium: false rumours, false scares, false cures, false hopes abounded. AIDS is the same today.

If a man had sex with a work colleague and three weeks later was dead, and that was repeated across the country, the impact would be dramatic. You would not need any health campaign because the coffins would be the campaign. But with HIV and AIDS the enormous time lag produces a credibility problem: the only people who really understand what is likely to hit us are the mathematicians. An invisible terror can be ignored.

If we have to wait ten years to see exactly what is happening, we will be too late. We need to learn now from what happened in San Francisco, a city I visited in 1987.

Estimated and projected annual AIDS incidences* by 'macro' region: 1980–2000

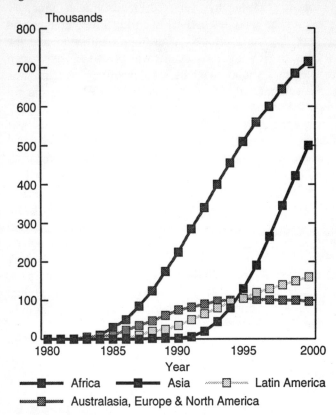

Africa
Asia
Latin America
Australasia, Europe & North America

*Number of new AIDS cases each year
Source: WHO 1993

San Francisco: the shape of things to come?

By as early as mid-1987 in San Francisco, nearly 3,500 people had been diagnosed as having AIDS. Just over 1,000 were still alive, with probably 10,000 others in a city of 800,000 already feeling unwell, and maybe 100,000 infected.[77]

Most gay men I talked with had buried between ten and twenty of their friends. A grandmother broke down and wept as she told me that her five-year-old grandson was dying. He had always been a somewhat sickly child, full of coughs and colds. One day he developed a rare chest infection and the doctors did an HIV antibody test: it was positive. They tested his mother and found that she was positive too. She was perfectly well but had led a somewhat risky life before she got married. She was devastated. She could not accept the doctor's diagnosis. The son of the woman I was talking to was fortunately still negative. She told me of another family she knew where Mum and Dad had both died, as had five of their children, one by one, until only the nine-year-old was left. 'She's doing fine, settled in her new school, with foster parents. She has got AIDS, of course, and she knows it, but she's a plucky little girl.' I found I was crying too.

During my stay in San Francisco I began to realise the overwhelming tragedy of the disease. I began to see why nurses and volunteers reach the point where they cannot go on. Many of them were personally involved: maybe they had recently nursed a friend with AIDS, or maybe they thought they were positive themselves.

The same has happened in the United Kingdom. In the late 1980s, on one ward close to a third of the male nurses were infected because of personal lifestyles.[78] Others may have had personal experience of the disease. It is understandable: cancer hospices have always drawn staff and volunteers from those who have been bereaved. However, hospices have known the dangers of giving in to pressures to accept help too soon. The recently bereaved soon find themselves reliving their own tragedy with every patient they see. Often the resulting grief and turmoil become overwhelming. They leave the ward in tears, have unpleasant dreams, are unable to sleep, or become convinced that they too are developing the disease. A complete break from this kind of work is usually essential to prevent serious depression. This can be hard if supporting friendships, identity and meaning in life are also tied up with the hospice.

I saw the same thing happening in San Francisco on a grand scale: whole communities becoming overloaded with grief, except that this is grief of a different kind.[79] With AIDS there is the second sinister dimension: if you become part of an AIDS ward team or volunteer programme because of nursing a lover with AIDS, there is the terrible possibility that you yourself are also infected with HIV. Not only do you then relive awful memories of the one you cared for as he died with each patient, but there is the hideous reality at the forefront of your mind that tomorrow it may be your turn. Every time you take a shower you find yourself checking all over for telltale signs of Kaposi's sarcoma—a form of skin cancer associated with AIDS. Every cough, cold or fever becomes a signal of possible disaster. Every episode of diarrhoea or feeling tired becomes a living nightmare. Every act of forgetfulness becomes a warning of dementia.

Sheer fright can produce the entire symptoms of early infection. A doctor in New York was convinced he had AIDS after a minor incident. He worried, became depressed and tired, stopped eating and lost weight. He had diarrhoea, produced a temperature, and finally developed rashes typical of early infection. Every test was negative—even the HIV antibody test. He then became convinced that he was in the fewer than one out of a hundred who never produce a positive test. This man has been followed up. He did not have AIDS or any other early signs, and his immune system is completely normal.[80]

A nurse, doctor or volunteer can find he is daily helping people dying of AIDS, supporting a colleague who is now becoming ill but wants to continue working (despite early signs of deteriorating brain function, encephalopathy), and then to cap it all, going home to nurse a dying lover of several years' standing. AIDS, AIDS, AIDS. No wonder so many are under a lot of stress. When you have already been to ten funerals of friends in the last year, you can reach the point of not coping any longer.

Then there is the terrible dilemma: what do you do when your colleague is becoming forgetful, clumsy and slowing up mentally? He is probably only too aware of what is happening and why. In one out of ten people this can be the first sign of AIDS.[81] Are you going to put him on permanent sick leave? Sick pay starts to run out after six months and stops after a year.[82] The person needs income and a stabilising routine. If you were to ask me what the first sign of encephalopathy is I would say it could be something like a pilot attempting to land with no undercarriage in place. I understand that British Airways is so worried about subtle loss of mental performance in airline pilots that it now routinely screens new pilots for HIV.[83] They have reason to be worried: by as early as 1987 nine of its male stewards were already dead and thirty-one more had AIDS.[84] A British newspaper published the nine death certificates because nobody believed the newspaper story.[85] Dan-Air, before its takeover, included HIV antibody tests as a routine part of medicals on cabin crew.[86]

A member of a nursing organisation in the United States of America told me they were thinking of introducing special intelligence tests for staff. When performance dropped below a certain level they would be suspended from duty and probably be fired.[87] With patient workload increasing every year they cannot afford to carry a growing number of mentally deteriorating staff on their payroll.

At the moment the gay community in San Francisco provides most of the volunteers. But the gay community could be overwhelmed, with many volunteers dead and increasing numbers unwell.[88] Fewer and fewer well people will be left to look after more and more who are dying. The same could be true of New York and London unless many more volunteers are recruited from outside the gay community. London hospital staff are already showing signs of severe stress due to heavy workloads and the intense nature of the disease.[89]

Another problem is that it can be less common to find supportive networks of friends around infected drug addicts.

One of the AIDS experts I met was shaking like a leaf. In the course of the one-hour interview it became clear that he was yet another person experiencing multiple losses: his lover had died at home recently, people in the office were ill or had died, and he had been to more than twelve funerals. He had no problems thinking, but his nerves were damaged by HIV, hence the uncontrollable shake.

If San Francisco faces a crisis, New York faces a nightmare since it has many more residents, many drug users and other groups without the emotionally supportive networks seen on the West Coast. The state of New York will have to play a much larger role in caring for those ill. By 1993, 20,000 children had been born in the city with HIV. These often unwanted babies pose a massive problem—just part of the picture of human suffering on a massive scale. An added complication in New York is that most with HIV are disadvantaged, poor, black and Hispanic people. Together with the gay image, it has meant that the white affluent middle class in the US has been able to dismiss AIDS as a welfare issue, a gay issue, someone else's problem—as we will see later. In many parts of the US, HIV is spreading most rapidly through ethnic-minority populations. Some black Americans feel AIDS is a conspiracy to wipe out the black race.[90] AIDS is now the commonest cause of death in Hispanic children in New York, and the second leading cause of death for African-American children in the city.[91]

Why San Francisco became a gay centre

In San Francisco I was welcomed by a senior churchman who was dying of AIDS. He explained to me how Europeans sailed west 200 years ago to get away from persecution in Europe and landed on the East Coast. Those who could not settle there drifted into the great plains. Those uncomfortable there drifted further west to the Rockies. Beyond the Rockies lay 800 miles of arid desert and beyond that lay the dream: San Francisco. A tiny collection of Spanish huts in the early nineteenth century, it was overtaken by the Gold Rush of the 1840s and then by the discovery of silver lode in the desert. A vast town sprang up where people risked and lost, loved and died.

A free-wheeling fantasy world was shattered by the vast earthquake of 1904 which destroyed four square miles and killed thousands of people. The new San Francisco was built over the ashes of the terrible fire that followed. The rebuilt city was populated by those 'going West', by Chinese from the East, and by immigrants from the South.

Part of the American dream has always been to opt out and escape by 'going West'. San Francisco was the centre for the beatniks of the 1950s and then the hippy movement of the 1960s. 'Make love not war' was the motto for prolonged anti-Vietnam demonstrations and drug-using 'free love' communes. The bubble burst in the 1970s with violence related to drug offenders. But then came a new migration West of people who felt they were unaccepted further East: homosexual men and women.

San Francisco has always had a reputation for carefree living, tolerance and sexual freedom—especially after the hippies came, cut their hair and settled down. Once a gay community was established, it grew rapidly. The gay districts used to be some of the poorest areas of downtown San Francisco; now they are becoming more fashionable. Gay consciousness became an important political force so that by the early 1980s it commanded 25% of the vote at elections for mayors and other local government officers.[92] Then the latest bubble was burst by a tiny virus.

Almost every Western nation has its own mini San Francisco: an area of a city which is particularly known for tolerance of homosexual lifestyles and becomes a centre of gay life.

The great cover-up

Why are so few people being honest about the extent of the problem and the risks? The first area of cover-up is in government because of intolerance and tightly controlled health budgets. In San Francisco people in the gay community talk of 'passive genocide' that they feel was practised by former President Reagan's administration for six or seven years. The problem of AIDS was barely acknowledged. Some have said that Reagan failed to implement in full the recommendations of his commission on the HIV epidemic, in particular on the issue of discrimination.[93] Reagan was quoted as talking about infected children as 'the innocent sufferers', so by implication the rest were guilty.

American society has always been rather intolerant of 'non-survivors' of the system. Those who are unemployed, chronically sick, or cannot afford health insurance are often in a desperate plight. The intolerance is especially magnified for problems considered to be directly related to a person's own decisions. Poverty is often considered to be the result of laziness. Diseases spread by sexual practices or drug abuse are condemned. There is a strong undercurrent of anti-homosexual feeling. Several conservative religious groups that helped elect Reagan are controlled by immensely powerful people with colossal grassroots support. Some of them are known for right-wing statements, on apartheid for example, but more recently for declaring that AIDS is the wrath of God on homosexuals.

Elsewhere in this book, these comments are examined and found to be unreasonable and absurd, particularly in view of what is now known of the disease in Africa, South East Asia and many other parts of the world. In some parts of the United States the feeling has been that homosexuals and drug addicts are being wiped out. The momentum to educate, plan, or treat them has been negligible.

Apart from the national lack of interest in what happens to gays, drug addicts or ethnic minorities, there has been a pressing economic reason for a great cover-up. In the early days when strange pneumonias and skin diseases were first noticed, these things plus several other strange infections were called AIDS. Unless you had one of these things you did not have AIDS. Even when the virus was discovered and people could be tested for antibodies, those who were positive and unwell could not be classified as having AIDS. Even if they were clearly dying as a result of the infection, they could not be labelled 'AIDS patients' if they did not have a second infection or tumour that counted.[94]

Clearly the definition had become meaningless. You can be either infected and feeling well, or infected and feeling ill. The sicker you get, the more likely it is you will die soon. However, the original, inadequate definition remained until very recently. Why? Because of money and politics.

The federal government only allowed certain benefits to be given, including free supplies ($6,500 per person) of Zidovudine (AZT) to those who 'officially' had AIDS. AZT is still the major drug used to slow down HIV in the body. All the statistics collected are for AIDS. Yet for every person who fits the AIDS definition, there are others feeling ill, so the problem is worse than statistics show.

In 1993, the US definition of AIDS was altered to include those with a low white cell count, even if not yet ill. This effectively doubled US AIDS cases and those eligible for benefits.[95]

Those closest to the problem can be numbed into silence, for example, over the problem of encephalopathy, or deterioration of the brain. Doctors are becoming better at treating strange chest infections and other illnesses. The length of life of someone newly diagnosed with AIDS is twice as long as it was. But now the more hideous problem of encephalopathy is emerging. When examined after death, brains of people with AIDS all show significant damage due to destruction of brain cells by the virus.[96] Sometimes this has been obvious during life, sometimes not. The brain damage

Western Europe: estimated HIV prevalence among the sexually-active population.[97] (See Appendix F.)

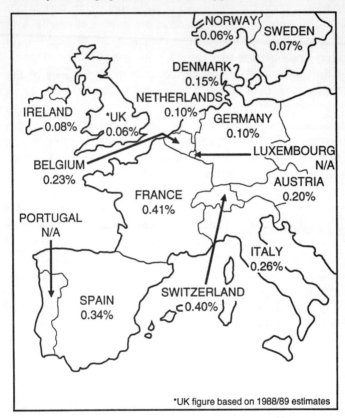

NORWAY 0.06%
SWEDEN 0.07%
DENMARK 0.15%
NETHERLANDS 0.10%
IRELAND 0.08%
*UK 0.06%
GERMANY 0.10%
LUXEMBOURG N/A
BELGIUM 0.23%
AUSTRIA 0.20%
FRANCE 0.41%
PORTUGAL N/A
ITALY 0.26%
SPAIN 0.34%
SWITZERLAND 0.40%

*UK figure based on 1988/89 estimates

can impair thinking, alter personality, change behaviour, rob people of dignity, and even affect movement. With careful testing it now seems that some evidence of mental deterioration can probably be found in most people who are about to die as a result of AIDS.[98] It is a terrible nightmare when you see it develop in your best friend, your colleagues and in yourself.

Remember that many people working in these projects at

the moment know that their own lifestyle means they are quite likely to be infected already. Being faced with possible progressive brain damage is so horrific that many people are unable to accept it. A state of denial is common in people with cancer and here we are seeing denial in AIDS health care workers and decision makers.

A third area of denial or cover-up is in discussions of the numbers of people likely to go on to develop full-blown AIDS. Statements that only ten out of a hundred would do so soon looked absurd, given the rate at which the numbers were increasing and the nature of the virus. Indeed the estimate was revised a year or so later to twenty out of a hundred. These figures persisted for years, being trotted out again and again.

One of the problems has been continued circulation of out-of-date leaflets that contain no date of publication. The proportion of those infected who were developing AIDS was clearly still increasing rapidly, so why didn't people say so? Soon the figures were revised again, and so on. The increases became obvious, inevitable, predictable—so why the strangely optimistic statements?

A senior official of the United Kingdom Department of Health told me unofficially that if he were honest he thought the final numbers dying—say after fifteen years—would be nearer 100%. The official version at the same time was a mere thirty-five or so out of a hundred, with the possibility of more. I think part of the reason was a desire to give as much hope as possible to those who were infected. Some of the people I met who quoted research papers so confidently were themselves infected. Seizing on these low estimates is a further kind of denial: a way of coping with personal fears.

The same thing results in wild claims being made for new drugs. 'Dementia won't be a problem now that we have AZT,' a senior AIDS counsellor told me several years ago. I wish that was what we were seeing at home and on the wards.

A fourth area of cover-up has been over the risks of infection by non-sexual, non-injecting contact. For example, statements have been widely circulated that HIV is very fragile and cannot survive except at body temperature for more than a few minutes.[99] It has also been said that it cannot withstand drying. These statements were made in good faith but were obviously wrong. Ask any haemophiliac who became infected from blood extracts. These extracts are obtained by freeze drying. The powder is then stored in a warehouse, transported to a hospital, and several weeks or months later it is reconstituted with sterile water before injection. The organisms causing gonorrhoea or syphilis would be destroyed instantly by such harsh treatment. But people can be infected with HIV this way.

Researchers took samples of HIV and placed them on a number of dishes to dry. After a day, the first sample was tested to see if it was infectious, and it was. The second day's sample was also infectious—and so on, right up to the end of a week. Some of the virus survived in dry dust for up to seven days. Then they repeated the experiment using the virus in water. They took samples each day and found that even after two whole weeks in water a few virus particles remained capable of causing infection. The public had been told pasteurisation (56°C for twenty minutes) destroyed the virus, but this same research showed that heating to 56°C must be continued for at least three hours to damage all virus particles.[100] (See also p 134.)

This research has been criticised. The amount of virus used was enormous. If the smaller amounts found in blood had been used, the results would probably have been different. In spite of this criticism it is still quite extraordinary that such a potentially important paper received so little attention, as it had vast implications for public health.

Although the study was included in Great Britain's Department of Health (DOH) circular on preventing cross-infection,[101] it was not widely reported. I think the reason was that medical personnel were scared that if everyone knew about it they would be even more reluctant to look after those with AIDS. A member of the DOH said the report had 'set the cat among the pigeons'. Sixty thousand copies were distributed to all the health districts in the United Kingdom, yet hardly anyone saw it. The DOH found that all thirty copies sent to one district were put straight into a filing cabinet and forgotten.[102]

The study has been repeated.[103] It has been found more recently that HIV survives at 275°C for six months or more. At room temperature, half the virus in a sample survives thirty hours in water, a quarter survives sixty hours and so on, with activity reduced a further five to twelve times by drying. In optimal conditions, researchers have found it can take over thirty days to reduce the amount of virus to less than 5% of the original quantity. In serum, HIV survives ten weeks.[104]

Heating at 48–56°C destroyed most particles after half an hour, although some survived even 64°C. Only a mixture of iodine and detergent at 2% left no detectable virus. Some virus in dried spills survived even treatment with 70% alcohol. Sodium hydroxide and acetone were less effective. HIV is therefore a very hardy virus, yet this important paper was not reported anywhere, or commented on, to my knowledge. What happened then to the truth about AIDS? The answer is that it was censored like the first paper because it was felt that you were likely to over-react and panic.

If the virus were really as fragile as people have said, destroyed after only a few minutes outside the body, then all surgeons in Africa would have to do to sterilise their instruments from HIV would be to hang them up in the sun for an hour. Not so—as the thick infection control guidelines in every country make clear.

It is true that a little knowledge is a dangerous thing, and it can be very worrying to think that infectious HIV particles could be quite widespread, until you realise, as we will see later, that HIV is quite difficult to catch, even if you jab yourself accidentally with a needle, or have unprotected sex with someone who is infected. In each example, the risk of transmission could be as low as 1 in 200. The risk of non-sexual, non-injecting HIV infection is therefore almost immeasurably small. This is a condescending cover-up, then, by people who think it best for you not to know. The trouble is that cover-ups backfire when people find out they have only been told half the story. People then reject or question everything else that is being said. No wonder there is confusion.

Likewise, other reports that break unspoken rules are not being given wide coverage. Many attempts have been made to keep doctors and nurses who have become infected out of the media's eye, together with a steady trickle of others who are being infected through unusual routes. At least six are already known to have become infected through skin contact with secretions or blood. The skin is full of special white cells, Langerhans macrophages and T-helper lymphocytes, which are particularly susceptible to infection by the virus if the skin is cracked or broken; intact skin is an excellent barrier to HIV. So the virus does not have to enter blood, but only the deeper skin layers.[105]

I want to emphasise again, as we will see in other sections of this book, the risk even to medical personnel of becoming infected other than through sex or sharing dirty needles is incredibly small. I am just pointing out that what has been said in public is often not the whole truth.

The fifth area of cover-up in some countries is the failure to acknowledge prominently two possible errors in all of the figures reported for AIDS.[106] We considered earlier the omission in the numbers reported of those sick but not having full-blown AIDS. However, another problem is failure by doctors to report cases. Reporting is totally voluntary in most countries. Voluntary reporting is always, by its nature, incomplete. Under-reporting can be significant—even in 'AIDS aware' parts of industrialised nations with excellent health facilities. A recent study in the UK showed up to 23%

of AIDS cases were not reported in an inner-city area of London.[107]

The second possible source of underestimating the numbers of AIDS cases is incorrect diagnosis. As the spectrum of the disease widens, more and more doctors will be asking themselves if AIDS was not in fact the explanation for that curious death some time ago. An example is pneumonia. Despite antibiotics, and before AIDS, people still occasionally died of pneumonia. As people get older, it becomes a more common cause of death. In the elderly it is very common indeed. Most people with AIDS are young so chest infections are more conspicuous, but there is the possibility that some older people may be dying of unrecognised AIDS-related pneumonias.[108] Missed diagnosis can be a serious problem in many developing countries. It is also true, as we have seen, that the AIDS diagnosis can be given mistakenly, especially where no laboratory facilities exist for HIV blood testing or for monitoring white cell counts.

Another example of missed diagnosis is death from an accident caused by unrecognised early brain damage. Even where the correct diagnosis is made, AIDS is often not recorded on the death certificate in the UK in order to save relatives distress. Pneumonia is often put down as the cause. This is yet another way that cases may not end up in the statistics even when diagnosed. A health department survey of young male deaths in the United Kingdom found an unexplained increase. Examination of records suggested that many of these deaths were due to AIDS although not recognised at the time.[109]

A sixth area of cover-up is the dishonesty of some who have become infected about how they came to be so. A man may say he slept with a prostitute once in 1983 but has otherwise been faithful to his wife. Several weeks later he admits he is a practising homosexual. Many of the 15% listed with 'no known risk factors' fall into this area. An extreme example is in the United States armed forces where up to three-quarters can give no explanation or only a heterosexual one.[110] The general unease about being honest makes it extremely difficult to monitor different methods of spreading.

A seventh area of cover-up has been over the large proportion of African AIDS cases hidden in AIDS figures in countries like the UK, as we saw earlier in this chapter.

I am not suggesting that these areas of cover-up are all the result of deliberate conspiracy; some aspects may be, others are part of a poor system of communication, and still others are non-deliberate distortions of a complex, confusing, and rapidly-changing picture. However, they all add up to a situation where what the average doctor, nurse, or member of the public understands is often only a part of the whole problem.

The African cover-up

The distortion of the real problem in the United States or United Kingdom is negligible in comparison to the almost complete silence of some African governments in the past. Confronted with a tragedy affecting their whole continent— and for once not related to war or famine—in an international atmosphere which they see as racist, many have been extremely unwilling to be honest. They are afraid of anti-black backlash if it is said that the problem started there. They are also afraid of economic ruin due to decisions of multinational companies to pull out, and the collapse of their tourist industries. Many of these countries desperately need foreign currency to prevent total bankruptcy. In addition it has often been difficult for doctors to be sure of the diagnosis. Testing is expensive, kits are hard to obtain, and sometimes hard to use. Indirect methods have to be used such as a negative skin reaction to the standard tuberculosis (TB) test.[111] Most AIDS-related deaths seem to be happening out in the bush, unnoticed and unregistered. The wards and clinics see mainly early cases.

So we have a bizarre situation where doctors in these countries are reeling under an impossible workload, and where even government members or relations of the country's leaders are dying,[112] but the problem is denied, or impossible to assess. Possibly twenty cases are admitted, or 100, or 1,000, or 10,000. The statements are usually meaningless. Scientists studying the epidemic in Central Africa are there under tolerance. Intensive research is going on all over Africa to understand the disease, but the results are censored. A scientist will often have to sign an agreement not to disclose publicly what he sees happening.

Information is leaking out all the time, but if it is traced back to a particular person or team the workers may be thrown out of the country or into prison. Fortunately, the situation is changing. It has to. The cover-up has had one appalling consequence which prevents an educational campaign. How can a country embark on mass prevention for a disease it says it does not really have? Once again we see denial for emotional reasons too, not just economic ones. How can you accept from a mathematician that maybe a third of your entire nation could die?[113]

South Africa has had its own reasons to cover up. It has an enormous problem, especially in the black townships where huge numbers of migrant workers come from countries further north in which AIDS is taking a terrible toll.

In places like Soweto, the town providing labour for the deep mines in Johannesburg, there have been up to 50,000 men living without their wives (officially). Their wives and children were all meant to stay in homelands like the Transkei. They didn't, of course, and drifted out in search of their husbands to build illegal residences made from corrugated iron, wood and plastic. Every now and then these 'shanty towns' were bulldozed to the ground and the women trucked back, sometimes more than 1,000 miles away.

Fifty thousand men on their own with a few prostitutes spells trouble—yet this situation has been common in South

Africa. The historic white government has had no political will to change anything. For them, a major disease that selectively hits black Africans and offsets the birthrate may have been convenient. However, South Africa is admitting an increasing problem in its white population. Since black prostitutes commonly serve white men, the white community may be stirred into action this way.[114]

The church cover-up

Although Britain's Lesbian and Gay Christian movement says there could be as many as 6,000 gay clergy in the United Kingdom, and although the number of clergy who are developing AIDS is steadily climbing,[115] the problem is not officially acknowledged.

To the non-churchgoing public it seems that at a time of inner crisis, the church reacts by closing ranks. No wonder clear definitive statements on family life and sexual behaviour have not been forthcoming—at least not until relatively recently.

In the United States the situation is further confused by many clergy's fear of discovery. This is not just a priest's fear of being recognised by a visitor or by the chaplain on an AIDS ward, but the fear that parishioners may suspect a hidden lifestyle.

At an Anglican conference in Washington, the church position on various issues relating to homosexuality was debated. A senior clergyman, who was a practising homosexual himself, told me how angry he had been to see priests whom he recognised from gay bars and other haunts voting in favour of harsh anti-homosexual statements.

Life after AIDS

Cover-up or no cover-up, honesty, secrecy, or confusion, one thing is clear: nothing will ever be quite the same again. AIDS is fundamentally altering fashions, behaviour, culture—in fact every fibre of our society.[116] In New York, fat is back in fashion: 'Who wants to look thin?—Perhaps he has AIDS.' Who would have thought that in 1987 James Bond would be portrayed as having a stable relationship? Sex three times with the same woman, not once each with three women! The Hollywood dinosaur of the movie industry is thrashing its tail and the ground is shaking. Television producers are stepping over each other in their zeal to include AIDS in soap operas, plays and comedies.[117]

Magazines like *Cosmopolitan* say that smart girls carry condoms. They hope that smart girls will not feel like loose girls when they produce the packet. They hope too for a new courage and honesty so that people will always tell of their unfaithfulness and promiscuity or drug addiction. They hope for new security in relationships so that when a girl or boy suggests using a condom, the other will not treat it as a terrible insult or lack of trust.

Whether such hopes will remain hopes or get built into a strange harsh reality of rubber-separated sex is unclear. But one thing is almost inevitable: out of the ashes of the crematorium will rise a new sub-culture which will affect a whole generation: a culture of stable relationships and marriages. A culture where a man and a woman find mutual sexual fulfilment for life.

The reality is that even an AIDS cure in 1998 or a remarkable vaccine in 2001 will not erase the traumas of a generation, nor eradicate the problem. As we have seen with the resurgence of TB and syphilis, low-cost treatment does not mean the end of the story. The message is burning home: sleeping around has always been unhealthy. Now it can be suicidal. Taking AIDS out still leaves the other epidemics untouched. The mid-twenty-first century will look at the 1980s, 1990s, and the early years of the next century as the 'era of AIDS'. The reasons for its spread, its origins, the apathy of governments, and the mistakes of scientists will be debated by historians for generations.

AIDS is likely to dominate the rest of our adult lives—especially the lives of doctors and nurses, and of young people becoming sexually active today. The question is this: will you be able to hold your head high? Will you be proud of the way you responded when you look back on it all?

Apart from a radical change of lifestyle in our society—which will not help those already infected anyway—our only hope remains in understanding this strange virus so we can fight it. But what exactly *is* a virus?

2

What's so Special about a Virus?

All viruses are dead. There is nothing alive in a virus at all. A virus is no more living than a computer game you can buy in the High Street. Bacteria are different: bacteria breathe oxygen or carbon dioxide, need warmth to grow, and they grow larger and divide into two. In fact bacteria behave like cells in your own body.

Some bacteria make poisons such as the tetanus toxin which causes rapid death. Others live quite happily on every corner of your body. An example is in your gut where bacteria help you to digest food. If you take antibiotics, some of these bacteria die and the result can be diarrhoea. So while some bacteria keep us healthy, others bring disease because of the poisons they make when growing.

You can see bacteria under the microscope. I have taken a swab from a man's penis or a woman's vagina and touched a microscope slide with it. You can see the red gonorrhoea bacteria easily and make an instant diagnosis. In most cases a single large dose of penicillin will kill the bacteria. Penicillin works by weakening the cell wall that holds the little organism together. The bacteria swell, burst, and die. A swab containing syphilis organisms is even more interesting: these creatures swim like little eels, thrashing about on the wet glass slide. Instant diagnosis. Immediate high dose penicillin. Immediate cure in most cases.

But AIDS is caused by a virus (HIV)[118]—see page 127.

Thousands of bacteria can fit inside a cell in your body, but virus particles are so minute that hundreds of thousands of them could fit inside a single bacterium. They are totally invisible under a normal light microscope. Viruses cannot grow and cannot divide. They don't breathe, don't need food, don't live, and never die. All our technology has failed to produce a single non-toxic drug that attacks and destroys a virus efficiently.

The kiss of death

The only real weapons we have against viruses are natural ones: antibodies which can also destroy bacteria. These are Y-shaped. The mouth of the antibody is shaped exactly to fit over part of a germ. Thousands of them lock onto a germ so that the tails bristle like a hedgehog. Sometimes that is enough to burst bacteria or to stop viruses from being able to touch a cell. Special white cells in the body stick on to these bristles and eat up the germ. These white cells are those that you find in pus, cleaning up an infected wound. The trouble with antibodies is that the body takes three days to produce the right antibody for the right virus. During this critical three-day period, the body is totally unprotected. Yet only an hour or two after viruses enter the bloodstream they have completely disappeared. You can hunt through the entire body cell by cell, with the best electron-firing microscope, and find nothing.

Why? Because every virus particle has disintegrated. Each one has burst like a soap bubble when it touches the ground.

The virus bag has disintegrated and vanished. What about the contents? They too have disappeared without trace, but the cell they touched has received the kiss of death.[119]

A sentence that kills

A virus is a bag containing a short piece of coiled-up 'string'. The string is formed entirely of four different chemicals

Diseases

Viruses	Bacteria
Colds	Boils
Flu	Pneumonias
Measles	(most types)
Chickenpox/shingles	Tuberculosis
Polio	Diphtheria
Herpes/cold sores	Tetanus
Smallpox	Cystitis
Glandular fever	Food poisoning
Rabies	Gonorrhoea
Hepatitis	Syphilis
AIDS	

arranged in an order. When stretched out, it reads like a language:

ABBDA   AABDACCC   ABDA   CCDAAAB   AA   CCDAA

This language is what we call a genetic code. It is the language used by the nucleus (brain) of every cell in your body. A cell of your body under the microscope looks a little like an egg. It has a central round core called a nucleus and a more transparent-looking outer area. The nucleus is black and is packed full of your chromosomes. You have forty-six chromosomes which determined everything from the moment you were conceived, including the length of your arms, whether you have black or brown hair, whether you will be bald by the time you are thirty, your height, gender, basic build, the shape of your nose. Everything.

Each of these chromosomes is tightly coiled up like a spring. If we stretched out the message and then typed out the sequence, and put all the messages from all the chromosomes in one cell in your body into a book, that book would be the size of *Encyclopaedia Britannica*.

These instructions program not only your outside appearance, but also every type of cell in your body. Have you ever thought how a skin cell learned it was a skin cell and not a nail- or hair-producing cell? How does a cell know it should produce bone and not hormones? If I cut my hand, how does a skin cell know to divide and go on dividing until the gap is covered and then stop? The answer lies in that vast book of instructions. The amazing thing is that *every* cell nucleus in your body carries a carbon copy of your entire genetic code.

Sinister experiments

If I take the nucleus (core) out of a single cell of a frog, and take the nucleus out of an unfertilised frog's egg, and put into that transparent egg a black dot which is the nucleus of that skin cell, a remarkable thing happens which you can watch under the microscope. (The procedure is easy in frogs because their egg nuclei are so big.) As you watch you will see that egg cell divide into four, then eight, then sixteen and thirty-two and so on. At this early stage any one of these cells, if separated, could go on to produce a twin frog. If the cells are left in a ball, each senses the presence of its neighbours, reads its book of instructions, and starts to develop different behaviour. One cell goes on to produce the brain, another the spinal cord, and so on. The result is a clone of the frog we took the skin from.

We may soon be able to do the same with human eggs. Scientists are very near being able to take a nucleus from a cell in my body, put it into an egg, and produce a clone or an identical twin of me. The only difference is that the twin will be years younger. The egg would develop to a full baby by being placed in the womb of a surrogate mother. We are already able to clone human embryos by separating cells from a dividing fertilised human egg.

Deadly secrets

Some scientists hate talking about this kind of work. A few years ago, I had a long talk with a leading research scientist in the UK, who confessed that he was nearing his lifetime ambition: the ultimate in spare-part surgery.

He was able now, he claimed, to clone a human embryo, place it in the womb of a monkey, and grow it. 'Unfortunately' these embryos were dying sooner than he would like. If only he could grow it as a foetus for a few weeks more he could 'cull' it, kill the monkey, kill the foetus and use—say—the young healthy kidneys as spare parts. He was not publishing his work in this area because he was sure his laboratory would be closed down, although his work was legal at the time. His laboratory is well known.[120]

I am telling you this for two reasons: first, to indicate how complex your genetic code is in every cell of your body, and second, to emphasise that as a race we are on the brink of terrible disaster—whether nuclear, biological as in AIDS, or through genetic tampering with life itself. This is the subject of a book I wrote in 1993 called *The Genetic Revolution*.[121]

Life-changing technology

We have already succeeded in altering the genetic code of a bacterium so it contains a small piece of code taken from a human being. This piece of code tells the bacterium not to produce poison but to produce human insulin—previously diabetics were dependent on insulin obtained by crushing the pancreas of a pig or cow. This new strain of bacteria grows and divides for ever, with each new organism containing a perfect set of instructions for making human insulin.

In 1991 over 62,000 genetically-mutated animals were born

in UK laboratories, each unlike any animal ever seen before. Human genes have been added to pigs to make them grow faster. The 'superbreed' is blind, impotent and suffers from severe arthritis. Human genes have been added to cows, sheep, rabbits, mice—and even fish. Scorpion poison genes have been added to cabbages—the list is almost endless. We urgently need the technology to cure disease and to feed the world, but its abuse to create, say, designer families for tomorrow's parents is just one nightmare possibility for the future.[122]

Various laboratories around the world are locked into a race to 'decode' the entire genetic material of a human. This enables us to say that:

ABCADDA = Insulin;
BCADDDD = Length of nose;
BCCABBA = Amount of pigment in hair.[123]

The correct bit for any part of a human can then be cut out and transferred, or be reprogrammed and put back into the cell.

So then, it is also possible to map out every single instruction a virus contains and understand precisely what it does in the cell it affects. Why can't all this remarkable technology produce a cure for AIDS? Consider what happens when the virus bubble touches its target cell.

How the virus kills a white cell

The surface of HIV is specially shaped so that it only fits onto a very small range of cells in the body. The flu virus latches onto cells in the nose, while HIV mainly latches onto one particular type of white cell (CD4 + T-lymphocyte), some brain cells, and one or two others.[124]

When HIV touches the cell and the bubble bursts, the genetic code (RNA) is injected into the cell. Within minutes the code is being read by the cell and the message carried into the cell brain, or nucleus. The message is then added permanently to that cell's 'book of life' as DNA. The process took only a few minutes and is complete. The cell looks normal in every way but is now doomed. It may continue to look normal for several years. During this time the white cell continues to travel in the blood looking for invaders while blissfully unaware of the invader within. If the attacked cell divides, the two daughter cells also carry perfect copies of the hidden message.[125] It is likely that the infected cells in semen or vaginal fluids are the main source of HIV transmissions during sex.

Biological time-bomb

Each cell infected by HIV becomes a biological time-bomb travelling in the bloodstream. Millions of them waiting to explode.[126]

One day a particular germ enters the body that this particular cell is geared to deal with. There are thousands of different white cells, all designed to kill different kinds of organisms. It just so happens that out of all the thousands of different infections a person could have caught, this particular one fits the role of this particular cell. It springs into action, programmed by its brain to react. It starts to produce proteins. The cell should help the body turn out finished antibodies that are the exact shape and form to fit the intruding germ and kill it. It's at this point that the effect of the virus is finally revealed. The virus message then overrides the entire cell system and orders a new product to be made: thousands and thousands of HIV messages in genetic code. These are then carried to the outside wall of the cell where each is wrapped and thrown out of the cell. So infected white cells become factories for more virus, instead of factories to help the body make antibodies.[127]

You can see special electron microscope photographs of hundreds of these viruses appearing as little bulges as they poke out from the cell. Eventually they emerge as little round balls, and the cell dies. Millions of virus particles are released into the bloodstream, each one floating in the blood until it touches another CD4 white cell, bursts, injects its message, reprograms the cell, and the process continues.

The trouble is that despite all our modern technology it is hard to detect an infected cell. They look identical from the outside until they are dying. Nor are we able to find the virus easily when it is floating in the bloodstream.

Antibodies don't protect you

The extraordinary thing about the virus is that its outer bag is formed from your own cell membrane. When it came out from the white cell, it was clothed in cell membrane, so its outer feel is in many ways just like a human cell. It is true that there are some distinguishing marks on the outside of the virus and the body does produce antibodies. However, when the antibody latches on to one of these lumps on the virus coating, the lump can break off, leaving the virus intact just as a lizard sheds its tail.[128]

The problem with HIV is *not* that the body cannot produce antibodies against the virus. On the contrary, almost every person produces antibodies. That is how we test for infection: not by looking for the virus, but by testing for antibodies. The sinister thing is that the virus appears to be *immune* to antibodies. No antibodies have yet been found in a human being that are effective in the long term against HIV. That is why a vaccine will be so difficult to find. It is easy to produce antibodies against the virus, but we don't know how to produce one that will prevent infection because we have no natural model from which to work.[129]

New strains of HIV appearing

The other worrying thing about this virus is its ability to alter its shape.[130] Earlier we saw that antibody-producing cells are specific. An antibody against one organism is only rarely effective against another. If an organism changes its outer coating at all, it is back to the drawing board to make a new antibody. HIV can change shape in subtle ways in the same person over the course of a few months, and a person can be infected with several differently shaped viruses at once, possibly with varying abilities to cause disease.[131] Even worse, HIV occasionally changes its shape radically. We are currently seeing new HIV-like viruses emerging every year or two somewhere in the world.[132] There are probably at least six HIV strains already.[133] Each of these major variants may have a slightly different ability to infect different groups. For example, in Thailand, the first strain which appeared spread mainly through injecting drug users and homosexual men. A subsequent strain from Africa is now spreading almost entirely through heterosexual relationships. While an alternative explanation is that HIV is spreading within different groups, it is a reality that new strains are continually emerging with different outer coatings and the potential to be more or less able to infect or cause illness.[134]

Some strains seem to have lower virulence, as seen in a group infected by blood transfusions from someone with HIV in Australia. Most are still well after years, and the virus cultured seems relatively mild.[135] An increasing number of people are infected with more than one type of HIV. Every time someone is infected, there is a minute chance that radical new changes will occur. As the number of infected people worldwide continues to increase each year, so does the risk of new strains emerging (see p 153).

The common cold virus is also unstable. That is why we are always getting colds. I probably have antibodies in my blood now to fifty or a hundred different shaped cold viruses. By the time one of those viruses has infected people between here, North America, Japan, Korea, India, Greece and back again, its shape has changed so much that I can catch the same cold

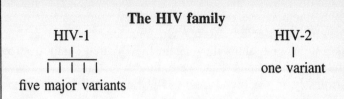

The HIV family

HIV-1   HIV-2

five major variants   one variant

HIV-2 prevalence mainly in West Africa. Produces similar disease spectrum to HIV-1, though possibly milder. Tests for HIV-1 detect all variants, but not HIV-2.

all over again. That is why we are light years away from a vaccine against the common cold.

The flu virus is also unstable, but less so. We can usually reckon on two or three different viruses causing most flu for a year or so before changing. We spot the new ones, make a vaccine, and give it to people each year. This annual vaccine has never been popular. Why? Because it often gives people a mild dose of the very flu they were hoping not to catch in the first place, and also because protection only lasts until the virus mutates.

AIDS vaccine could give you AIDS

Even if—and a big if—we could create a new vaccine radically different from any other we have ever made, one that somehow could make the body produce antibodies that latch on to any kind of HIV, whatever its shape, there is the worry at the back of people's minds that it could have some serious side effects.

Vaccination of animals against viruses similar to HIV made some of the animals ill. A shortage of chimpanzees and lack of a true animal model for HIV infection mean that animal testing does not tell us much. Vaccines have to be tested at an early stage on humans.[136] Even if vaccines do not give people AIDS, there is the possibility that they might get ill more quickly if infected later.[137]One reason for this is the suggestion that antibodies against HIV may help destroy infected white cells that were otherwise circulating quite harmlessly in the bloodstream. The immune defences of the body against HIV may actually be part of the reason for illness developing.

Imagine giving 10,000 New York school children the new vaccine. How many years do you think it would take before we could be 100% sure that none of them would ever go on to develop problems with the vaccine? The answer is probably five to fifteen years because that is the time scientists now think it can take to develop AIDS. Testing of vaccines requires human guinea pigs. On whom are we going to try it? The answer is that UK trials are being planned to take place in countries like Uganda. This raises big ethical questions, especially as those vaccinated may think they are now protected. First generation vaccines do not work, although they do give us useful information.

There is the possibility that we could make millions of virus particles without the damaging genes inside.[138] This should be safe but may not be effective. Damaged virus particles tend to produce a very poor immune response and are usually very poor vaccines. Almost all the effective vaccines we possess depend on a milder form of the virus actually infecting the body. Polio vaccine is an example. But there is no milder form of AIDS that we dare risk giving people.[139]

Attempts have been made to take a mild virus used in another vaccine (called 'vaccinia') and change it so the outside looks like HIV but is relatively harmless. This may eventually be our best hope. However, as we have seen, the virus may still turn out to be immune to the antibodies produced. Any vaccine, whether effective or not, will cause all those vaccinated to give 'positive' test results, making detection of infection more difficult in those vaccinated.[140]

How flu vaccine works

Without vaccine	With vaccine
virus particles enter nose or lungs	virus particles enter nose or lungs
virus particles enter cells	antibodies ready
reproduce	most virus particles destroyed
increasing number of cells killed	few cells infected
symptoms of flu	mild symptoms
antibodies start to form in three days	massive increase in antibodies within twenty-four hours
virus numbers start reducing	infection never gets a chance
infection over	

The vaccine gives you the same protection as if you have already had this particular flu a few months before. Your white cells usually have a memory for life. Response is rapid second time around.

So then, in summary, we are a long way from a widely available, effective vaccine. In the meantime you will continue to read of countless spectacular claims. Even if a vaccine existed today that was 100% safe and reasonably effective, it would probably take five years to become widely available at reasonably low cost. When it does come, it will almost certainly be useless at treating those millions already infected. However, work is also continuing into different kinds of vaccines which might help an infected person fight infection.

Hope of drug cure?

Our only other hope lies in a drug that could destroy viruses in the body. We have none that is effective. For forty years we have searched in vain for a single drug that would work well against a virus without killing the person who takes it. When such a drug appears it will almost certainly cure polio, chickenpox, flu, and a host of other diseases from which our only protection at the moment is vaccination. We will undoubtedly find such a drug one day but it is a long, long way off. How do you kill something that does not breathe, does not need food, does not live and never dies?

There are four target areas where HIV might be open to attack in the body:

1. Before it touches a cell and its genetic code is injected through the cell wall.

2. When the genetic code has been unravelled inside the cell and the message is being transferred to the cell brain (nucleus) using a special enzyme called 'reverse transcriptase'.

3. When the cell starts to make new viruses.

4. When the viruses start budding out of the cell wall.

All the newspaper reports of so-called 'AIDS wonder drugs' over the next few years will fall into one of these groups.

Attempts have even been made to flood the bloodstream with small pieces of cell wall (CD4) so the viruses are unable to touch living CD4 white cells. Another method being tried is to inject antibodies ('neutralising') from HIV-positive people to give extra protection to people with AIDS.[141]

Others are now looking closely at the virus to try to find any important piece of 'machinery' which is unique to virus production and cannot be found in a normal human cell. Machines in cells are called enzymes.

Enzymes are what are found in biological washing powders. We understand what they do very well. Like antibodies they are very specific indeed and each enzyme is capable of only one thing. Enzymes either split large molecules into two smaller ones—which is how they loosen dirt in clothing—or take two smaller ones and join them together. There is a particular enzyme that reads the genetic code of HIV to form the message that reprograms the cell. It is called 'reverse transcriptase'. The body does not usually make it, and only viruses use it. If we could find a way of jamming it effectively *without bad side effects*, we could prevent viruses from reprogramming cells.

We are able to jam various other enzymes in the body. For example, aspirin and arthritis drugs jam an enzyme which makes the most painful substance known to man: prostaglandin. This is produced whenever cells are injured in the body. Nerves are irritated by it and fire thousands of electrical impulses which your brain understands as pain. By jamming this enzyme, prostaglandins are reduced and pain is lessened.

Poison for life?

There would be one terrible problem with all such potential drugs. If they can be found, they will have to be taken for life. If some cells in the body are already infected, then a drug preventing entry of new viruses into unaffected cells will need to be taken until every reprogrammed cell and its descendants are dead—which could take fifteen years or longer. If we stopped the drug after ten years and a single reprogrammed white cell were to be activated to make more virus particles, the disease could start progressing all over again. This applies also to drugs preventing reprogramming, virus manufacture, or budding from the cell.

Almost all drugs have side effects and this particular range of drugs has more than its fair share of them. Zidovudine (AZT), for example, which works by jamming the enzyme reverse transcriptase, is also a poison to the bone marrow of the body which produces all your blood cells. You can die from taking too much Zidovudine for too long, and Zidovudine-resistant strains seem to be developing rapidly.[142]

Many people need regular blood transfusions to keep going with the treatment. Every other drug currently being tested has either been found to be poisonous to some degree or other or to have little or no anti-viral effect. In fact, some are so obviously dangerous that the only way a licence can be obtained to give them to human beings at all is because it is on the strictest understanding that all the 'human guinea pigs' are going to die soon anyway from AIDS so a death from the drugs is less serious, even if the hope of cure is remote.

The United States federal government is usually extremely strict on new drugs. Drugs have to be tried on vast numbers of animals for years before they can be tried on humans. The United States federal government has never approved so many half-developed products so quickly, propelled by a ghastly sense of urgency for the million or more United States citizens already infected.[143] The same is likely to happen in the United Kingdom.[144]

So the drugs currently being tried are usually suitable only for those already affected by AIDS, and while some may be suitable for those who have only become infected, they are completely unsuitable for giving to the whole nation.

However, as doctors are now seeing such a large proportion of those infected go on to develop AIDS, the pressure is growing to try using these drugs on more and more people at an earlier stage.

The use of AZT on those who have HIV who are in the pre-AIDS stage has always been controversial, with recent disappointing results from Concorde, a large combined British and French study[145] disputed by some US scientists who feel they have shown some benefits, in five early-use trials involving 3,002 patients. The reason for confusion has been that AZT treatment improved CD4 white cell counts—a sign usually associated with increased survival. It was found that in those on AZT, CD4 counts were not an effective predictor. AZT may help prevent mother-baby infection.[146]

Vaccines—a high risk business

Drug companies are pouring billions of dollars into research to find better treatments and much less into vaccines. With a lot less work they can rush through testing and licensing and bring a new drug onto the market.[147] Advertising is unnecessary. Media hype does most of it, and pressure becomes irresistible from patients who are desperate for any hope of cure. Doctors and governments are forced into using drugs which are very expensive—possibly $4,000 per patient—but may hardly work at all and may actually make the patient worse.

Of course we need research trials but they need to be carefully regulated. You can spend millions on a treatment for 500–1,000 patients, or maybe for the same money get 500 full-time health educators on the road into schools, clubs, colleges, factories and offices, preventing maybe 20,000 or more extra AIDS deaths a year. New treatments available in many industrialised nations have increased the cost of caring for someone with AIDS from diagnosis to death.

Vaccines are a different matter altogether: they are very complex to make and many doubt we will ever be able to make one for AIDS that works and is safe. A long period of investment is required over five to ten years before the drug company that develops a vaccine is likely to earn any money. Even if a company creates an effective vaccine, there is a risk of financial ruin if the vaccine turns out to have serious side effects. In the United States, public liability laws and the vast size of lawsuit claims make drug companies vulnerable to bankruptcy if they market something which turns out to be unsafe.[148] As a result, a new Bill has been introduced to US

Congress designed to protect researchers and manufacturers from liability in testing AIDS vaccines.[149]

AIDS is big business and many other organisations stand to gain or lose millions of dollars over what happens. A furious argument over who first discovered the AIDS virus took place between French and American scientists. At stake were world rights to royalties from every blood test for AIDS.[150] The row took years to resolve.[151]

Some companies also fear that they would have to make their new product available 'at cost' if it turned out to be a wonder cure or an effective vaccine. Public reaction would be great if profits were seen to be made out of tragedy.

Governments need to look at this urgently. No one expects drug companies who operate on behalf of shareholders to go bankrupt in the public interest. They need to be reasonably sure of a return, or if the risks of heavy losses are too large, they need some kind of financial inducement such as low taxation on profits from AIDS vaccines. Failure to address this fundamental issue could set back progress by a decade.

The United Kingdom Wellcome Foundation, which dates back to the yellow fever vaccine developed by Sir Henry Wellcome, is the world leader in vaccine research and production. Currently, millions are being poured into the development of new vaccines—for malaria, for example—but rather less money into AIDS vaccines. On the other hand, a vast investment by Wellcome has produced the world's main anti-AIDS drug, which is still selling over £170 million a year.[152] For many drug companies the risks of failure are considered too great to justify a search for an AIDS vaccine. The problems of finding suitable human volunteers in sufficient numbers are also considered insurmountable.[153] Many companies are waiting for government laboratories to come up with a good vaccine they can test. They might then be interested in marketing it.[154]

Unfortunately, in the absence of large numbers of volunteers for vaccines in places like the UK, trials are taking place in Uganda, Rwanda, Brazil and Thailand.[155] One might question the ethics of this. The vaccines being used today are useless at preventing AIDS. They produce a degree of immune response, but are only a very first step. Yet in a developing country, an injection of 'the latest experimental vaccine' may well create a false sense of security in those taking part in the study. The result could be their deaths.

The vaccines are so unproven, and have such a high risk of potential side effects that it is highly unlikely that parents of children or teenagers in developed countries would want to volunteer members of their family. So are we so sure it is right to proceed in other nations? It can be argued that no adult takes part without giving consent, but it is easy to underestimate the huge faith many villagers place in a Western doctor with high-tech equipment offering the very latest in medical research. At the moment there is nothing to stop someone in a country like Canada or the UK from going over to Africa and doing research there which would be illegal at home. There are huge ethical issues here tied up with inequality of resources and exploitation of developing nations.[156]

Altogether fifteen experimental vaccines entered early trials between 1987 and 1993. Thirteen of these have been tested on uninfected volunteers as preventative vaccines, and eight in infected individuals as therapeutic vaccines designed to slow down the development of illness. The vaccines in uninfected people seem to be generally safe, but only produce an immune response after several doses. The level of antibodies made are low, short lived and specific to only one strain of HIV. Vaccines tested on infected people seem to cause few problems, and increase the immune response to HIV. Whether or not this will improve survival has yet to be seen.[157]

Most of these vaccines are made using 'recombinant' genetic engineering. Cells are programmed to make millions of harmless virus fragments which are then injected into people. Antibodies to the fragments should then cross-react with intact infectious HIV. The World Health Organisation is worried that a vaccine might emerge which is very expensive and works only against certain strains in specific areas, useless and unaffordable to developing countries.[158]

The World Health Organisation is now encouraging the development of an infectious non-lethal form of HIV as a vaccine, similar to the vaccine for polio.[159]

There are many examples where people may be making money out of AIDS in various ways.[160] Pacific Dunlop (condoms and surgical gloves) profits grew by 31% in six months of 1987 due to the AIDS scare.[161]

Viruses as drugs by the year 2000?

There is a fascinating possibility that by the turn of the century scientists and doctors will be able to program back to normal any cell that has already been reprogrammed by a virus. Suppose a cell has been taken over by a virus and the book of life is now altered. In the laboratory they painstakingly write a new message and put it into genetic code. Then they (somehow) place the new code into an empty virus bag. The test-tube virus is now allowed to touch a white cell. It enters and releases the new message which programs back the book of life so it reads normally.

If you are familiar with computers, it is a bit like recreating a corrupt disc. We are a long way from this, not least because most viruses get cells to produce a special chemical called interferon as soon as they have entered, preventing a second virus from entering the same cell, whether a wild one or a test-tube virus.

A major step forward in human reprogramming was taken in 1990, with children who had adenosine deaminase deficiency. This gene defect is something children are born with and means white cells fail to work properly. The result is an illness like AIDS, with early death.

In a remarkable breakthrough, scientists at the US National Institute of Health located the correct gene, inserted it into viruses built in the laboratory, removed defective white cells from the child, infected the cells to program them back to normal, and then replaced the cells. The child was cured. To do the same in HIV-infected white cells would mean overcoming the interferon locking system HIV activates once inside a cell, designed to prevent other viruses from entering.

When these tools for tinkering with genetic code of cells in our bodies become widely available we will begin to see cures for other genetic diseases—for people with cystic fibrosis and many others. Perhaps you will one day be able to buy a bottle of hair colour that works permanently. You take it as medicine and the viruses in it reprogram all your hair-producing cells to produce jet black hair instead of red hair.

Like most major discoveries, it could also turn into a terrible curse: the ultimate in biological warfare. An infectious organism that causes all newborn babies to have no brains, or no legs. A drug that causes children to grow one foot taller by adult life.

AIDS as biological warfare?

Some have suggested that AIDS is the result of a laboratory accident. HIV was made, they say, in a search for new germs for use in wartime and escaped, or was tried out on a few human guinea pigs and spread wildly across the world.

Although we now possess the means to make viruses far more deadly than HIV, we know that HIV virus first appeared at least as far back as the early 1970s and probably as early as the 1950s, at a time when such technology did not exist.[162] Similar naturally-occurring viruses are common in some animals in some countries and have probably been around in one form or another for centuries.[163]

Fifteen years ago we hardly understood anything about viruses and could not even locate the human code for insulin, let alone anything else. It is extremely unlikely that this virus was first made in the laboratory, although it is conceivable that it mutated in a laboratory from an animal virus used to infect human cells in a test-tube experiment.

Testing claims for 'wonder drugs'

When you read a newspaper report, take great care. Medical journals are full of papers which contradict others published only a month or two before. This happens because some studies are badly designed or have very few patients in them. If you throw two dice three times and get three sixes, two ones and a three, you could write a little report saying that you conclude that the dice contains lots of sixes, no twos, and no fours or fives. Everyone would laugh at you because they can pick up the dice and look at them. So what went wrong with your research? You threw the dice too few times to comment and you failed to understand how dice work.

Now if, on the other hand, you threw the dice 10,000 times and half the time they came up with sixes, you might correctly conclude that the pair of dice behave as if they are weighted. If you wrote a newspaper article telling people that all dice from a particular shop are weighted people might believe you—particularly when they hear you threw the dice 10,000 times. You and they would be wrong. How can you generalise about all dice when you tested only two?

You may think these illustrations are an insult to your intelligence, but research workers all over the world make classic blunders every day in the same way. You may not think it possible, but it is.

Take the pill, for example. A very effective contraceptive—but is it safe? Every now and then there is a large increase in the number of pregnancies, many of which unfortunately are ended by abortion. These usually follow some report or other from somewhere in the world that the pill may cause some rare cancer or problem with blood or whatever.

Even if the reports are true—and they are often contradicted by others published months before or after but *not* reported in the press—there is a vital fact missing. None of the reports points out that to be pregnant carries a risk to life. A small risk, but a risk nonetheless. Abortion also carries a risk. The risk to most women is *far* less from continuing to use the pill than from changing to the notoriously unreliable condom[164] with the possibility of a new unwanted pregnancy.

So then, how do we assess the newspaper scoops on new wonder drugs? Ask yourself what the drug does. Where does it act on our scheme of things earlier in the chapter? What are the risks of taking it and how long do you need to take it? How many patients has it been tried on and how many of them have died? Have the results been published in a reputable scientific journal? Many so-called treatments turn out to be elaborate hoaxes or frauds. Recently a woman in the UK was jailed for providing a useless preparation for a fee of £95.[165] People feel better after taking a chocolate Smartie if you tell them it is a wonder drug. This is called the placebo effect. Did these patients know they were being given a wonder drug? If they did, then no wonder they reported feeling better. Your own doctor will be able to advise you on these things. The vast majority of so-called wonder drugs are nothing of the sort, so do not be too disappointed by the negative reaction of your doctor when you show him a press clipping.

When several research papers say the same thing, when each study contains a large number of people with objective results, eg, numbers still alive after five years, then we can start to feel more confident.

New approaches to therapy

In the last year or two, several new approaches have been developed, all of which are highly experimental, yet could offer hope for the future.

1. Combination therapy

Using anti-HIV drugs in combination, so that the dose of each is kept low, side effects are reduced and the virus is hit hard. This approach may also help prevent drug resistance developing in new virus mutations, although early results have been disappointing.[166]

While the results of using AZT early, before people are ill, are confused and contradictory, with many physicians expressing great caution except in those with full-blown AIDS, the real future is likely to be in using two or even three similar drugs at the same time, or in sequence. Trials are particularly looking at:

(a) AZT (azidothymidine)—also known as Zidovudine/Retrovir, made by Wellcome;

(b) ddC (dideoxycytidine)—also known as Zalcitabine, made by Hoffman-La Roche;

(c) ddI—also known as didanosine/Videx, made by Bristol-Myers Squibb.

2. Liposome delivery of drugs

Liposomes are protein bags similar to ones which occur naturally in the body. They fuse with cell walls, so the contents of the liposome (genes or medication) end up inside the cell. This could be helpful in the future, and is becoming a method of delivering new genes to the lungs of people with cystic fibrosis.

3. Gene therapy

This covers a very large number of different approaches, all designed to help the body fight HIV by adding new genes to human cells. These genes can be designed to help cells block infection, or to help prevent virus multiplication.

4. Virus competition

This approach uses another relatively harmless virus to control HIV. For example, scientists have found a human herpes virus (HHV7) that only targets CD4 cells, the same ones that HIV infects. When CD4 cells are occupied by HHV7, there is some evidence that HIV is prevented from access. Inactivated HHV7 shows some effect too. There is a possibility then of a live vaccine one day: a mild virus targeting CD4 cells, spreading in the same way as HIV.[167]

5. Preventing auto-immune reactions

There is some evidence that many dying white cells are destroyed not by HIV directly, but by the body's own defences which have been made aggressive by HIV. For example, an attack on infected white cells can easily damage 'innocent' uninfected cells. Indeed, one part of the HIV structure looks and feels very similar to part of a CD4 cell, so a reaction against HIV could also wipe out white cells directly. It might seem a strange approach in someone with an immune deficiency, but there may be a rationale in some cases in the future to dampen down another part of the immune system using drugs, in order to keep someone well. It all depends which bit of the immune system is dampened down. As we have seen, HIV damages just one part. The rest functions normally, or is even overactive.

6. Blocking cytokine production

We know the cancerous Kaposi's sarcoma is caused by HIV operating together with another agent we have yet to identify. It is a serious condition in people with AIDS and a common cause of death. It seems that HIV makes some white cells overactive so they produce a large amount of a chemical stimulant called cytokine. As a result, cells lining small blood vessels begin to divide and the sarcoma develops. By blocking cytokine production it may be possible to help prevent Kaposi's sarcoma. (For further avenues, see pp 125–126.)

7. Developing a spermicidal cream

For those seeking to avoid sexual infection with HIV, there is an urgent need to develop a new spermicidal cream which is highly active in destroying HIV. This could be used in addition to a condom.

In summary, then, HIV infection is highly complex, involving new, dangerous genes being added to white cells. As gene technology advances rapidly we may hope to see real progress towards a safe, effective, low-cost vaccine or cure. However, the advances being made at present are painfully slow, despite a vast global research effort. This must focus our energy all the more urgently on prevention.

Having seen what a virus is, and how HIV enters and destroys a cell, we can now begin to look at what happens to the body when large numbers of these cells start to die.

3

When Cells Start to Die

The virus causing AIDS enters the blood and quickly penetrates certain white cells (called 'CD4' cells) in the body. As we saw in the last chapter, they program the white cells after which there is often little or no trace of the virus at all. This situation usually lasts for six to twelve weeks. During this time the person is free of symptoms and antibody tests are negative.

First signs of illness

The first thing that happens after infection is that many people develop a flu-like illness. This may be severe enough to look like glandular fever with swollen glands in the neck and armpits, tiredness, fever and night sweats. Some of those white cells are dying, virus is being released, and for the first time the body is working hard to make correct antibodies. At this stage the blood test will usually become positive as it picks up the tell-tale antibodies. This process of converting the blood from negative to positive is called 'sero-conversion'. Most people do not realise what is happening, although when they later develop AIDS they look back and remember it clearly. Most people have produced antibodies in about twelve weeks.

Latent infection

Then everything settles down. The person now has a positive test, and feels completely well. The virus often seems to disappear completely from the blood again.[168] However, during this latent phase, HIV can be found in large quantities in lymph nodes, spleen, adenoid glands and tonsils.[169] We do not know how many people will go on to the next stage. As we saw in an earlier chapter, at first doctors thought it might only be one in ten, then two or three out of ten. Now it looks as though at least nine out of ten will develop further problems.

San Francisco studies show 50% with HIV develop AIDS in ten years, 70% in fourteen years. Of those with AIDS, 94% are dead in five years.[170] The rate of progression can be faster in those with weakened immunity from other causes—drug users[171] or those in developing countries, for example.

Some scientists and doctors are convinced that if we follow up infected people for long enough—maybe for twenty years or more—then all or nearly all will die of AIDS.[172] How long can someone live before some infection triggers production of more virus and death of more white cells?

The next stage begins when the immune system starts to break down. This is often preceded by subtle mutations in the virus, during which it becomes more aggressive in damaging white cells.[173] Several glands in the neck and armpits may swell and remain swollen for more than three months without any explanation. This is known as persistent generalised lymphadenopathy (PGL).

Early disease progression

As the disease progresses, the person develops other conditions related to AIDS. A simple boil or warts may spread all over the body. The mouth may become infected by thrush (thick white coating), or may develop some other problem. Dentists are often the first to be in a position to make

---

Died from AIDS

Rock Hudson	Film star 1985
Freddie Mercury	Rock star 1991
Ian Charleson	Actor 1990
Liberace	Entertainer 1987
Roy Halston	Fashion Designer 1990
Rudolph Nureyev	Ballet dancer 1993
Miles Davis	Jazz musician 1991
Tina Chow	Model 1992
Tony Richardson	Director 1991

Over two million others somewhere . . .

'One death is a tragedy, a thousand deaths is just a statistic' Joseph Stalin 1879–1953

---

the diagnosis.[174] People may develop severe shingles (painful blisters in a band of red skin), or herpes. They may feel overwhelmingly tired all the time, have high temperatures, drenching night sweats, lose more than 10% of their body weight, and have diarrhoea lasting more than a month. No other cause is found and a blood test will usually be positive. Some call this stage ARC, or AIDS related complex.

You can easily panic reading a list of symptoms like this because all of us tend to read about diseases and think instantly we've got them. Chronic diarrhoea does not mean you have AIDS. Nor do weight loss, high temperatures, tiredness and swollen glands. These things can be particularly common in many developing countries.

At the moment in places like the UK there is an epidemic of viral illnesses which cause fevers, tiredness and other symptoms that last a long time, always go away completely, and have nothing to do with AIDS. See your doctor or go to a clinic for sexually-transmitted diseases (STD) or genito-urinary medicine (GUM) if you are unsure.

Late HIV illness—AIDS

The final stage is AIDS. Most of the immune system is intact and the body can deal with most infections, but one or two more unusual infections become almost impossible for the body to get rid of without medical help—usually intensive antibiotics.

These infections can be a nightmare for doctors and patients. The desperate struggle is to find the new germ, identify it, and give the right drug in huge doses to kill it.[175] The germ may be hiding deep in a lung requiring a tube (bronchoscope) to be put down the windpipe into the lung to get a sample. The person is sedated for this. It may be hiding in the fluid covering the brain and spinal cord, requiring a needle to be put into the spine (lumbar puncture). It may be hiding in the brain itself. It may hide in the liver or gall-bladder or bowel. It can hide anywhere.

Chest infections are common

The most common infection is a chest infection. A twenty-three-year-old man walks into his doctor's office with a chest infection not responding to antibiotics. He is flushed and has a high temperature. He has been increasingly short of breath with a dry cough for several weeks. He becomes breathless and has an emergency chest X-ray. The X-ray is strange. No one has seen anything like it before. Could this be AIDS? Samples are taken from the lung. The man is rushed to intensive care and is too ill to ask if he would agree to a blood test. Within two days he is dead. A strange germ is found in his lung: pneumocystis carinii. This is incredibly rare except in AIDS.

He may or may not be reported as a statistic to the centre

collecting information on AIDS. This is voluntary and doctors are busy. If he had died a day or two earlier, the cause of death would have been thought to be pneumonia. Yet another silent victim, unnoticed and unrecorded. Our statistics may be incomplete, and remember, no test was done for HIV.

He was unlucky. Average life expectancy if you develop your first pneumocystis pneumonia is just over two years. 78% survive the first episode, only 40% survive the second.[176] You could live for over three years, or you might be dead in three months. Each new chest infection could be your last. Often people seem only an hour or two from death, then pull around, recover completely, and go home for several months until the next crisis.

We know that eighty-five out of a hundred people with these chest infections in Western nations are infected with pneumocystis carinii, but many are infected with several things at once. Worldwide, the commonest HIV-related chest infection is tuberculosis. As HIV spreads, TB is on the increase, with possibly 600,000 extra cases worldwide by the year 2000.[177] Latent TB infection is common in the general population. HIV damage to CD4 white cells allows reactivation, rapid deterioration and death.

A man is being treated for his second pneumocystis pneumonia. He is really thin now and is developing the hard blue marks in his skin of the Kaposi's sarcoma. He also has a sore mouth because of thrush and boils all over his face. He has a tube in his vein for his high-dose antibiotics. He is feeling ill and tired. Although his chest is improving, one morning he complains of headaches and feeling giddy. He is violently sick and becomes confused later in the day. He gets up in the night and asks for breakfast. He falls over and has to be put back to bed. The following day urgent brain scans are ordered and samples of spinal fluid are taken. Is this meningitis—an infection of the brain surface?

Every test is negative and he rapidly gets worse. He becomes very sleepy and weak and his chest gets worse again.

He dies peacefully four or five days later. What caused it? Who knows? A strange infection of his brain? Was HIV directly attacking his brain?[178]

Damage to nervous system

Half of the people with AIDS will develop signs of brain impairment or nerve damage during their illness. In one person out of ten it is the first symptom.[179] HIV itself seems to attack, damage and destroy brain cells of the majority of people with AIDS who survive long enough.[180] The virus is probably carried into the brain by special white cells called macrophages, which then produce more virus there.[181] Brain cells have a texture on their surfaces similar to CD4 white cells which enables the virus to latch on and enter.[182]

The damage happens gradually and often is not noticed until a significant part of the brain has been destroyed: a brain scan shows a shrunken appearance with enlarged cavities. The signs can be threefold: difficulties in thinking, difficulties in co-ordinating balance and moving, and changes in behaviour. Sometimes the problems are caused by other infections spreading throughout the body, or by tumours, all brought on by AIDS.[183]

A thirty-year-old man is fighting hard to get home again and be independent. He has known about his infection with HIV for over three years, ever since he went to the STD clinic complaining of constant diarrhoea, weight loss and tiredness. Having recovered from one chest infection, he is now learning to walk safely without falling over. He is becoming forgetful, cannot remember a telephone number for even two seconds, and is very aware of his shortcomings. With the help of two loyal friends, and our support team of nurses and volunteers, he manages to go home and stay there for a few months. A volunteer rings one day, because he has become gradually more unwell over the last week, is fighting for breath, and has become very frightened. He is readmitted and, despite all therapy, dies a week later.

AIDS—why do people die?

People with AIDS die because of many complex problems such as infections and cancers. The spectrum varies from country to country and from group to group. Here is a survey of autopsies on seventy-five men who died with AIDS in the US from 1982 to 1988:
They showed:
   Cytomegalovirus (CMV) 81%
   Candidiasis (thrush) 69%
   Pneumocystis carinii pneumonia (PCP) 68%
   Kaposi's sarcoma (KS) 65%
   Herpes simplex diseases 39%
   Mycobacteria diseases (including TB) 35%

Many had more than one of the above. The most frequent causes of death were PCP, CMV of lung, adrenal glands or bowel, toxoplasmosis, KS in the gut, bacterial pneumonia. Most deaths were due to difficulties in treating these conditions rather than missed diagnosis. Patterns of illness are changing as people survive longer. For example, in the UK, deaths from cancers have overtaken deaths from pneumocystis pneumonia.[184] In African nations TB would have rated far more highly.

A sixty-three-year-old man spends all day asleep at home. He has been unwell and has lost weight. He is sent to the emergency room of the hospital. He has been a practising homosexual but has not had sex with anyone for six or seven years. He agrees to an HIV test when all other tests are negative. The test is positive. He is extremely confused, and he becomes incontinent of urine and is catheterised. He lives with a friend who cannot manage him at home. After several weeks, he is transferred to an AIDS hospice unit. Apart from dementia, he develops few other problems and dies peacefully of pneumonia some four months later.

Brain damage affects children as well. In one study, sixteen out of twenty-one children with AIDS developed progressive brain destruction (encephalopathy).[185] But any part of the nervous system can be damaged in adults or children, not just the brain, and AIDS can mimic just about any other disease of nerves.[186]

Children with HIV

Worldwide, over a million children have HIV infection and half a million may have died. In the US alone, around 2,000 babies are born with HIV each year.[187] Altogether, 83% of children with HIV will show some kind of abnormality in their white cells, or will have symptoms, by the time they are six months old. Problems seen can include large lymph nodes, enlarged liver and spleen, failure to thrive (small for age), small head, ear infections, chest infections, unexplained fever, encephalopathy (brain deterioration).[188]

Children with AIDS[189]
10% with HIV die before one year old
73% with HIV still alive by fifth birthday
50% alive after eighteen months ill with AIDS
28% alive after four years with AIDS

Of those showing symptoms within the first year of life, half die before the age of three.[190] However, with improved treatments children are surviving longer. A common pattern is beginning to emerge of a child who becomes unwell in the first year or two of life with different chronic or acute infections, yet with treatment carries on for many years, possibly even into adolescence with many ups and downs. Pain and other symptoms are often overlooked in these children.

Blood tests are often confused by the presence after birth of the mother's own antibodies. All babies of infected mothers will test positive for around the first year, whether infected or not. There is a very slight risk that children who later test negative may still carry HIV. If first infected in the womb, the child may regard HIV as part of itself and not react to it.[191] We are still in the early stages of learning about HIV in children.

Skin rashes and growths

The majority of people with AIDS develop skin problems which are usually an exaggeration of things common to most people, such as acne and rashes of various kinds.[192] Cold sores and genital herpes may develop, or warts. Athlete's foot in severe forms, ringworm and thrush are common. Rashes due to food allergy are also common—no one knows why. Hair frequently falls out. Drug rashes frequently occur, often due to life-saving Septrin (co-trimoxazole) used for treatment or prevention of the pneumocystis carinii pneumonia.[193]

Kaposi's sarcoma develops in about a quarter of the people with AIDS (depending on the country and route of infection). This produces blue or red hard painless patches on the skin, often on the face. In the majority of these people it is the first sign of AIDS. Tumours can spread to lymph nodes, gut lining and lungs where they can be confused with pneumocystis pneumonia. The growths may be caused by a second virus that is allowed to grow more easily if you have AIDS.[194] Treatment consists mainly of radiotherapy and chemotherapy, including injections of the lesions.[195]

Because it often affects the face or may be visible elsewhere on the body and is so distinctive, people who develop Kaposi's sarcoma often feel especially vulnerable. In fact people usually live longer if they first develop this tumour than if they first develop a pneumocystis pneumonia.[196] Kaposi's sarcoma is less common in drug users with AIDS, presumably because it is caused by a second virus also found in gay men, which is then activated by HIV. Some researchers have suggested that the sarcoma is also associated with the use of nitrate inhalants (poppers) often used as a muscle relaxant by gay men.[197] However, this has been disputed.

The other common cancer is a tumour (lymphoma) which develops in the brain or elsewhere in the body.

Problems in gut, eyes and other organs

Almost all people with AIDS have stomach problems from strange infections[198] and cancers caused by AIDS and HIV attacking the gut directly. All three cause food to be poorly digested resulting in diarrhoea and weight loss. Stool samples can be examined or samples can be taken from within the gut using special tubing (endoscopy) to see if there is a second treatable infection in addition to HIV.

AIDS can also seriously affect sight in up to a quarter of all those with HIV by allowing an infection of the back of the eye (retinitis).[199] This is usually caused by cytomegalovirus and is sometimes amenable to treatment.[200] In addition, the virus can cause damage to other organs of the body such as the heart.[201]

Changing disease pattern in adults

In different parts of the world, AIDS tends to have its own characteristics. This may be due to the pattern of other illnesses present in different communities, which explains why TB is the commonest cause of death from AIDS in Africa. Different patterns may be related to different co-factors (gay men compared to drug injectors, for example), viral differences or possibly genetic differences.

However, patterns are changing. For example, the incidence of Kaposi's sarcoma is falling among gay men with HIV in a number of countries, while it is rising among drug users. Some of these changed patterns are because of altered treatments; others are due to other factors. In the UK, there has been a dramatic shift in the pattern of illness, partly because of improved treatments.[202]

The proportion of people with AIDS who developed pneumocystis pneumonia fell from 56% in 1984 to 24% in 1989. One UK study found this infection killed 46% of those dying with AIDS in 1986, but only 3% in 1989—a dramatic drop explained by the use of AZT, other medication given to help prevent the pneumonias, and prompt treatment.

Partly as a result of longer survival, deaths from Kaposi's sarcoma rose rapidly during the same period from 14% to 32%, while lymphoma deaths also rose from 5.8% to 16%, usually because of a tumour developing in the brain. Survival expectancy increased from ten months (1984–1986) to twenty months (1987), and is probably over thirty-six months today.

As survival times have increased, and as cancer has become the commonest single cause of death in those with HIV, other problems have emerged which are far more difficult to treat. These include blindness due to cytomegalovirus, progressive multifocal leucoencephalopathy (weakness, muscle wasting, difficulty thinking), cryptosporidiosis (causes various infections), mycobacterium infections and cryptococcal meningitis.

In addition, as we have seen, advanced Kaposi's sarcoma can bring its own problems, with lung involvement causing shortness of breath and triggering chest infections, gut involvement causing obstruction or sudden bleeding, and with blockage of lymphatic drainage causing swollen limbs or face, skin ulceration and infection.

In a study of 347 people with AIDS in the UK the following problems were seen:[203]

Pneumocystis carinii pneumonia	51%
Kaposi's sarcoma	25%
Cytomegalovirus in eye or gut	25%
Candida (thrush) from mouth to stomach (oesophageal)	13%
Cerebral toxoplasmosis	10%
Mycobacterium avium infections	10%
Cryptosporidiosis (diarrhoea)	9%
TB elsewhere than the lungs	7%
Cryptococcal meningitis	4%
Lymphoma	5%
Progressive multifocal leucoencephalopathy	2%

In a quarter of those dying with AIDS, the exact cause of death may be difficult to establish, with profound weakness, loss of weight and multi-system failure. Many infections can be chronic, low grade and difficult to diagnose, and when diagnosed can be hard to treat. Indeed, post-mortem examinations show that half of all HIV-related diseases found at autopsy have not been diagnosed during life.[204]

In the early days in many countries, those with AIDS often spent a long time in hospital as doctors battled to get to grips with the complex spectrum of illnesses. Now people with AIDS are usually able to spend more time at home, with many treatments given in clinics or in the home. However, many have multiple problems and need practical help, backed by nursing care and symptom control, to stay at home in comfort and in control of their own lives. Later on in this book we will look at the practicalities of setting up community care programmes.

Many people who are ill are now opting not to have every symptom investigated, when the price is valuable time spent in hospital, unpleasant tests, and treatments that may have side effects.

AIDS diagnosis in developing nations

In developing countries it can be hard to make an accurate diagnosis of AIDS because of the lack of HIV testing facilities. The World Health Organisation proposed a clinical case definition, combining symptoms and signs common in AIDS (see table below). This has been used as the basis for AIDS statistics in many countries, but is inaccurate.

Old World Health Organisation clinical case definition of AIDS for use in Africa (up to 1991)

AIDS in an adult was defined by the existence of at least two major signs associated with at least one minor sign in the absence of known causes of immunosuppression such as cancer or severe malnutrition or other recognised aetiologies

Major signs
- Weight loss > 10% body weight
- Chronic diarrhoea > 1 month
- Prolonged fever > 1 month (intermittent or constant)

Minor signs
- Persistent cough > 1 month
- Generalised pruritic dermatitis
- Recurrent herpes zoster
- Oropharyngeal candidiasis
- Chronic progressive and disseminated herpes simplex infection
- Generalised lymphadenopathy

The presence of generalised Kaposi's sarcoma or cryptococcal meningitis were in themselves sufficient for the diagnosis of AIDS

A study of hospital patients in Zaire showed that the case definition missed 31% of AIDS cases (definition not very sensitive), and 10% of those it identified as having AIDS were errors.[205] The case definition misses people dying with severe HIV illnesses which do not fit the definition. For example, deaths from streptococcal pneumonia are far more common in those with HIV, yet such deaths were not included.

The commonest manifestations of AIDS in Africa are gross weight loss, chronic diarrhoea and chronic fever—the picture of 'slim disease' as AIDS is known in African countries. However, it is difficult to exclude other causes for the same symptoms and signs.

Deaths from tuberculosis are another problem. TB is probably the most important infection in those with HIV in Africa. High rates of TB infection are found in those with HIV and the risk of death from TB is greatly increased in those with HIV. However, it is questionable whether all those with TB and HIV can be diagnosed as AIDS cases, since many have TB anyway. Many with TB lose weight and have fever as well as a cough. Therefore in the absence of HIV testing, many with advanced TB are likely to be labelled as AIDS cases using the WHO case definition.

In the light of all these problems, a revised case definition has been agreed (see table).[206] You may wonder how it is possible to be sure of the right diagnosis at all without laboratory facilities, and the answer is that it is very difficult.

Some have pounced on this difficulty to suggest that there is no AIDS in Africa at all. As we see elsewhere, this is not very convincing for two reasons. First, death rates have soared in the sexually-active age groups as HIV infection rates have risen. TB and other illnesses have been around and studied in detail for decades. Something new is happening. Secondly, when people with AIDS from African nations are cared for either in countries like the UK, or in very well-equipped hospitals nearer home, it is clear that there are gross abnormalities of their immune systems indicative of AIDS, with positive antibodies for HIV and damaged white cells.

New WHO case definition for AIDS in Africa[207] (1992)

For epidemiological surveillance an adult (> 12 years) is considered to have AIDS if:

The Centers for Disease Control surveillance case definition for AIDS is fulfilled*
　OR
A test for HIV infection gives positive results
　AND
One or more of the following are present:

- > 10% body weight loss or cachexia, with diarrhoea or fever, or both, intermittent or constant, for at least one month, not known to be due to a condition unrelated to HIV infection
- Tuberculosis with the features given above, or tuberculosis that is disseminated (involving at least two different organs) or miliary, or extrapulmonary tuberculosis (which may be presumptively diagnosed)
- Kaposi's sarcoma
- Neurological impairment sufficient to prevent independent daily activities, not known to be due to a condition unrelated to HIV infection (for example, trauma)

* Certain diseases indicative of AIDS under the CDC surveillance case definition, such as Kaposi's sarcoma, may have a high background incidence or prevalence in Africa, independent of HIV infection. Such conditions should be considered to indicate AIDS only in the presence of a positive HIV test result.

AIDS-related illnesses in Africa

The spectrum of illness seen in AIDS in African nations can vary, particularly in places where HIV-2 is more prevalent. The pattern is very different from developed countries:[208]

Candida (thrush) in the mouth	80–100%
Oesophageal candidiasis	30–50%
Tuberculosis	30–50%
Cerebral toxoplasmosis	15–20%
Herpes zoster (shingles)	10%
Cryptosporidiosis (diarrhoea)	6–50%

Most people have several problems. (For further discussion on needs of those with AIDS and how to meet them, see Chapters 10, 11 and 14; also Appendices A, B and C.)

So, now that we have reviewed how the virus attacks cells and causes diseases associated with AIDS, we are in a position to look at some of the ways the virus can enter the human body and how we can prevent it from happening.

Classification of HIV illness

This classification of HIV disease is now replacing the terms ARC and AIDS. The term AIDS is less and less helpful, but in most countries is defined as a combination of group 4 below.[209]

Group 1: Acute infection—transient illness.

Group 2: No symptoms or signs.

Group 3: Persistent generalised lymphadenopathy.

Group 4: a. Constitutional: fever > one month; weight loss > 10%; diarrhoea > one month.

b. Neurological: encephalopathy, myelopathy or peripheral neuropathy.

c. Secondary infections:
  c1. Pneumocystis, cytomegalovirus, toxoplasmosis, recurrent pneumonia.
  c2. Oral hairy leucoplakia, widespread herpes zoster (shingles), salmonella, tuberculosis, oral thrush.

d. Secondary cancers: Kaposi's sarcoma, non-Hodgkins lymphoma, primary cerebral lymphoma, invasive cervical cancer.

e. Other conditions.

However, many doctors are now finding it more helpful simply to divide those infected into two groups: HIV well and HIV unwell.[210]

On 1 April 1992, the US centres for disease control issued a new case definition for AIDS: all HIV-infected people with cell counts of less than 200/NL. This effectively doubled US AIDS figures, and makes comparisons with many other nations meaningless. The EC made small changes in July 1993.

4

How People Become Infected

Different groups of people tend to become infected with HIV for different reasons. Children, drug addicts, sexually-active homosexuals, and heterosexual men and women are all developing AIDS in particular ways. Whole family groups are now becoming ill.

How children get infected with HIV

By 1993 some estimated that there had been 20,000 HIV-infected children born in New York City alone.[211] A friend of mine who is a family doctor cared for his first 'AIDS baby' recently. The UK had 354 children alive with definite or possible HIV by February 1994, with sixty-three deaths.

1. Infection before or during birth

HIV can cross the placenta in the womb, and can also infect during labour, when the baby swallows amniotic fluid and blood. Some people used to think pregnancy could shorten the life of a woman with HIV. Doctors now think the risk of rapid deterioration is not very great.

The baby of a woman who is infected has a 15–30% chance of being infected and dying within a year or two (estimates vary).[212] The number of infected babies is rising fast in the United States as the number of infected female drug addicts rises. In New York one in sixty-one newborn babies is born to an infected mother. Survival also varies, as we have seen: many infected babies die in the first year, but an increasing number grow up into their teens with intermittent problems.

2. Infection just after birth

Mother's milk can carry the virus from mother to child.[213] This may account for up to half of all infections from mother to baby. One critical factor may be when the mother becomes infected, since virus levels are highest shortly after infection. The risk of infection to baby could be 29% if the mother is infected while breastfeeding, 14% additional risk if the mother is infected before delivery.[214] As a result, many hospitals in the United Kingdom have discontinued milk banks for sick babies. Questions have been raised over what advice to give mothers in developing countries. Conventional wisdom is that the risk of death from diarrhoea and vomiting due to contaminated bottle feeds is too great to allow mothers to stop breastfeeding (artificial feeding is a major factor in deaths of 105 million infants a year).[215] The balance of risk may vary according to the individual and the local situation, especially if the mother is known to have HIV.[216]

3. Vaccinations/injections

In Eastern Europe and Africa infection has spread through using the same needles between patients. If there are only a few needles left which are not hopelessly blunt, the temptation is great to immunise a whole clinic with a single needle. Blood from one infected child can spread the disease to others in the group. In some parts of Africa and Eastern Europe many medicines are injected rather than swallowed. Mothers seem to prefer it.

4. Transfusions and blood products

Unfortunately some children in the UK received blood or products made from blood before testing and heat treatments

were started in 1985. A terrible tragedy is that over half the
people in the United Kingdom who have a severe form of the
rare haemophilia bleeding disorder and were given blood
products in the mid-1980s were infected (around 1,200
people), many of whom were children (around 240). As we
saw in an earlier chapter, many Romanian children also
received infected blood. In some parts of Africa, up to one in
ten of all new infections is thought to be related to blood
transfusions. Although the cost of testing is less than a dollar a
unit, this is still beyond the budgets of many countries.
Education of health care workers is critically important: to use
fewer injections, less blood, and take great care.

5. Incest/sexual abuse/child prostitution/early teenage sex/ drugs

A thirteen-year-old girl shyly came up to me with a friend
after a talk I gave to her class. I had to ask her teacher to leave
before she could bring herself to speak. She wanted to know if
someone could get infected with HIV through being raped.
She was thinking of someone in particular. I had to say yes.

I was talking to a church leader recently who has an eight-
year-old boy in his church who is infected. No one knows
how. We are going to see an increasing number of these
tragedies. In New York, a self-appointed orthodox rabbi fled
to Israel after being accused of assaulting 100 children under
the care of his private psychology clinic. Nearly a third of
these children are now infected.[217]

A child has become infected after sexual abuse by the
mother's boyfriend.[218] A child in Trinidad has become
infected following sexual abuse.[219] Five children in Australia
have developed AIDS after being sexually abused.[220] The risk
of HIV infection in sex abuse cases is such that some have
suggested HIV testing for all sexually-abused children who
develop infections or weight loss.[221]

Child prostitution is a major worry in London. A professor
of paediatrics at a London teaching hospital resigned recently

after a child pornography business was discovered (photographs and magazines), although there was never any suggestion that he had acted in anything other than a fully professional way with his patients.

The message is that many adult men from a wide variety of backgrounds find children sexually exciting, leading to activities ranging from reading child pornographic magazines to seduction of children to violent molestation. These things have terrible and permanently devastating effects on children and also expose them to the risk of AIDS. Children are also becoming sexually active very young and are not changing their behaviour.[222] Street kids are at high risk in countries like Brazil. Gonorrhoea and syphilis are common in fourteen- to sixteen-year-olds in New York detention centres.[223]

One unfortunate trend in high-incidence countries such as Thailand or Uganda has been the targeting of young teenage girls for sex by older men, who hope they will be less likely to be carrying HIV than adult women. This is one reason why the ratio of infected teenage girls to boys can be as high as five to one.[224]

Child prostitution is becoming a global problem. In Taiwan there are an estimated 60–200,000, while around a million children are thought to be traded as sex slaves each year in South East Asia. UNESCO estimates that 800,000 children work as prostitutes in Thailand alone,[225] while child prostitution is also growing in other parts of the world.

How drug addicts get infected with HIV

Drug addicts become infected by sharing syringes and needles.[226] A common habit is to rinse the last dregs of drug out of the syringe using your own blood—drawing blood out of your vein and injecting it again. This means the next person injects a lot of virus into the bloodstream if the previous person is infected with HIV. It is far more dangerous than if a doctor pricks himself with a bloody needle. In that case the amount of blood involved would be much less.[227] In Edinburgh, the virus spread from one addict to infect between 1,000 and 2,000 other people in eighteen months. In Thailand, 50,000 drug addicts were infected in two years, with other countries likely to become similarly affected.[228]

The drug addict population is hard to estimate. Addicts do not like to stand up and be counted. Those with children are often scared their children will be taken into custody. Others are just shy of any official contact.[229] In the United Kingdom the only ones known about are those who enrol in government programmes to wean them off heroin and other narcotics. Even though this often gives an addict regular drug supplies for life, many are still reluctant to come forward.

Estimates vary from 50–100,000 daily using heroin or similar drugs in the United Kingdom,[230] which includes 1–3,000 in Edinburgh.[231] In the United States the estimate of drug addicts is thought to be around 1–2 million.[232] But this may be a gross underestimate. No one knows. AIDS has the potential to spread quickly in this group, although in the UK at least there has been a very encouraging drop in needle sharing, and infection rates among drug injectors have stabilised. A growing number are starting to inject drugs other than heroin, such as amphetamines.[233] The risk is still the same.

The United Kingdom government is willing to give free drugs to addicts to cut out the growing power base of drug bosses. In the United States some say money from drug dealing now exceeds the entire defence budget. Funds channelled by drug dealers in dishonest ways can destabilise a country; dealers own people, companies, factories, weapons, and they buy votes. Needle-exchange schemes are running in New York and many other cities. Volunteers visit 'shooting galleries' where addicts share needles, giving out bleach and condoms. Methadone treatment centres are expected to increase in number from 4,000 to 8,000 just to accommodate the huge rise in the drug addict population. Washington, DC, also has a severe shortage of places for its 16,000 addicts.

The United Kingdom government is providing free needles at twelve centres and has found that addicts will be less likely to share them, despite the suggestion that issuing needles may actually accelerate the growth of drug abuse.[234] In Italy where needles have been available from chemists for years, over half the addicts are infected. It certainly makes things hard for the police: 'My men are being asked to turn a Nelsonian eye while the addicts uplift their needles,' said one police inspector.[235]

Drug abusers (including alcoholics) have an increased risk of becoming infected with HIV in other ways. When they are 'under the influence', judgement is impaired and risks can be taken. Safer sex, discretion and caution can be thrown to the wind. The same with safe injecting practices. Drug addicts are often thought to be hard to educate, not only because they are hard to find and possibly hard to motivate (some addicts can have a kind of death wish), but also because, even if they decide to be careful, they may forget in the rush of the moment. However, education has worked, to the surprise of many.[236]

The third extra risk is that by injecting all kinds of foreign substances—including dirt, germs, and powdered chalk[237]— the immune system is weakened. Addicts frequently come into clinics with huge septic boils, rashes, or strange fevers (septicaemia). They are in no fit state to fight HIV. Infection is more likely and deterioration probably more rapid. An infected addict should be encouraged to stop. It seems that poppers (nitrites) used to increase sexual arousal may also be associated with greater risks of infection, probably because they weaken the immune system directly.[238] We are going to hear a lot more about drug addicts and AIDS over the next few years, because a large number infected in the mid to late 1980s have yet to become ill. Also because so many of them are women, and the women then give birth to infected babies or sometimes work as prostitutes. Because of drugs, half the prostitutes in Edinburgh and 13% in New York are infected.[239]

Drug users may also be at risk of becoming infected when they are in prison. Most addicts end up in prison at some time in their lives. In the UK, for example, this means that some 12,000 out of 100,000 are behind bars at any one time, an increasing number of which are infected.[240]

Containing spread in prisons is difficult, with many calls not only for condom issue (could be illegal as prison is technically a public place, so condom issue may encourage public sex), but also for needle provision. However, a bloody needle and syringe make a formidable weapon in the hands of someone who may be infected. Prison officers fear attack. In the meantime, injectors may be at greater risk of sharing in prison than in the community. In most prisons a wide range of drugs are freely available from illicit sources.[241] In the absence of needles, even greater risks may be taken. An ACET prison worker recently talked to a man who had shared parts of a ballpoint pen as a 'needle' to inject drugs into his neck.[242] The needle provision issue is discussed more fully on page 322.

Legalisation of drug use

The spread of HIV and the emergence of needle exchanges, in addition to the system of registration in countries like the UK, mean that addicts can now obtain medically prescribed opiates and injecting equipment. Such countries are possibly already halfway to legalisation of drug use.

With some national economies increasingly destabilised by the massive power of drug-dealing co-operatives, there are increasing calls for some system of licensing for personal possession and use of drugs. The head of Criminal Intelligence and of London's Scotland Yard said recently that 'the time had come to think the unthinkable'.[243] Other nations may do so first. The argument is that such a move would cut out the drug pushers, the criminal trading activity, reduce drug-related theft and violence, and allow police resources to be diverted elsewhere. Once the percentage of drug users in a population reaches above a certain level it becomes increasingly difficult to enforce the law. The counter-argument is that legalisation will greatly encourage experimentation and addiction.

Drug users infected with HIV could become a major source of infection in the heterosexual community of some nations. A study at London University published in 1993 showed that 70% of drug injectors were sexually active, 70% never used condoms with their main partners, 48% had non-injecting partners, 33% never used condoms with casual partners—even if they were infected too. Of the sample of 534 people, 13% were infected.[244]

How practising homosexuals get infected with HIV

In the United States of America and the United Kingdom, HIV has spread rapidly through gay communities. Why? There are two reasons. First, it does appear that someone who allows a man to push his penis into his rectum and ejaculate there has a particularly high risk of getting the infection.[245] The lining of the anus is fragile. The lining of the rectum is also likely to bleed during anal intercourse, especially if a pre-sex douche (enema) or a dildo (artificial penis) is used. It is possible that some cells in the rectum have surfaces particularly suited for HIV to latch on to and can become a reservoir for infecting the whole body.

Anal intercourse has always been known to carry a health risk: as we have seen, hepatitis B virus is spread easily by this route and many active homosexuals appear to have chronic low-grade infections of various kinds that may then lower their resistance to HIV.

Many people have jumped on these suggestions to reinforce their quite mistaken belief that AIDS is a gay disease. It is part of their mental defences—a desire to turn AIDS into someone else's problem. The fact is that the characteristics of anal sex are not enough to explain what has happened to the gay community and, in any event, as we have seen, over the last twelve months 90% of new HIV infections worldwide have been heterosexually transmitted.

Anal sex is not unusual among heterosexuals in the United States and the United Kingdom. Up to one in ten of women questioned report having had anal as well as vaginal sex in some surveys.[246] Anal sex alone is not the reason for the spread of HIV. The biggest reason of all has to be found somewhere else, which brings us to perhaps the main reason why the gay community is experiencing an epidemic.

If you are an active homosexual, a major predictor of infection has to do with the number of different men you have had intercourse with over the last few years. This is only a generalisation. There are people who have become infected after having had sex with only one man. However, in general, the same rule holds true—the greater the numbers, the greater the risk.[247]

It is true that some practices carry a particular risk of trauma and infection, eg 'fisting', where the hand and sometimes the forearm are inserted into the rectum.[248]Surveys show many surprises. For example, the frequency of oral/anal contact and use of urine in gay sex.[249] The trouble is that in the days when only one in a hundred gay men was infected, reducing your numbers of different partners from, say, fifty a year to six a year was likely to reduce your risk of sex with an infected person considerably. But once infection levels rise, the advice breaks down. If every third person you sleep with is likely to be infected,[250] what starts to matter is the number of times a year you have sex with someone who is positive.

You might have only three different partners in a year, but if you have sex with one of them for four months, and he is positive, you are very likely to get infected. The very promiscuous person who slept once each with 100 different men, may in fact have been taking a lower risk: only one episode of infected sex a year compared to the second example of maybe fifty episodes a year. These are reasons why the spread of HIV will continue even if drastic changes in behaviour occur. The changes need to be even more drastic.[251]

The AIDS epidemic has forced social psychologists to ask some basic questions about human behaviour—questions that may be embarrassing and have been hidden behind closed doors for decades. Questions like: How many people have you had sex with in the last ten years? Do you have sex with more than one person regularly, or are you frequently unfaithful to a regular partner? What sexual techniques do you practise? Have you ever had sex with a man if you are a man, or with a woman if you are a woman? If you are married have you had homosexual sex since marriage? If you consider yourself a homosexual, have you ever had intercourse with the opposite sex?

These questions are extremely hard to get honest answers to,[252] but are extremely important to enable us to predict how the disease might spread in order to plan effective education. In a clinic for sexually-transmitted diseases some of these questions are asked routinely. The fear of answering can stop some coming for treatment, which is why these clinics have to go out of their way to provide an accepting non-critical atmosphere. Many studies to get further information have been based in these clinics because people have already opened up simply by attending. The results are fascinating.

One of the big surprises to emerge from a recent large sexual survey in the UK was how few men said they had homosexual partners. The UK study interviewed over 18,000 people.[253] While the famous Kinsey study in the US (1948) had given figures of 37% of men having had a homosexual experience to the point of orgasm, 10% exclusively homosexual for more than three years and 4% lifelong homosexuals, the UK study showed a different pattern. Less than 5% had ever had a homosexual experience, and only 1.7% had had sex in a homosexual relationship in the last five years. When the latter result was separated out, great regional differences were found: 5% in London and only 1% in the rest of the country.

The results caused uproar because they challenged the established view that about one in ten of the male population was a sexually-active homosexual. However, the figures were not so much of a surprise to those running sex disease clinics, or working in the AIDS field. For some time people had been quietly saying that the sexually-active gay community seemed to be far smaller than originally thought. This was vitally important in making forecasts about HIV spread and numbers of AIDS cases. After all, if a London clinic found that a quarter of all gay men attending were HIV-infected, it was vitally important to know if that was a quarter of a total of 2,000 men, or a total of 10,000.

Within a few weeks similar surveys were published in France and the US. Both confirmed the basic findings, contradicting the critics who said the surveys were misleading because gay men were afraid to answer honestly.[254] It is true, however, that the surveys may well have underestimated homosexual activity to a degree, but most experts on sexual behaviour have now concluded that the enormously influential Kinsey study was flawed.

One of the things that shows up is that sexual behaviour is far more chaotic than many people imagine. Many of us have stereotyped impressions which are miles away from what is actually going on in people's homes, or in the streets.

For example, a United States study has shown that possibly one in four men who have sex with men also have sex with women.[255] Considering that up to seven out of ten homosexual men in San Francisco (depending on number of partners) are infected with HIV, this is worrying indeed for women in the area. No wonder an increasing number are becoming infected. In the UK, a national sex survey showed that 59% of men having anal sex with men had also had female partners.[256]

Sexual preference sometimes changes with circumstances. A starving man on a desert island will eat strange foods. The reason why there are serious outbreaks of all sexually-transmitted diseases (including HIV and AIDS) in prisons is that many men who behave heterosexually outside prison practise homosexually in prison. I have been on two occasions into Wormwood Scrubs to see new prisoners being admitted. All are routinely tested for gonorrhoea and syphilis because if they're not, the diseases could spread throughout the prison in a few months. The same risks for HIV exist in prisons.[257]

Incidentally, in some prisons dominant prisoners will, with the assistance of others, force new prisoners to receive anal sex.[258] This form of initiation brings fear, humiliation and respect of the boss.[259]

Surveys show that some homosexual men go on to marry and maintain exclusive heterosexual relationships.

However, the most startling fact to emerge from many different studies both in England and in the United States has been the enormous number of different partners some homosexual men used to have in a year. This is in fact no surprise to anyone who has worked in an STD clinic. Dr Fluker, consultant in charge of West London Hospital Martha and Luke Clinics, said in a lecture before he retired[260] that in his experience it was not unusual for some of his homosexual patients to have had 300 or more different partners in a year—most of whom were met only briefly on one or two occasions.

Over half those attending a London clinic said they had had between six and fifty partners in a year. Many had between fifty-one and a hundred—how do you keep an exact count? Common meeting places are certain well-known public toilets, gay bars and other known venues.[261]

In one US study, some gay men claimed up to 5,000 previous partners.[262] San Francisco officials were so worried about the horrendous risks being taken daily at the bath houses that they were all shut down by law. One senior churchman, himself part of the gay community, told me the reason bath houses had originally been so popular was to ensure that an anonymous pick-up was at least going to be safe. Not safe from AIDS—this was before all that—but safe from violence or murder.

I have attended several post-mortems of people in West London who have been cruelly and savagely mutilated and murdered by an unknown partner. Male rape is increasingly common,[263] either by surprise attack in a public place or by a trusted father-figure such as a teacher, youth worker, priest, or stepfather. Sometimes the attacker is alone, sometimes in a group.[264] It is not that gay people are any more violent—you only have to look at the female rape, abduction and murder figures to see that.

Why the extreme promiscuity by some? The contrast with the heterosexual group is enormous. Very few men will claim to have slept with more than fifteen women in a year. The vast majority claim to have had only one partner in any year.[265] Incidentally that is still unsafe. Each different partner each year is a new risk—even assuming faithfulness on both sides for twelve months. Serial monogamy is very common and is not the answer to AIDS.

When a prominent churchman was appointed as an Episcopalian bishop recently, he was shocked and outraged by what he found in the gay community. What made people do this? What happened to a sense of belonging or relationship? The answer he discovered was that, in 'coming out', many gay men had felt able to leave behind conventional restraints such as marriage, home, pregnancy, or anything else.

By deciding to sample 'the fruits of the earth', with no relationship ties, they had found a 'wonderful new freedom'. Even people living together in stable homosexual relationships for years were expected to explore regularly outside that relationship.[266] Public disapproval of gay partnerships also tended to make stable relationships difficult to form and maintain.

In San Francisco, studies have clearly shown that the more partners a homosexual man has had over the previous ten years, the more likely he is to be infected. Those with the most partners are the worst affected, with up to 70% testing positive.[267] Remember, though, the people with AIDS whom you meet may have had only one or two partners. The best man at the wedding of a friend of mine died of AIDS. He was an active churchgoer. He had thought seriously about monastic life. He had had only one short homosexual relationship before AIDS was even recognised as a disease and had never been to an STD clinic. You see, just one person can infect many others in a year, some of whom may never have had homosexual sex before and may never do so afterwards.

The other popular misconception is that because many gay men have multiple partners, they are uncaring. One of the most impressive things about the Shanti project[268] in San Francisco, or the Terrence Higgins Trust in London, or Body Positive, is the warmth of care, love and compassion among the volunteers and friends of the person with AIDS.

I think that this is where one of the stereotypes may be true: many gay men have a gentleness and softness that people usually expect to find in women. That is why so many women make such excellent nurses, mothers and comforters. Shanti is full of such female characteristics despite the virtual absence of women. The quality of caring is exceptional and is similar in many ways to that which exists in a church like the one I belong to. The paradox is that in my church it is in the context of faithful happy marriages, extended families, positive celibacy, or waiting for the right person. In the gay communities in the past, it has often been in the context of multiple casual sexual encounters.

It is important to understand the reason why. Gay people have felt totally ostracised and rejected by society. Beaten up in alleyways, labelled as perverts, and victims of relentless low-grade discrimination, they have often felt misfits. Rejected by family and former close friends, many have found tremendous security and self-acceptance among others who have been through an identical experience. The feeling of togetherness is strong. At last they can be themselves without fear of rejection. This fear is often of heterosexual men. Women are usually more tolerant.

This feeling of intense rejection, isolation, loneliness and vulnerability is then magnified a thousandfold by AIDS. The illness suddenly blows the cover off a quiet homosexual man. Everyone knows he is gay. 'That queer deserves every bit of it,' is on people's lips, even if unsaid. The person may feel so guilty anyway about his lifestyle that he suspects this is what everyone is saying behind his back, or thinks that he deserves it.

This totally false 'gay-plague' label has stuck and reflected on a whole community which has responded with an amazing mobilisation of talent, resources and kindness to support and surround people with AIDS with love. Victims, as they see it, not of AIDS, but of horrendous prejudices and discrimination.

No wonder the gay community is so sensitive to the hostile attitudes of some parts of the church. Many people in the gay community have seen AIDS as something that has generated openness and an unprecedented care and concern from people who are not gay: 'Things will never be the same again.'[269] However, others have predicted a possible backlash.[270]

Police arrived at a man's house to arrest him for a suspected crime. They were wearing 'space suits' because they were warned he had AIDS (totally unnecessary). Neighbours saw the suits and set fire to his house leaving his family homeless.

A man went into a hospital for an operation. He was tested for AIDS without his knowledge or consent. He was found to be positive and the result was sent to his doctor. He went to his physician's office one day and as he walked in the door, the receptionist, who opens and files all letters from hospitals to the practice, whispered to a colleague, 'Look, it's the man with AIDS.' The comment was overheard. That night his home was burned to the ground.[271] Why? Just another form of 'queer bashing'. Both these cases happened in London in the late 1980s. Attitudes have softened a lot, but fear and isolation often remain.

A cinema projectionist in England was fired without warning after seventeen years' employment. The reason given was that he was known to be a practising homosexual. He appealed, of course. Since when has a man's sexuality been grounds for dismissal? In the army, yes, in many countries, but in a civilian job? The industrial tribunal made history. They actually upheld the decision on the grounds that he was gay and would therefore be more likely to develop AIDS.[272]

This decision has had devastating implications for every other gay person in any job in the United Kingdom. The decision was overturned by the Court of Appeal.[273] But the fact remains that he was fired, and his appeal to the industrial tribunal was rejected. Do you think he will ever be able to enjoy working there again? His employer has won. Even after winning his second appeal he was entitled to only a few months' wages as compensation. But for what? A devastated life with terrible public exposure of a private lifestyle.

A survey of 321 UK companies showed that four out of a hundred would sack people with AIDS immediately, and twenty out of a hundred would ask them to resign. So in a quarter of jobs, someone with AIDS may find themselves on the dole. Only sixteen out of a hundred would take disciplinary action against those refusing to work with someone with AIDS.[274] In the US, employment attitudes may be more tolerant, perhaps because of strict legislation and the fear of lawsuits. A recent survey showed more than 66% of companies employing 2,500–5,000 workers and about one in twelve smaller companies have employed someone with HIV or AIDS. However, the outcome was unclear from the survey.[275] It is hard not to employ people with HIV on a regular basis when a million of your potential workforce are infected.

We have double standards. In our society we say, 'Do what you like,' but if you are caught there is an outcry. 'It's OK to be gay,' the papers say, until a government official or a spy is caught having an affair with another man. 'Disgraceful,' the

papers declare. 'He ought to be sacked or put in prison.' The
elderly homosexual man is brought to testify under the bright
lights. He hangs his head in humiliation. So much for our
tolerant society. The same is true of any sexual indiscretion or
hint of one. They all become front-page, full-blown
scandals.[276] If you cannot grasp even a hint of the emotional
devastation wrought on many gay people by our society, you
will never remotely understand why the response to AIDS
now from the gay community has been so overwhelming in
terms of practical care, time and financial help.

How women get infected with HIV

Women become infected in several ways. Historically in many
societies women have been disadvantaged sexually and
vulnerable to sexual abuse. It is still true today that it is
very difficult for women in many parts of the world to protect
themselves against HIV from a dominant male partner.

Their main risk in some Western countries in the 1990s is
sleeping with a man who has had sex at some time in the last
ten years with another man, or who has injected drugs.[277]
Once may be enough for him and for her. They will probably
never know because the man will never say. Married women
all over the country are discovering that their husbands have
been having sex secretly with other men for years. The
average interval between marriage and the wife discovering
her husband's homosexual preferences is between five and
fifteen years. The wives usually first discover when full-blown
AIDS is diagnosed. This can happen, too, to a church leader's
wife.[278]

Women can also become infected from a heterosexual man
who has been infected by another woman—commonest in
developing nations—or who is a drug addict.[279] Very rarely a
woman can catch HIV from nursing her child with AIDS.[280]

In African countries such as Malawi or Kenya, the majority
of infected women in some groups have been celibate before

marriage and monogamous since, yet have been infected because of the unfaithfulness of their partners, or because partners were infected before marriage.[281] Some experts have expressed concern at the effect of new Western influences, undermining traditional family values in developing countries, and encouraging higher rates of partner exchange.

Long-term relationships can also clearly carry a great risk where no precautions are taken. Often women may have no idea their husbands are infected, but even if they suspect so, they may be unable to do anything about it.[282] One woman I spoke to after an open-air presentation on AIDS in Uganda told me she was certain her husband was infected because he was continually unfaithful with a large number of partners, but she was unable to make him change to using a condom with her. She was powerless and lived in fear of her life. These are important issues in prevention, but may lead to confronting cultural norms in a way which could be accused of imperialism. Sensitivity is needed (see Chapter 14).

Sensitivity is also needed to tackle dangerous traditional practices in some countries, such as widow cleansing, where the brother of a man who dies is required to have sex with the widow. This is hazardous if the man died of AIDS after infecting his wife with HIV.

Women can be particularly at risk through anal sex, which is far more common among heterosexuals than many people realise. As we have seen, a number of surveys of young women have suggested that up to one in ten have experienced anal intercourse at least once.[283] This carries possibly twice the risk associated with vaginal intercourse, partly because of the possibility of trauma to the delicate anal and rectal lining, but also because there are cells in the wall of the rectum that have receptors for HIV, so can be infected directly.

Women are at high risk through prostitution, particularly as clients may insist that no precautions are taken, or may indulge in violent sex or anal intercourse.

Lesbians are one group of people, apart from those who are

celibate,[284] where HIV infection is almost unknown. I know of only one or two cases where a lesbian woman has infected another.[285] However, there may be many more infected who are as yet unknown. Lesbians are at risk if they inject drugs and have heterosexual relationships as well.

How heterosexual men become infected with HIV

A heterosexual man becomes infected by having sex with a woman who injects drugs, by injecting himself, or by sleeping with a woman who has previously had an infected partner, the latter being the commonest reason worldwide.[286] You will never know unless she tells you. Sex on a single occasion with an infected partner can be enough to infect you, although the risk from a single act is very small (see Chapter 6).

In some developing countries initiation rites such as male circumcision with a communal knife or ritual mutilation can risk HIV spread. Such practices need to be discussed sensitively, as we will see on page 343.

Heterosexual syphilis is increasing in the United States as heterosexuals continue risky lifestyles.[287] Circumcision reduces risk of HIV transmission, probably because the risk of other sexually transmitted diseases is lower.

AIDS and the church

Some churchgoers contracted HIV before they became Christians. It can surface after they have begun new lives and are happily married, infecting their wives and possibly their children as well.

Others who regularly attend church lead double lives: a person can pretend to be one thing for an hour or two a week, and probably at work too, while beneath the respectable veneer he has a drug problem or is sleeping around with men or women. The result may be AIDS.

For some today there is no double life. The risky lifestyle is maintained openly in defiance of traditional church teaching, perhaps in a church led by someone with liberal views.

And tragically, as we will see in Chapter 14, a small but increasing number of church members are becoming infected as missionaries in places like Africa where they are exposed frequently to medical hazards.[288]

5

Questions People Ask

Every day I am asked questions about AIDS, usually the same ones over and over again. Some are based on reasonable fear—of getting the disease from sleeping around, for example. Others are based on unreasonable fear—maybe a fear of going swimming. Here are some common questions and some answers to enable your fears to be reasonable.

Q. How is AIDS caught?

You cannot catch AIDS. You acquire infection with HIV, the virus which after several years can produce the condition we call AIDS. The virus is spread almost entirely through sex and sharing needles or syringes. Other routes are extremely rare, except infection through untested blood in some developing countries, broken or faulty equipment, or inadequate supplies of reagents. Spreading the virus through normal social contact or even through kissing is unknown.

1. Vaginal, oral, or anal sex can transmit the virus from a man to a woman and a woman to a man. Oral (orogenital) or anal sex also transmits in both directions from man to man, and oral sex from woman to woman.[289] In the words of the previous United States surgeon general: 'Sex may be hazardous to your health.'

2. Other sexually-transmitted diseases will make infection more likely.[290] Wherever sores (which may be hidden and

painless) or pus are, there the virus will be in large amounts. These areas are also entry points.

3. Tears, saliva and urine do contain virus, but almost always in tiny amounts. The amount is greatly increased by eye, mouth, or urine infection. White cells in saliva carry the virus in up to nine out of ten people with AIDS.[291] The virus needs to enter the body to cause infection. Swallowed virus particles are kept first in the mouth by gum and cheek linings, and do not enter the blood unless you have mouth sores or cracked lips, then in the continuous pipe we call the gut. They are destroyed by stomach acid. They cannot enter the blood once they enter the stomach. Virus particles inside your gut tubing are no more a part of your body than a plastic bead pushed up your nose. (See question on communion cup below.) Urine will not usually contain much virus unless there is a urine infection.

4. With the exception of sweat, all other secretions from the body may contain virus—especially from wounds. The virus cannot enter the body through the skin unless you have a wound, a rash, or some other cracked area on your skin. The most vulnerable place for this is your hands. Gloves are the best protection.

5. If you are going to 'take a risk', a condom will reduce the risk. Condoms do not give you safe sex. It is safer, true, and condom use reduces your risk enormously if properly carried out.

6. Injecting drugs with a shared needle is dangerous. Non-injected drugs including alcohol may impair judgement and make risks more likely. Poppers may directly damage the immune system, as may other drugs.

7. Safe sex means one thing: for two people who are currently uninfected to enter into an exclusive faithful relationship for life, with neither injecting drugs with shared needles. The trouble is you may never know. If someone wants to sleep with you that badly he or she may never tell you about previous risks or a drug habit.[292]

Q. Should I take the test?

Remember that it is no good turning up at the STD clinic or your family doctor the day after you have taken a risk. You need to wait at least six weeks, ideally three months, for your blood to have time to become positive if you are infected. During this time you must not be in any further risky situations.[293]

Why are you wanting the test? Are you ready for a positive result and all that could mean? Who would you tell? Could you keep it a secret? Remember it could result in a strong reaction against you from people who know. Will you be able to live with that? Are you sure your family doctor will be able to prevent the result from leaking out? It has happened before.[294] Is the receptionist going to know? Are they discreet? A positive result could prevent you from getting a mortgage and will prevent you getting life insurance cover. People should think through these issues, with professional help. It is often easier to change behaviour after a test result.[295] Tests save lives and allow treatment.

Q. What are the insurance implications of having a test?

Insurance company rules vary from country to country. In the UK the Association of British Insurers has laid down guidelines that only those testing positive for HIV or those with a past of drug injecting should be refused cover. Those testing negative should be allowed life insurance. However, premiums are often higher if the risk of HIV is seen to be greater than average, as revealed by a lifestyle questionnaire. For example, one company quoted a monthly premium of £13.43 for an HIV-negative, thirty-year-old, married non-smoker wanting £50,000 of life cover, but £28.70 if he was a single heterosexual, and £48.70 if he was gay with more than five partners a year. An alternative is to agree an AIDS exclusion clause. Insurance companies are nervous about this because it is so difficult for them to find out if someone died from AIDS.[296] (See pp 187–194 for ethics of testing.)

Q. How accurate is testing for HIV?

HIV testing is now very accurate, but it is important to realise that HIV tests often need repeating and can occasionally be wrong. There are two main ways of testing for HIV: indirect and direct. Because HIV is so small and difficult to find in the body, the cheapest and simplest way to detect infection is to look for antibodies that people make to fight the virus. These are very specific to HIV, like a spanner shaped to fit a nut.

The most widely-used test is called ELISA.[297] Results are usually confirmed using a second test called Western Blot, but can be confirmed in some cases by a second slightly different ELISA test. In most cases the antibodies can be detected after about six to eight weeks from the time of infection. In newborn babies there is an added difficulty because the test is confused by the presence of maternal antibodies until around the first year of life.

The first ELISA tests were not as accurate as the ones today, with higher false positive results. There is some evidence that malaria antibodies may have produced a significant number of false positives in some African countries in the mid-1980s,[298] and that the tests were also muddled by other infections. However, the tests are now much more specific, although it is true that if someone has HIV infection, the antibodies against HIV can produce a false positive result when testing for malaria.[299]

ELISA is designed to be ultra-sensitive, picking up every person with HIV antibodies, but the more sensitive the test, the more likely it is to react positively to other things. In a population where the level of infection is very low, up to 70% of all those testing positive with the latest ELISA tests will turn out to be negative when the ELISA is repeated. Proportions vary with the exact tests used.

An initial false positive result can be caused by many

things. For example, recent vaccination against influenza will produce a positive ELISA test in around 1% of uninfected people.[300] Hepatitis B vaccine can also confuse the test. In almost every case, these incorrect results are sorted out by a Western Blot, which is highly specific to HIV. In many countries second or even third tests are carried out on the same sample so that false positives are eliminated immediately. If you wish further technical detail, read on, otherwise skip to the next question.

In the Western Blot test, virus building blocks are made in the laboratory. A number of different fragments of viruses are separated and 'blotted' onto a special surface which is then cut into strips and exposed to the serum sample. Core proteins (p24, p55 and p17) and envelope proteins (gp120, gp160 and gp41) are used. People with HIV tend to produce antibodies to all these bits of HIV. When serum is added to the membrane, together with special markers, you can see a series of colour bands where anti-HIV antibodies have reacted.[301]

A person is only diagnosed as HIV-infected using Western Blot if antibodies are found to at least two of the bands p24, gp41 and gp120/160. Depending on the population group, between 20% and 70% of repeatedly positive ELISA tests are confirmed using Western Blot.

ELISA:[302]
99.3% of infected people are identified (very sensitive)
99.7% of uninfected people correctly test negative (specific)

Western Blot:[303]
98.9% of infected people are identified (sensitive)
97.8% of uninfected people correctly test negative (very specific)

Combining the results of both tests increases accuracy. However, it can be seen that if 10,000 people are tested with ELISA, we can expect that 0.3%, or thirty people, will test positive even if none of the 10,000 is infected. The proportion could be higher if the test was carried out only once, and if testing facilities are poor, as is the case in some countries.

Some samples show a slight reaction to one or two bands. These are called 'indeterminate results'. There are three reasons for this. First, some people may be in the very early stages of infection, so antibodies are not yet fully present. A repeat test a few weeks later will sort that out.

Secondly, some may be infected with HIV-2, which is similar enough for antibodies to cross-react against HIV-1 to some extent.

Thirdly, it may be a true false-positive result: the person may be completely healthy and not infected with any kind of HIV strain. This is very rare.

People with very early infection, or infection with HIV-2, usually show a reaction to the viral core protein p24 first. Between 60% and 90% of HIV-2 infection is picked up with an HIV-1 ELISA test.

Although the 'window period' between infection and antibody detection is usually regarded as about six to eight weeks, around 95% will test positive after twelve weeks and 99% by six months.[304] International standards are maintained at a very high level by the World Health Organisation which regularly sends out test samples to over 100 laboratories.[305]

Some can be ill or dying with AIDS and test negative. The reason here is that their immune systems are so severely damaged that they have lost the ability to form antibodies. The diagnosis is usually obvious from symptoms and other laboratory tests looking at their white cells.

It is possible to test for HIV directly, not waiting for antibodies to develop. This method looks for viral genes—the DNA instructions that the virus inserts into white cells to hijack them into virus factories.

A special chemical reaction is used called PCR (polymerase chain reaction), which can multiply a million copies of viral DNA in three hours, and combined with other equipment can detect as little as one piece of viral DNA in ten microlitres of blood. The test has been useful in some situations to detect possible infection far earlier than antibody tests. More than 90% of antibody positive people also test positive by PCR, but not all. The technique is extremely sensitive to cross-contamination from previous samples. It is very easy to get false positive results.

Viral culture is another method of testing, where attempts are made to obtain HIV from white cells. It can detect 50% of HIV-infected children at birth, unlike antibody testing.[306]

In conclusion then, HIV testing is now very accurate indeed, although the initial test result always needs to be confirmed.

Q. Can saliva be used instead of blood to test for HIV?

Saliva testing is convenient and fast, and depends on finding antibodies to HIV in the mouth. A few drops of saliva are absorbed onto a special pad inserted into the mouth for a few minutes.[307] The length of collection time is important. The fluid can then be tested using exactly the same equipment as for testing blood. Saliva collection has been used to screen prisoners,[308] drug injectors, and now applicants for life insurance.[309] However, studies show the results are not yet quite as accurate as for blood, for two reasons. First, the collection method may not adequately collect antibodies, particularly if the collection period is too brief. Secondly, food residues and other proteins in the mouth may confuse the test, although this is less of a problem as testing methods improve.

By packaging a simple saliva collection device with one of the latest 'instant' testing kits, the technology now exists to market a do-it-yourself home test for HIV, available from chemists.[310]However, there are grave concerns about this. While there may be a market from people who do not want anyone else to know their result, or from people wanting to test new partners or prostitutes in the bedroom, there is a real danger that people will misunderstand the implications of the result, or even take their own lives if the test result is positive and they are not given adequate counselling (see pp 186, 335).

Q. Are all those with HIV going to develop AIDS?

We do not know whether all with HIV will develop AIDS because we have not been following people with HIV long enough. As we have seen, half are ill within ten years and 70% in fourteen years. Long-term survivors are an interesting and important group because they may have within their genetic makeup some kind of enhanced ability—complete or not—to contain HIV infection. Unfortunately, when we study the immune systems of long-term survivors who are well, we find the majority show some signs of immune damage. Of course, the longer people survive, the more likely it is that they will die of some other cause in the meantime before AIDS develops.

Q. Is it possible for people to get rid of HIV once infected?

There have been possibly one or two cases where there has been good evidence of HIV infection, but after a year or two, no trace of virus anywhere in the body can be found. Although it is still too early to be sure, some experts believe that these individuals may have succeeded in eliminating HIV.

It also seems possible that a certain group in the population with particular genes may have some kind of constitutional protection against HIV infection.[311] This should not surprise us. Just like bacteria develop resistance to antibiotics because susceptible bacteria die, leaving one or two variants with natural protection, so we would expect to find among millions of different human beings, a few with gene variations which protect.

By focusing on how the genes work, we may be able to find a way of protecting the rest of the population. For example, one man studied since 1984 is still alive and well with HIV. It seems certain white cells in his body (CD8) are producing a substance which locks HIV inside CD4 cells. The substance is active against all variants of HIV. It is a small protein which has yet to be identified. It could turn out to be a key to therapy in the future.[312]

By analysing people's genes we may also be able to predict in the future what treatments will be most appropriate and at what stage.

Some individuals exposed to HIV show no sign of HIV infection by antibody tests or by PCR viral antigen testing (see previous question on test reliability). However, their white cells show signs of sensitisation to HIV, suggesting that their immune systems have encountered HIV but have eliminated it within days of exposure.[313]

As we will see later (questions on mosquitoes and kissing), it may be that one reason why HIV seems not to be very infectious might be that many people have an ability to destroy a limited number of HIV particles. A small exposure would then fail to infect many people. One US study has suggested that up to 65% of HIV-negative gay men, 45% of negative drug users and 75% of health care workers accidentally exposed, all show evidence of sensitisation, but not infection. The same research workers found strong evidence of HIV sensitisation in around 2% of the US population—not surprising if the official figure of 1 million HIV-infected is correct.[314]

Q. Are some types of condom safer than others?

There are hundreds of different brands available, ranging from latex to animal membrane.[315] The ultra-thin/sensitive varieties are most likely to tear, although any condom may tear during anal sex.[316] All latex condoms will rot rapidly if oil-based lubricants are used, and will deteriorate with storage in high temperatures. Animal membrane condoms may permit virus to pass through more easily.

In summary, if you are taking a risk you need to use a thick latex condom. This will reduce your risk enormously if the condom is correctly and carefully used. (See next chapter for further details on condoms.)

Q. Do the results of an HIV antibody test go on my medical record?

In many countries you can go to a clinic and get a completely anonymous test done. However, the results of named tests are very likely to go on your medical records.

Q. I have heard some say HIV does not cause AIDS and that AIDS in Africa is a myth. What is the evidence?

There has been a lot of confusion in the British press, with suggestions that HIV may not be the cause of AIDS, and that the AIDS epidemic in Africa is a myth.[317] This has in part been due to the claims of a US scientist, Professor Duesberg, who has promoted the view that HIV is relatively harmless, and that AIDS is caused by recreational drugs or other causes of immune damage.[318] Connected with this has been the claim that AZT is useless, even in those with AIDS—indeed that AZT actually *causes* AIDS.[319]

Considering how poorly these claims are supported by scientific data, how few other scientists take them seriously and how damaging the claims are to the health campaign, it is surprising they have been given such sympathetic media coverage.[320] Underlying some of these claims is a conspiracy theory involving alleged multinational fraud by research workers and drug companies, with the collusion of governments and the World Health Organisation.

I am asked for clarification almost every week by well-informed people who are deeply puzzled. The confusion is dangerous too. At the 1993 International AIDS Conference I was handed a leaflet by an AIDS activist titled 'HIV is good for you'.

Here is a brief summary of some of the reasons why almost all scientists working in the AIDS field are convinced that HIV is a highly dangerous infectious virus causing AIDS.

1. The appearance of AIDS always follows HIV spread. In every group studied we have seen the rise in numbers ill with AIDS closely linked to the increasing spread of HIV infection some years earlier.

Example: In Edinburgh rapid spread of HIV among drug users was followed by a steady rise in those ill or dying. In Glasgow, drug users of similar age, background and lifestyle were much less affected by HIV (HIV hit Glasgow later and behaviour changed in time) and death rates have been much lower. Incidentally, scientific studies have shown that nitrites and other recreational drugs do not cause AIDS.[321]

Example: In many parts of Africa people have died from illnesses such as tuberculosis in large numbers for decades. However, a large rise in deaths in the sexually-active age group has followed spread of HIV into this group, with death rates in two years sixty times higher in those with HIV.

Some have claimed that HIV has been present at similar levels for decades. This is nonsense. HIV levels in most towns and cities in many nations show rapid year-on-year rises took place during the 1980s and early 1990s. Indeed, one study in 1986 found HIV levels as low as 1 in 1,000 in some groups, rising since.[322]

Some have claimed that there is no massive AIDS epidemic in Africa and that HIV is being blamed for deaths of people who would have been dying anyway. It is true that diagnosis of AIDS in an individual in Africa can be difficult, as we saw in Chapter 3, but the fact is that death rates in the younger age groups are unexpectedly high—and among babies of those infected too. Many Africans arriving in countries like the UK with HIV, who become ill and die, clearly have an identical illness to those with AIDS infected in industrialised nations.

Some say there is a cross-reaction between malaria antibodies and HIV tests. As we saw in the earlier question on test accuracy, this was a problem in the mid-1980s, but not today. It is obvious anyway that malaria confusion is not taking place on a wide scale. The numbers in the population with malaria antibodies have remained relatively constant, while the numbers testing positive for HIV have soared.

Great weight has sometimes been placed on comments by African specialists and politicians that the AIDS problem has been exaggerated by the West and that the actual size of the epidemic is far less significant than has been made out. Unfortunately, almost all doctors and nurses from European and other nations working in government and mission hospitals give a different story, based on first-hand experience of the unfolding catastrophe. Many African experts are not free to talk about AIDS, for reasons we saw in Chapter 1. Indeed, many Western doctors in these nations may also find it difficult to talk until they go home on leave.

Example: Those with haemophilia have received blood extracts for many years without problems. However, once HIV contaminated their supplies they began to grow ill and die. Some have claimed that these haemophiliacs are only ill because the blood extracts of Factor VIII are rejected as foreign to the body and damage their immune systems. Evidence quoted in favour of this is from unpublished early reports that haemophiliacs with HIV are progressing more slowly to AIDS when converted to pure genetically-engineered Factor VIII. However, if Factor VIII is the sole explanation, why are uninfected people who have been receiving impure blood extracts for years not developing AIDS? We would also expect those receiving HIV in a blood transfusion to remain perfectly well when the fact is that they become ill and die too.

Example: As we have seen, mothers can transmit HIV to their babies through the womb, during birth and in breast milk. These babies get ill and die of AIDS. Those who do not become infected remain well throughout life. Remember of course that we are not talking here about babies falsely testing positive to HIV because the result is confused by maternal antibodies.

2. *The pattern of HIV spread fits AIDS patterns.* If HIV is

the cause of AIDS, we should expect to find that HIV shows evidence of spread through sexual activity and through the blood, since we know people with AIDS are linked by such contact. This is indeed what we find, with overwhelming evidence of person-to-person spread of HIV by these routes.

3. *HIV targets the cells which are damaged in AIDS.* Some have tried to make a case that HIV is just an innocent passenger, not causing illness but just travelling with whatever does do the damage. However, the more we study HIV the more we understand how dangerous it is.

We know that HIV gets inside the same white cells whose death results in AIDS. We know that after an initial brief illness, HIV goes on multiplying in lymph nodes, where large numbers of infected cells can be found throughout the symptom-free period. We know that as virus levels rise, the person becomes more ill. We know that HIV attacks some cells in the brain and in the gut directly, explaining why people with AIDS can have damage to both organs. Although early studies have suggested that only one target white cell in 10,000 becomes infected, more sensitive tests have now detected HIV infection in one in ten cells.[323]

4. *Anti-HIV treatments benefit those with AIDS.* If HIV is the cause of AIDS, then we would expect drugs used to fight HIV to produce an improvement in those who are ill. As we have seen in Chapter 2, there are a great number of independent studies which show that the anti-HIV drug AZT improves the condition and survival of those with AIDS when used appropriately. It is true that AZT has side effects, in particular causing anaemia, and it is also true that resistance to the drug can make treatment less effective after a while. As this happens, CD4 cell levels fall, virus levels rise and the person often begins to deteriorate. This is all evidence of linkage.

Great play has been made by a minority on the discovery of a very small number of people who seem to have an AIDS-like illness with no evidence of HIV infection. I am not referring here to those who for various reasons lose or never develop an antibody response, but those in whom HIV is never found, even with many different detection methods.[324]

There are two explanations for this, neither of which destroys the HIV basis for AIDS. First, we sometimes fail to look hard enough. Even in an illness like TB, it is not always possible to find the organisms. In other very rare cases it appears we are looking at a very rare form of immune problem that has probably been around for centuries, and is nothing to do with AIDS.[325] Such cases account for only a few in a million of what gets diagnosed as AIDS.

In summary then, there is overwhelming evidence that HIV causes AIDS, although, as with the link between smoking and lung cancer, much of it is circumstantial, based on large-scale studies of disease patterns. As we have seen in earlier chapters there are undoubtedly other factors which can cause acceleration or slowing of disease which might include other infections such as mycoplasma[326] and the genetic makeup of the individual.[327]

Q. Is it safe to share pierced earrings?

No. Inserting an earring can cause a tiny amount of bleeding and the earring can accumulate dried debris. Earrings should not be shared. They should be regarded in the same way as needles. Clip-on earrings are safe. Many stores in New York and several in London no longer allow pierced earrings to be tried on. Liberty's of Regent Street have also banned trying on clip-on earrings after an unpleasant scene when a customer noticed a small cut on another customer's ear.[328]

Q. Is a communal bucket and sponge safe for athletes to wash bloody injuries?

The sponge could transmit the virus by allowing blood from one player into another player's wound. Clean the bucket and sponge with antiseptic between players. The virus can survive in water for several days (see p 47).

Q. Are contact sports safe?

You are far more likely to die from a broken neck or be paralysed for life during rough contact sports than catch HIV. For this to happen, blood from an infected player's body would have to be rubbed into a wound on your body. This is extremely unlikely, but may have occurred once.[329]

If the whole of one team was infected, obviously the risks to members of the other team would be greater, but at present the number of infected athletes must be very small, except in certain developing countries.

Q. Are swimming pools safe?

Swimming pools are safe. Some councils took the absurd step of banning all those infected with HIV from using pools.[330] This produced widespread alarm.

The only way you could possibly catch HIV at a swimming pool would be if someone carrying the virus cut themselves— say on glass at the side of a pool—and left a puddle of blood which you stepped in, cutting yourself on the same piece of glass. In the pool itself the dilutions are so enormous that I am sure that even if you poured ten fresh pints of blood full of virus into the pool scientists would be hard pushed to find a single blood cell, let alone a virus particle. My wife and I go swimming regularly with our children and we have no intention of stopping.

Q. What about going to the barber?

This is safe as long as disposable razor blades are used—and preferably disposable razors as well. Shaving tends to draw tiny amounts of blood—maybe too small to see. The old cut-throat razor blade could transmit virus from one client to another. For the same reason, razors should never be shared in a household. British government guidelines were sent to 60,000 barbers and hairdressers in September 1987, but doubts have been expressed about whether they are always followed.[331]

Q. What about contact lens solutions and cases?

The bottles of solution may be shared but lens containers may become contaminated by tears. The plastic or glass lens inserted into the eye could help the virus then to enter the body.

Q. Can the virus survive outside the human body?

People used to think that all the HIV particles became severely damaged after only twenty minutes outside the body. If this were the case, surgeons would only need to hang up their instruments in the sun for an hour before safely carrying on with the next operation. Infection control guidelines are several centimetres thick in many countries. Sterilisation is vitally important. An important paper shows that although most virus particles do become damaged after a few hours, a few may survive after three to seven days in dry dust, and over two weeks in water, although only under unusual conditions. In freeze dried Factor VIII, HIV survives undamaged for months, hence the problems for those with haemophilia before heat treatment began in 1985 (see p 47).[332]

Q. Does the virus survive in someone who has died?

As HIV survives reasonably well outside the body, it is not surprising to find that it also survives in those who have died. A recent survey of post-mortem blood examinations showed that HIV could be found in half of those who died, depending on the length of time between death and the examination.[333]

Normal infection control measures used while the person was alive should therefore be continued—for example. wearing gloves to prevent contact with body secretions.

Q. How can we disinfect things?

The most important thing is to make sure that instruments and equipment are washed clean of blood and other body fluids before disinfection, as blood residue is a powerful neutraliser of almost all disinfectants. People used to think that a temperature of 56°C for half an hour or so would destroy the virus.[334] This has now been questioned. One study shows that some virus may remain infectious for up to three hours at this temperature.[335]

A solution of one part bleach to nine parts of water (10%) will destroy all virus in sixty seconds[336] unless there are thick deposits of blood or dirt. These may inactivate the bleach, or require longer for the bleach to work.

For some medical purposes 70% isopropyl alcohol destroys virus very quickly, as does a 2% solution of glutaraldehyde[337] or betadine (povidone-iodine 7.5%).[338] The virus is *not* destroyed by gamma irradiation or ultraviolet light—both used to sterilise.[339]

Although it is alarming to think that HIV may sometimes remain active outside the body, cases where this has resulted in infection are almost unknown and are confined entirely to puncturing of the skin with blood-covered medical instruments and other accidents.

The general rule still holds true that outside of sex and shared needles, HIV does not spread.

Q. If I scratch myself with a needle, after it has been used to take blood from someone who is infected with HIV, what are my chances of becoming infected?

Probably much less than one in two hundred from one accidental needle stick injury exposure.[340] We know this from following up the results of a large number of such accidents. You are far more likely to get hepatitis B (up to one in five chance) for which you may need a protective injection within the next few hours, unless you have been vaccinated previously.

Q. Is it safe to go to the dentist?

Yes—assuming your dentist sterilises or disinfects equipment after each consultation. The risk is not to you, the risk is to the dentist. Every time dentists give an injection or draw teeth there is a slight risk that they will puncture their own skin. If the patient is carrying the virus there is a slight possibility the dentist could become infected. This has already happened in New York.[341] For this reason dentists are now using gloves, masks and glasses when treating people known to be infected.[342] Some dentists are using gloves and masks when treating all their patients. There has been one well-publicised case where a dentist with HIV infected several patients.[343] Despite intensive investigations, we are still no nearer understanding how this occurred.

Some pieces of dental equipment are very delicate, containing fibreoptic cables as light sources and are difficult to sterilise. They should be cleaned carefully, then disinfected, following normal infection control guidelines—eg 70% alcohol or 2% glutaraldehyde for four minutes (although glutaraldehyde can cause tissue reactions and fumes can be unpleasant).[344]

There is some evidence that the internal air chambers of high-speed dental drills can become contaminated, with material slowly dislodged by air during subsequent procedures.[345] Like many of the other risks we consider such as kissing, the risk must be very small indeed since a case has never been described of infection by this route (patient to patient transfer at a dentist using such a device). Equipment needs to be well maintained and thoroughly cleaned before disinfection or sterilisation between patients.

Q. What about the risk to doctors and nurses?

Doctors are particularly at risk when they take blood. I have accidentally jabbed myself with a needle many times when trying to fill a blood bottle. Needles should never have their sleeves replaced before being disposed of. A third of accidents occur this way.[346] Casualty doctors are in the frontline when sewing up wounds. Again I have scratched myself with needles several times while stitching injuries—gloves give only partial protection. At risk most of all are surgeons whose hands may be deep inside a patient with a lot of bleeding, sharp needles, and poor visibility. A friend of mine who is an experienced surgeon at a leading London teaching hospital tells me that he frequently tears his gloves during operations. Blood can also spurt from a small artery into the eye. More than thirty occupational infections have already been reported, but the real numbers must be much greater—not yet detected (see p 191).[347]

Ideally surgeons would like to know before starting an operation whether the patient is a virus carrier or not so that they can be especially careful during the operation and in cleaning up afterwards. At present doctors are usually denied this information for ethical reasons. (See pp 187–194 for further discussion.) As a result a number of surgeons may die over the next decade. At least three surgeons have already died from an infection passed on by patients.[348]

Nurses could become infected by cutting themselves on broken blood bottles. There are very few cases recorded so far of nurses contracting the infection from dirty needles or blood contaminated 'sharps'. One case has occurred where the virus is thought to have entered through cracks in a nurse's hands caused by severe eczema. She was attending a patient with AIDS, without using gloves, and her hands were regularly covered in the patient's secretions.

There are several reports of people who have become infected from blood or secretions coming into contact with their skin—usually on the hands, face and mouth.[349] It is certain that many such incidents have resulted in infections which have not yet been detected. Some of these reports were of people who had no reason to suspect a risk from their patients and were unaware of any accident until they went to give blood and were found by routine testing to be infected.

This is quite different from the situation where a doctor pricks his finger with a needle used on a patient in an AIDS ward. In this situation a report is made out and the doctor is tested. Few such incidents are missed.

In the normal course of nursing or doctoring, the risk of HIV infection is minimal.[350] Care should be taken with needles, and good quality gloves should be worn if there are cuts or abrasions on the hands.[351] It is true that several medical staff in the United Kingdom, and a greater number in the US, are now infected through caring for patients, but this is a tiny number out of the vast numbers involved in looking after these individuals. (See Chapter 7 for further discussions of ethics and risks.)

Q. Can artificial insemination transmit HIV?

Yes. Artificial insemination carries a risk. To help reduce this, donated semen is usually frozen and stored for several weeks—not used until the donor has returned for a blood test to make sure he was not infected at the time of donation. As we have seen, normal HIV antibody tests only detect infection after a 'window period' of a few weeks.[352]

Q. Can I get HIV infection from a human bite?

Bites can probably pass on the infection, but the risk is almost certainly very low. I have before me a report[353] where a boy infected his brother. It is thought that he bit him and that was the method of transmission. There is a small but variable amount of the virus in saliva which, it has been suggested, entered through the teethmarks of the bite. In the past, New York police have been seen regularly wearing bright yellow rubber gloves when arresting gay rights demonstrators. There have been a number of instances where infected people, or people likely to be infected, have deliberately bitten police to frighten them. But the risk from a bite is very low indeed.

Q. Where did HIV come from?

Scientists cannot agree on the origin of HIV, and any discussion of the subject generates great heat in those who fear a backlash against certain groups or nations—particularly those in Africa, if it is suggested that HIV originated there. This is unfortunate. The question of origins is a purely scientific one of the greatest importance in preventing the emergence of further plagues like AIDS.

We know HIV has been in existence since at least the 1950s because we find antibodies to HIV in serum samples going back this far. We know HIV is very similar to SIV in monkeys.[354] These animal viruses have probably been around for centuries, particularly in Africa. In the light of this, many scientists have suggested that HIV mutated at some stage from an animal form. However, the animal viruses are equally different from HIV-1 and HIV-2, indicating that if HIV strains are derived from monkey SIV, then the mutations must have happened many decades ago.[355] If the mutation were recent, we would expect HIV-1 and HIV-2 to be much more similar to each other than to SIV.

A form of SIV would need to have entered a human being at the same moment as mutating—not inconceivable if humans were regularly exposed to these animal viruses. Exposure could have taken place in a variety of ways: fertility rites or rituals involving monkey blood, bestiality, laboratory accidents or germ warfare research (a KGB theory used to try and discredit the US),[356] contamination of vaccine preparations using animal or human cells, transplantation of monkey tissues,[357] or even conceivably insect transmission.

Each of these possibilities has been thoroughly explored. While we have the technology to make viruses like HIV today, we did not in the 1950s.[358] A special investigation has failed to find a firm link with vaccine programmes,[359] and insect transmission seems extremely unlikely.[360] Rites using animal blood, or accidental contamination of a laboratory worker both remain possibilities.

Q. Can you get HIV from mosquitoes?

This suggestion is worrying people all over the world[361]—especially in Africa where the number of people infected with HIV is large and people are used to catching another disease, malaria, from the Anopheles mosquito. This was the most common question asked at the big open-air education meetings I spoke at in Uganda in 1988, and also in 1990.

It is almost certain that no one will get HIV from a mosquito.[362] The needle-like mouth of the insect is so fine that white cells carrying the virus cannot be carried in it or on it from one person to another. Scientists have studied outbreaks of AIDS and malaria: malaria is no respecter of age or sex. If you are bitten, you can get malaria. However, there are particular age groups that rarely get infected with HIV—older men and women and older children.[363] These people are not immune to HIV—they simply have never been exposed to the virus. They have often been bitten by mosquitoes and may have developed malaria. Tests on a variety of insects show that HIV cannot multiply inside them.[364]

It is likely that several virus particles need to be transmitted simultaneously for there to be any significant risk of infection—something unlikely to happen from a bite. In summary, it does not seem to be happening, and given the very low risk of transmission, even from a medical needlestick injury, we can see why.[365]

Q. What is the risk from a single episode of unprotected sex?

We are unsure. Various attempts have been made to quantify the risk. It may be as low as one in 200 for non-traumatic heterosexual vaginal intercourse without a condom (see next chapter). Risk is higher for male to female, anal intercourse, first vaginal intercourse in a woman (bleeding), higher during menstruation (for a man), higher if other sex diseases are present.

A calculation can be made that in a low-incidence area

where only one in 3,000 heterosexuals are infected, the chance of infection from a single encounter could be as low as 200 multiplied by 3,000, or one in 60,000 against. 'Not a lot to worry about,' many heterosexuals might say. In practice, the risk may be higher because someone willing to have sex in a one-off encounter may have had sex with many others before in similar situations.

However, let us compare this theoretical estimate of risk with the risk for a gay man with a new partner in an area where up to one in five is infected, with anal sex taking place on one occasion. The risk of infection here might be one in 500. These estimates might seem very low, but the lifetime risk becomes very significant when you add up the total number of risk exposures—say 100 a year for sexual risk. (See next chapter for condom risk calculations.)

We also need to remember population size. Ten million people taking a risk on average twenty times a year gives an annual total of 200 million risk episodes—and HIV spreads.

The overall message is that HIV is relatively uninfectious compared to many other disease-causing organisms. This helps us put the even lower non-sexual, non-injecting risks into context. The biggest danger can come not perhaps from a chance one-off encounter through sex or needle sharing, but through regular day-in, day-out exposure from someone who is not known to be HIV-infected. Hence the situation in Malawi, where it is reported that a third of infected women in some groups were virgins before marriage and have been faithful since (see Chapter 14).

Q. If the risk to heterosexuals is so low in low-incidence countries, what is the point of general health campaigns?

Clearly it makes sense to target those most at risk—sexually-active gay men and drug injectors, for example—while also targeting those likely to be the risk-takers of the future: those still in school. Teenagers today are the AIDS generation. In their sexually-active lives they may well see one in fifty of the global adult population HIV-infected, with very high infection rates in many parts of the world.

Since it may take a generation to change the cultural expectations and behaviour of a generation, we have to start now. Surveys show it is harder to change established behaviour than to prevent it in the first place. However, it could be argued that, say, campaigns targeted at middle-aged heterosexuals in the UK are currently likely to be a waste of money, unless they are directed at business travellers and sexual tourists (see Chapter 12).

We must be forward thinking. In Scotland, new heterosexual infections have overtaken those from homosexual sex or from drug injecting.[366] The writing is there on the wall.

Q. What about tattoos or ear piercing?

Both of these procedures can be hazardous unless properly sterilised equipment is used. The hepatitis virus has been spread by these methods in the past. Always go to a reputable establishment.

Q. What about hot wax treatments and electrolysis?

The wax should be properly heated between treatments to destroy any virus. The electrolysis needles must be sterilised or discarded. Again, use a reputable establishment. If in doubt, ask what they do to sterilise equipment.

Q. Can you get HIV from acupuncture?

Not if the needles are sterilised or discarded each time. There is currently no legislation in the UK to enforce good standards during tattooing, ear piercing, acupuncture, or other things which could transmit HIV. This may change.[367]

Q. Is it safe to kiss someone on the lips?

Yes. The risk of infection from a dry kiss is almost zero, and since the number of infected people in the general population is low, the risk of catching HIV from kissing someone on the lips must be absolutely minute. A 'French kiss' where tongue and saliva enter another person's mouth carries a higher risk, especially if one person has sores in the mouth, cracked lips, or bleeding gums. However, we have never yet seen a single case of 'mouth to mouth' spread. Even if one or two cases are found, it would not alter the advice that the risk is infinitesimally small.

Q. Is the communion cup safe?

Yes! An Anglican canon in South London remarked to me once that by the time communion is over, the cup is sometimes full of bits of saliva, saturated bread, and spittle floating in the remains of the wine.[368] He said it had always given him a strange sensation to drink it all, and then to drink all the water used to rinse it, as is the Anglican tradition. He was not the only one to feel uneasy.

Several elderly women in his congregation had recently started returning to their seats after taking the bread only—because of their fear of AIDS.[369] This was in a church with no gay people known to be a part of the congregation, let alone someone actually carrying the virus. New Revised Anglican guidelines now permit the wafer to be dipped in the wine as a response to the fear.[370] When I visited Uganda, I found many churches had abandoned the common cup. After some teaching we shared communion together—a very moving experience as it was the first time for over a year for many.

Fear, fear, fear—threatening to split congregations. But what are the facts?

True—the virus can survive in water for up to two weeks under exceptional circumstances.

True—the alcohol content in communion wine is not enough to damage the virus.

True—the virus can sometimes be found in the saliva of an infected patient.

True—the virus particles from one person could be swallowed by another member of the congregation.

BUT the number of virus particles in a sip of wine is likely to be extremely small and you are extremely unlikely to get an HIV infection, even if a number of virus particles do enter your mouth. This is because saliva itself inhibits HIV to some extent[371] and because of an amazing protection your body possesses. It is called epithelium or gut lining.

Viruses or bacteria in your mouth are kept out of your blood by a continuous lining of internal skin which lines your tongue, gums, cheeks, back of your mouth and throat. Swallowed virus enters a continuous pipeline between your mouth and your anus. There is no break in the lining of the pipe. Nothing can enter your bloodstream from inside the pipe (gut, stomach, etc.) without being digested first. This breaks up what you eat into tiny fragments, and then into molecules of protein, fat and sugar. The first part of the pipe is stretched out into a bag full of deadly acid (the stomach) which kills the virus anyway in a few seconds. Even if the virus was made of steel it could not enter your blood—it would just pass out the other end.

So the communion cup is safe and I will continue to drink from it. We are not going to see a great epidemic of AIDS through church congregations because of the communion cup. It just will not and cannot happen.[372] We would first need to see a serious outbreak of HIV through kissing before we began to worry about the communion cup.

Q. Can my children catch HIV from another child at school?

Some schools are now sterilising the mouthpieces of wind instruments, etc. I think that is a courtesy to other children and parents. The main items to watch are the reeds of oboes, bassoons and clarinets which should be washed and then soaked in a chlorine solution.[373] Playground knocks and scratches are extremely unlikely to spread HIV. To do so, blood from one child would have to be rubbed into the wound of another. (See earlier question on contact sports.) A 'bloodpact' between two children could spread HIV and secondary school children could spread HIV if they are injecting drugs and sharing needles. This is much more common than parents or teachers often realise. My wife and I would be happy for our children to share a class with an infected child. We are not going to see an outbreak of AIDS spread by school children—except through teenagers injecting drugs or sleeping around. (See p 149—HIV from skin contact.)

Q. Can I get HIV from a discarded condom?

The first time many young people ever see a condom is in the street. There it is lying in the gutter, chucked out of a car window the previous night. There is a small but growing risk that the semen it contains is full of virus. However, it is not going to infect you unless its contents come into contact with your broken skin—hardly likely.

Q. Are female condoms safer than male ones?

Female condoms are made of tough vinyl held inside the woman by an inner and outer ring, so they might be expected to be safer. However, surveys have shown failure rates almost as high as with male condoms.[374] The reason for failure can be that the condom is hard to keep in place. In a study of 106 women, only 29% completed six months' use. The devices slipped out, were accidentally pushed inside, the penis entered outside the condom, they were uncomfortable, the product rustled, was noisy and felt cold.[375] A World Health Organisation spokesperson said at a recent AIDS conference: 'It lurks, slurps, glucks and slicks.'[376] However, half the study group said they enjoyed sex more when using them!

Q. Is it true that nonoxynol-9 spermicide cream protects against HIV when used with a condom?

Experts disagree about the use of spermicidal creams such as nonoxynol-9 in the fight against AIDS. While some preparations show anti-viral activity in the laboratory, this is difficult to test in practice. On the one hand they give added protection against pregnancy and sexually-transmitted diseases such as chlamydia or gonorrhoea. On the other, there are many reports of vaginal or cervical irritation, which could provide entry points for the virus.[377]

The World Health Organisation has announced a major research effort to develop an anti-HIV spermicidal cream which could be an effective weapon against infection. However, it will have to be non-irritant to be safe.

Q. Can I get HIV from being raped?

Yes, it is possible. The risk can be higher because the violence used can make abrasions and bleeding more likely, creating entry points for the virus.

Q. Is it safe to have blood transfusions?

Routine testing of all blood has been carried out to detect HIV since 1985 in the United Kingdom. Unfortunately a number of people were already infected by this time from transfusions. From 1985 to the end of 1986, sixty-four pints of infected blood were detected and thrown away. The risk is now very low.

However, the test does not pick up, for example, the man who gives blood five weeks after sleeping with an infected prostitute while on a business trip abroad. The test can take three months or more to become positive, during which time a donor could give lots of infected blood to the Red Cross. Very rarely it never becomes positive, even though the person is dying of AIDS. This is because it sometimes happens that people never produce antibodies. At the moment the risk is very low in countries like the UK because gay men, drug addicts and other people who might have been exposed to HIV have been deliberately asked to stop giving blood, and almost all have ceased to do so. However, as the number of infected people in the general population rises, the number of infected units that pass through undetected also rises.

If I were about to have a major operation, I would ask for as few units of blood to be used as possible. Blood is not so essential as many people sometimes think. We have some excellent blood substitutes now which can replace the first two or three pints of blood lost unless you started off very anaemic. In the United States there are large numbers of Jehovah's Witnesses who refuse blood transfusions for religious reasons. Few die, however. Major surgery without the use of blood transfusions is now a well-practised art in the United States.

It is sometimes possible to arrange to give your own blood which can be stored before your planned operation.[378] This makes you slightly anaemic, forcing your body to make a lot more blood cells.

By the time your operation takes place, your blood is normal again and two or three units of blood are ready for you in the blood bank. The shelf-life of stored fresh blood is only thirty-five days, which is one reason why not many hospitals yet offer this facility.[379] The other reason is cost.

As soon as we have a widely available blood test for the virus itself, not the antibodies to it, we will be almost 100% safe. In the UK, out of 15 million blood donations between 1985 and 1991, 190 were found to be infected.[380] During the same period it is possible that around fifteen infected blood donations were missed due to the 'window period' (see question on reliability of testing).[381]

Try to avoid having a blood transfusion outside Europe, North America, Australia, or other countries where medical facilities are good. Many other countries have inadequate facilities for testing, although the situation is changing rapidly. However, in high-incidence countries such as Côte d'Ivoire in Africa, even with testing, up to 1% of blood transfusions may be infectious, due to undetected recent infection of blood donors.[382] In some countries, the machines that screen blood are often broken, and it takes months for technicians to mend them—therefore screening does not take place. Testing kits can also run out (during civil wars, for example).

For a long time, people in the UK who are too embarrassed to go to a sex disease clinic for a test for HIV antibodies, have been going along to give blood. They know that all blood is tested there. This happened a lot until the Blood Transfusion Service woke up to what was happening and tried to stop it. It is terribly dangerous: someone infected last week who goes to give blood gives infected blood expecting it will be detected, but it isn't. The test will not be positive for weeks. The blood slips through and is used in a hospital.[383]

This is still going on. A doctor friend of mine told me that he had heard of a group of friends who trooped down to the Red Cross hoping to get a secret test. They had all been at risk. They all gave blood. Some of that blood may get through and infect a patient.[384]

More than a thousand people in Britain may die as a result of infected blood or blood products.[385] The government should probably have taken precautions earlier when it was first alerted to the dangers of importing blood products from the United States. It has now agreed that all those infected as a result of this treatment should receive automatic compensation. For those having to cope with chronic bleeding problems due to haemophilia, the knowledge they may now develop AIDS is an even more terrible curse. There was also a big scare in Germany in 1993 over failure to test supplies adequately—several million people were potentially at risk over the previous few years.

Q. Can I get HIV by giving blood?

Not at all. Some people are afraid of infection and are staying away.[386] But there is no danger at all in giving blood. There is no risk to you at all, so long as all the needles used are sterile.

Q. What about babies of infected mothers?

We know that between 15% and 30% of babies born to infected mothers may turn out to be infected themselves, although all will test positive for the first few months (see question on testing and Chapter 4). Breast-feeding significantly adds to the transmission risk, although advice in developing countries is to continue because of the dangers of death through gastroenteritis from bottle-feeding. New tests may detect HIV within three weeks of birth.[387]

Q. What is the risk from oral sex?

The risk from oral sex is unclear. To be sure that orogenital contact is the route, it is necessary to find couples where other methods of intercourse have not taken place, and this can be difficult. Among gay men there can be a tendency for some to admit to oral sex, but not to anal sex, although both have taken place.

Studies available suggest orogenital contact can transmit HIV, so care should be taken.[388] There is much we do not yet understand. For example, spread from saliva is unknown from kissing, although the virus is present in saliva. The lining of the mouth and gut of an adult seems to give some protection, yet a newborn baby is very much at risk from HIV in breast milk.

Q. Can I get HIV from a toilet seat?

For this to happen there would have to be fresh blood on the toilet seat in contact with breaks on the skin or genitalia of the next user. The more likely scenario might be an infection from one of the organisms causing diarrhoea in someone with HIV. This can be prevented by normal washing of hands after use.

Q. Can I get HIV from sharing a toothbrush?

This is theoretically possible, but we have never seen infection by this route despite careful studies of many families where one person is infected. Brushing causes tiny amounts of bleeding from the gums so a toothbrush should be used by only one person. Likewise, articles such as towels or razors (even electric razors) should not be shared.

Q. Can I get HIV from the skin of someone with AIDS?

If the patient has weeping boils or other skin problems causing the skin to crack, bleed, or produce secretions, then care should be taken. The secretions may carry virus. Remember, however, that virus on your own hands is not going to infect you unless there are breaks in your own skin. Hands are especially vulnerable, so cover cuts with waterproof bandages and if in doubt, use gloves. Several cases of infection have occurred following heavy contamination of broken skin by blood or secretions. Infected blood on the face of a person with acne or a skin rash has been known to transmit the virus.[389]

Q. Is HIV present in sweat?

Although HIV can be found in many body fluids including blood, tears, saliva, semen, cervical secretions and breast milk, extensive tests have failed to detect HIV in sweat. However, all other body secretions should be regarded as potentially infectious.[390]

Q. Am I more likely to get HIV from an infected person if my hands are cut or sore?

People with eczema should be especially careful to wear gloves when likely to come into contact with secretions from someone with AIDS. The thousands of tiny cracks and itchy blisters are entry places for the virus. Cuts should be covered with a waterproof plaster. Gloves should be worn by all people whenever handling anything covered with secretions or when lifting or turning a person in bed.[391] Obviously gloves are *not* necessary for normal social contact, handling of crockery, or unsoiled clothing.

Q. Can I get HIV from mouth-to-mouth resuscitation?

The same principles apply as for French kissing or communion. I once found a man who had collapsed three minutes previously on the pavement outside Liverpool Street

Station in London. I gave him mouth-to-mouth resuscitation for twenty-five minutes until the ambulance arrived. By the end I was covered with his saliva. It was over my face, in my eyes, in my mouth and in my lungs. Every time I lifted my mouth after giving a breath he spluttered back at me.

You can reduce the risk enormously by covering the mouth with a handkerchief and breathing through it. Hospitals and ambulances carry a special tube connecting your mouth to the dying person. It has a valve preventing air and secretions blowing back in your face. Many police cars now carry these too. They should be standard issue but since they make resuscitation more difficult[392] it probably would not make sense to use one unless you were already familiar with it.[393]

That man walked out of the hospital despite it taking forty-five minutes from his heart stopping to his arrival in the emergency room. Mouth-to-mouth resuscitation saves lives, and if you do not do it because you are afraid of getting infected, you may have to live with your conscience for the rest of your life. The good Samaritan was the one who took the risk of being mugged or robbed to stop and help a dying man lying in the road.

For a man in the street, in a low-incidence country, the risk of the other person carrying the virus is low. The risk of catching the virus would be more for someone who knew that the person who had collapsed was positive, had AIDS, was a drug addict, or was a homosexual.

Q. Can you pick up any other infections from looking after someone with AIDS?

Yes. There are three possibilities: TB which can develop rapidly in someone with AIDS,[394] cytomegalovirus and other infections causing diarrhoea.

People with AIDS are 100 times more likely to have TB than the average person, although the kind of TB they have is often less infectious to others.[395] If someone walks into a hospital and has widespread TB, one of the first questions doctors ask now is: Does this person have AIDS?[396] In healthy people tuberculosis is usually easily treated.

As we have seen, tuberculosis is the commonest reason worldwide for someone with HIV to die. The natural immunity that most people have to the microbe is destroyed, so people die quickly of TB. Therefore it comes as no surprise to find that worldwide TB cases are on the increase, even in industrialised nations such as the US or the UK.[397]

One worrying problem has been the recent emergence of new strains which have resistance to most drugs used against TB. Someone with HIV needs to take antibiotics for long periods. It is difficult to eradicate the infection without some natural immunity to help. If medication is taken intermittently, there is a risk that resistance will develop. So far this has only been seen as a significant problem in New York and Miami, particularly among drug users. If health care workers become infected with these strains, treatment can be difficult, although fortunately many have protective immunity due to exposure to TB as a child, or from vaccination.

To reduce the risk to care workers, it has been recommended that people with HIV who have unidentified chest infections should be regarded as potentially infectious for TB. It is also suggested that in areas where multiple drug resistance is a problem, staff should be tested for TB every three months.[398]

The other hazard, the cytomegalovirus infection, is very common and usually quite harmless, but can be crippling to someone with AIDS.

Some ask if pregnant women are at risk from cytomegalovirus (CMV) infection picked up from someone with AIDS. CMV infection is very common in the general population. Some 50% of women of childbearing age are actively infected at any time, without any signs unless the immune system is damaged. About 1% of uninfected women become infected with CMV during pregnancy. CMV can cross the placenta and infect the unborn child, almost always after new infection. In

1,000 UK births around three to four babies are CMV-infected. Of these, 10–15% have a CMV-induced abnormality such as brain damage and/or deafness. In the UK between 200 and 300 out of 650,000 infants are permanently damaged at birth by CMV each year.[399]

A few hospitals offer screening for CMV antibodies to nurses working in high CMV incidence areas, eg AIDS wards. If antibodies are absent, women are advised to work elsewhere. However, there seems to be little hard data to support this advice, and the additional risk to the unborn child appears to be extremely small. The Royal College of Nursing official advice is that no special precautions are necessary for the care of HIV-infected people excreting CMV, but that good personal hygiene should be followed, especially hand washing, after contact with respiratory secretions or urine.[400] This advice is also confirmed by the UK Advisory Committee on Dangerous Pathogens: 'There is no scientific reason why women of childbearing age or pregnant women should be excluded from contact with known secretors of CMV. There is no indication for routine serological screening of female staff . . . because there is no evidence that CMV is an occupational hazard.'[401] Similar recommendations exist in the US and Canada. Good personal hygiene will prevent other bowel infections being transmitted. Apart from TB, the risks are entirely the other way around, as the simple cough or cold a well person has could make someone with AIDS seriously ill.

Q. I have heard that cats can give toxoplasma infections to those with HIV. Is this true?

It used to be thought that toxoplasmosis in those with AIDS might be linked to cat ownership—so much so that one person I visited with AIDS at home used to call his cat Toxo! Fortunately, a study has shown that where toxoplasmosis develops it is almost always the result of activation of infection many years previously. No cases were found of recently acquired infection.[402]

Q. What is the importance of a 'doubling time'?

The doubling time is the time it takes for the number of those with AIDS or early infection to double. It used to be six months in many countries first experiencing the disease but is now averaging three years or more in countries like the UK.

A story is told of a famous chieftain who was agreeing the price of a piece of land: he had a chessboard in front of him with sixty-four squares. He said his price was a grain of wheat on the first square, two on the second, four on the third, eight on the fourth, and so on. The deal was agreed. What the other man did not realise was that by the time he got to square sixty-four, all the grains of wheat in the entire world would not be enough! In around ten doublings you reach a thousand, but by twenty doublings you reach nearly a million. By thirty doublings the number is impossible even to imagine.

A doubling time of six months to a year means it only takes a generation to multiply current numbers by billions. But current numbers infected worldwide are already reckoned as millions.

Another way of looking at it is that all doubling times have to slow down.

Q. Could we all be wiped out by AIDS?

No. The spread is likely to slow down as many of the people with multiple partners and drug addicts become infected.[403] The length of time for the number of new cases to double is getting longer in most countries. At the start of an epidemic the doubling time is often six months. After a few years it usually lengthens to more than a year or two. This is still very serious, but at least it shows some sign of hope. The United States took nine months to double from 3,500 to 7,000 cases, eleven months to double from 7,000 to 14,000, and thirteen months to double from 14,000 to 28,000 by December 1986.[404] In Africa, South East Asia, and parts of Latin America other factors such as other sex diseases are encouraging the spread in ways we do not fully understand. Outside these areas the spread throughout the general population will continue, but almost certainly more slowly. Eventually we hope there will be a cure (although conceivably not for ten to twenty years).

The only way the whole of mankind might die would be if this highly adaptable, unstable virus were to change its method of transmission. Other similar viruses can be spread through droplets, coughing and sneezing. We really do not understand fully why this does not happen with HIV. We are all hoping this will never happen in the future, but it could, and the more people who are infected each year, the greater the chance of such a mutation (p 64). If it happened, the whole of mankind could be destroyed rapidly unless we found a cure in time.

Q. Is early treatment with AZT effective?

When studies showed signs of benefit to those with AIDS from AZT, in terms of length of survival and general wellbeing, there was enormous pressure for licences to be extended allowing those still well to receive the drug also. Unfortunately, the first studies were terminated early after initial promising results, with only a few patients followed up for a limited period. A much larger and longer study (Concorde) then followed, with very disappointing results suggesting that there is no long-term benefit in those who have early HIV infection.[405] However, by the end of 1993 the situation was still unclear, with some US researchers convinced there is a benefit. Having heard both US and UK/French teams debating their different results, it is clear that all the studies have their own strengths and weaknesses. Since we know that viral resistance develops quite quickly, it may be that is part of the explanation for a benefit of limited duration. More research is urgently needed. In the meantime, the emphasis is shifting to a multi-drug approach (see Chapter 2).

Q. Why not test everyone and separate infected from uninfected people?

I am horrified when people ask me this question. This is a recipe for concentration camps. Also it will not work: many infected people will be missed due to the test not becoming positive for up to nine months after infection. Many who think they are positive will disappear and go underground. The days when any country could close its borders are over—particularly EC countries with abolition of border controls. Millions of people travel to other countries each year, many illegally. Someone would have to enter quarantine after being abroad even for twelve hours because that is long enough to share a needle or have sex. Quarantine would be for up to nine months. During this time the person would have to be kept in solitary confinement in a prison cell so there could be no possibility of sexual intercourse or sharing needles. What would happen to business trips? No tourist could travel without being in a 'sex-free' prison for up to nine months first. What are you suggesting? An iron curtain even more effective and destructive than was the one in the East? Husbands and wives separated on one side or the other? Children never able to see an aunt or an uncle except in a room with a television camera?

Even if the epidemic is controlled in one country, if all neighbouring countries have rapidly increasing problems HIV will find its way in. That is why even if I agreed with the concentration camp idea—and I find it utterly repulsive—I would think it stupid to try it. The answer has to be a worldwide answer. The only alternative is to close all borders, airports and sea ports, and blow up any ship, pleasure boat, or plane that approaches the coast.

Q. What is the cause of same-sex orientation?

I am often asked after AIDS talks why people turn out to be heterosexual, homosexual or bisexual. I often wonder what is behind the question—a reaction against gay sex as perverted or abnormal, a desire to promote gay sex as natural and acceptable, or just curiosity? I am going to attempt to answer the question because misconceptions continue to inhibit a compassionate response to gay men with AIDS, with statements like, 'He chose to be gay' linked to an 'own fault' attitude.

Although, as we have already seen, most HIV infection worldwide is heterosexual, people's views of gay sexuality can be profoundly important in the response to AIDS in countries like the UK where gay men comprise the majority of those ill or dying.

At the risk of being rather simplistic, it could be said that in the past many of those approving of homosexual relationships may have tended to the view that people are 'born gay'. Many disapproving of such relationships may have tended to the opposite view that people 'become homosexuals' either as a result of upbringing, or as a result of individual choice.

What are the facts? There is certainly evidence that sexual orientation can be profoundly affected by what happens to people as they grow up, but there is also growing evidence that our genes may have a degree of influence too.

Classical psychoanalytic theory has pointed to the family dynamic and a common pattern of a weak or absent father and a powerful or dominating mother being more likely to result in a homosexual son.[406] Another model has suggested that sex abuse can either drive the person towards same-sex relationships or away from them, depending on the circumstances. The model breaks down—as do all the simple models—because there are many with a same-sex orientation whose childhood and adolescence were quite different.

In the 1950s and 1960s two studies were done of identical twins reared apart.[407] These kinds of studies are very interesting because they help us settle the nature/nurture argument, as each pair of twins has identical genes. Any differences must therefore be due to factors operating after birth. If sexual orientation were purely preprogrammed, then such twins would always have the same sexual feelings. The studies found there was a link, but not a complete one. Many, but not all, of the twins were found to have the same orientation as the other.

In 1991, a study was made comparing the brains of homosexual and heterosexual men at death. It was found that a small region of the brain called the hypothalamus showed differences, with a larger area of tissue present in most heterosexual brains. Some criticised the findings on the basis that potential presence of HIV in some of the homosexual brains could have caused brain damage and have affected the results.

In 1993 it was announced that scientists had managed to locate a region on the X chromosome that seemed to be associated with a higher than expected incidence of gay orientation in adult life. Again, evidence suggested the link was partial, indicating a degree of influence.

These findings should not surprise us. The more we understand about the way our bodies work, the more we come to realise that most aspects of human existence are multi-factorial, influenced by many things.[408]

This is particularly true of illness. For example, there are only a few diseases like cystic fibrosis which are entirely caused by a gene, while most have a mixed basis. Asthma and eczema can pass through parents to some of their children, yet are both heavily influenced by environmental factors. Blood pressure, height, weight, cancers, arthritis and hundreds of other things are genetically influenced. What about basic temperament, personality, intelligence, or personal preferences?

The nature/nurture debate can get very heated. On the one hand some may say that a genetic influence on sexual orientation justifies homosexual relationships as normal. Others may say that if there really is a gene, it must be just as abnormal as the one causing cystic fibrosis and should be eliminated from the population. My own view as a Christian is neither of these two extremes. My understanding is that God loves us whatever our genetic makeup. Genes in themselves are morally neutral, yet a part of our fallen world. The real question seems to be how we choose to live with them.

Some Christians get very agitated over the issue because they feel that an environmental explanation based on 'unfortunate experiences' is easier to cope with than the thought that our Creator might have 'designed us like that'. However, to be consistent, if we take the line that all genes in all people are as God designed and originally intended, then we are forced to the odd conclusion that God intended people to have haemophilia, cystic fibrosis, or a host of other conditions programmed by genes.

The traditional Christian view on illness and suffering has been that God created the world perfect, but gave us free will. When man fell, sickness and decay entered the universe. This makes sense of the observation that we probably all contain rogue genes, useless genes, harmless genes, beneficial genes, dangerous genes and genes which are just part of the varied normal human condition. It then becomes a matter of heated theological and biological debate to decide which category so-called 'gay genes' might fall into.

This is something which needs sorting out, since a tough secular world has a knack of quickly destroying embryos which do not fit the fashion of normality. Christians have been remarkably united in condemning such a utilitarian approach to life. In this there is a strong consensus between Evangelicals, traditional Catholics and the Gay Christian Movement. All are utterly opposed to the possibility of destroying embryos on the basis of a possible gay gene, although perhaps for different reasons.

Some are troubled over the question of choice. Some make the suggestion that if sexual orientation is environmental, people can choose. Since people do not choose their parents, the circumstances of their upbringing, or to be sexually abused, I cannot see it makes any difference if sexuality is more or less genetic or environmental.

I cannot find any evidence that people choose to have homosexual feelings. On the contrary, many are troubled by them and wish they were heterosexually inclined. People can, however, choose how feelings are expressed in terms of behaviour. This is a deeply sensitive, complex and controversial area, and one which has caused confusion in the church to the detriment of those ill with AIDS. Confusion and uncertainty mean people are unsure of how to respond.

As we will see in a later chapter, personal views have to be laid aside in order to care unconditionally. The day your views or mine—on politics, lifestyle, religion, race, sexuality or any other factor—begin to affect the care we give is the day we should stop trying to care for people. Doctors, for example, should be struck off the medical register for refusing to look after someone on the basis of race, lifestyle or because they have an unacceptable illness. If we cannot accept, love and care for people as people, then our care is almost worthless.

You do not have to agree in order to care. You might have a completely different outlook on life, but that does not take away the possibility—or indeed the obligation—of giving loving sensitive help to another human in great need. Some fear that expressing care condones behaviour they may consider immoral. If that is the case, then nursing someone with alcoholic liver cirrhosis would also be unacceptable, or helping someone who fell under a car when drunk—or is it just a special judgement to be imposed on those who are practising homosexuals? For further discussion see Chapter 8.

Q. What should I do if I'm worried about infection?

If you are concerned about HIV infection, the first thing you could do is change your lifestyle: have one partner (currently uninfected) for life and do not inject drugs.

If you are a heterosexual, living in the West and not injecting drugs, the risk that you could be infected is very small unless you have been taking risks in the last six to eight years. People are often worried about things they were doing in the late 1970s or early 1980s. Almost all those infected during that time were gay or bisexual men in those nations.

You may feel you have good reasons to be worried. You need expert advice from a physician with experience in this area as a result of which you may want to be tested. You need to think this through carefully. The decision to be tested is not straightforward and you need good preparation if you decide to go ahead. If the test comes back positive things can happen very fast. In the upset you can end up sharing the result with someone who then lets you down by telling other people. The result can be a lost job or worse, so you need to have thought through what you will do if the result is positive.

You may have been required under US state law to have a test because you are about to get married. Many people are choosing to get married somewhere else to avoid a test. But this is one area where testing is especially important: here are two people committing themselves to each other for life and probably intending to have a family. I know people who have decided to be tested because of their past lives, out of courtesy and respect for a future spouse or partner.

A positive test result needs checking a second time to be absolutely sure. The result can occasionally be wrong. A confirmed positive result means your body has been exposed to the virus. Some of your soldier cells will have been reprogrammed. We have to make sure that those soldier cells stay asleep for as long as possible before being stimulated by other infections into producing more virus particles.

Anything that would improve the health of an uninfected person is also likely to give the very best chance of health to someone who is infected. Boosting your immune system will also help your body keep well if some of your soldier cells are starting to die.[409]

Eat a balanced diet, avoid physical exhaustion, and pace yourself in what you do. Exercise regularly and be careful about situations you know are likely to leave you completely drained emotionally. It seems that some people can live for many years—even decades— with this virus. The longer you live, the more likely it is that we will find more effective treatments or even a cure.

A lot of people may try to exploit your fears by selling you all kinds of treatments or remedies. Before you spend your savings on these things, just remember that every drug company in the world would love to find a natural substance that could work well for people with AIDS. Every folk remedy you hear about has already been examined and rejected by scientists or is as yet unproven. Most of these things gain their reputation because people who take them often seem to improve. However, as we have seen, what makes people with AIDS ill is usually the other infections that invade when the soldier cells are damaged. The natural course of the illness can be a series of dramatic ups and downs. People then credit a folk remedy for an improvement that was bound to happen anyway.

I do not want to stop you from trying these things but many people have wasted a lot of money on 'cures' that are totally worthless.[410]

You may panic because, having read this book, you think you are suffering from the early stages of AIDS. This illness is a great mimic of other less serious conditions. For example, a fever together with swollen glands for a while is quite likely to be caused by glandular fever. All kinds of things can produce rashes or diarrhoea. If you are worried, you should see a physician.

However, you may know that you are a carrier of the virus, and your physician has confirmed that the virus is now making you ill. Exactly the same things apply as for those infected but feeling well: basically, take care of your body to give it the best environment to protect you.

If you are infected with AIDS, you have probably already become an expert on the disease. Some days you may feel able to handle it and other days you may feel you are not coping at all. However you became infected, and whatever your background, not far from where you live there are other people in the same situation who may be able to help you. AIDS is too big a burden for anyone to have to carry on his or her own. Sometimes you will find yourself caught between facing the practicalities of dying and wanting to build plans for the next two decades.

Whatever your situation, there are a number of agencies available to help you practically, emotionally and spiritually. A few are listed at the back of this book.

Often it is more harrowing to watch someone else suffering than to be in the situation yourself. You can feel helpless and frustrated. On top of all that can be the exhaustion that comes from giving care twenty-four hours a day, seven days a week. There can also be a lurking unease that your partner may have infected you or that you infected your partner. All these things can produce high levels of anxiety and stress.

Again I urge you to link up with various agencies where they exist, for practical and emotional support. You may be encouraged to know that many partners have not infected each other even after long periods of unprotected sex. You will need to think through that whole area now in the light of the next chapter in this book about condoms and the advice to partners of infected people.

Q. Is there an answer to AIDS?

A simple answer to AIDS is, in the words of a doctor from Northern Ireland, an 'epidemic of faithfulness'. An epidemic of faithfulness will have a major impact on the epidemic of AIDS—together with testing blood donations, taking care over sterilisation and disinfection, and discouraging sharing of needles and syringes by drug addicts.

In the words of the World Health Organisation: 'The most effective way to prevent sexual transmission of HIV is to abstain, or for two people who are not infected to be faithful to one another. Alternatively, the correct use of a condom will reduce the risk significantly.'[411]

All these questions are important. However, the biggest question in my mind is this: Are condoms really as safe as everyone seems to think they are? Is the emphasis on condoms for safer sex simply because we can't think of anything better to say—or is it really grounded in fact? If it is safer, how much safer is it?

6

Condoms Are Unsafe

Whenever I talk to young people about AIDS I find the same thing: they think that using a condom will prevent them from getting HIV. The truth is that it may greatly reduce the risk, but I wouldn't trust my life to a condom.[412]

Condoms are unreliable. If a hundred couples use condoms for contraception, up to fifteen of them could be in clinics *each year* asking for abortions.[413]

Condom demand is growing because of AIDS. Total global sales were 5–6,000 million a year in 1992 (150 million in the UK). A survey of 50,000 condoms from 110 brands on sale in Europe, Brazil, Indonesia and Thailand showed only 3% to be 'very good' (strength, aging, no holes), 48% 'poor' or 'very poor'. No condoms on sale in Italy, Portugal or Spain were 'very good'. The EC is now proposing a new stricter standard for the 'eurocondom'.[414]

In one UK survey, holes were found in up to thirty-two out of a hundred condoms of the least reliable makes. These holes were gross defects, not microscopic holes seen in some latex (5 micron, HIV is 0.1 micron), which are worrying but probably far less significant.[415] The British Standards Institute permits up to three out of a hundred to have holes in them when they leave the factory.[416] In the US, government standards are much higher, tolerating only four condoms out of every thousand to have leaks. But even with this standard, users still experience a failure rate of between 3% and 15%,

164

which is the percentage of women who have an unwanted pregnancy using this method of birth control over a year.[417]

A spokesman from the London Rubber Company (Durex) admitted that if incorrectly used, the failure rate of condoms could be anything from 25% up to 100%, and there are real problems with teaching people how to use them—not least because of illiteracy. Problems of illiteracy are so bad in the United States (one in five adults) that the army printed manuals in cartoon form for the Gulf War. In the United Kingdom, Durex instructions now contain illustrations for the one in ten who cannot read.

The condom is the least reliable contraceptive in wide use—it's as bad as the diaphragm or cap with spermicide. The only thing less reliable is the sponge (up to 25% pregnant each year).[418] Many violently disagree. They say it is a superb contraceptive, it is *people* who are unreliable: they put it on too late or inside out, tear it, forget it, let it fall off. They say people are unreliable but the condom is reliable, if properly used. Condoms may be too small for one in five men.[419]

Condom failure (UK)[420]

138 women wanting pregnancy advice

Reasons pregnant:

Split or leaking condoms	93
Condom fell off	13
Intermittent use of condoms	32

Recently there was an outcry about how dangerous three-wheeled invalid vehicles were. 'Unsafe,' people said. No one went on TV to say that the vehicles were perfectly safe, it's just that people need to be careful when driving them when going round corners. On the contrary, I think most people saw that average drivers could very easily have accidents through no fault of their own. It is easy to have an accident with a condom. Condoms are unreliable compared to, for example, the pill. That is why the pill is so popular—not just because it is a more convenient method.

Things are worse than they appear from the pregnancy rates. Out of 100 couples, ten will have great difficulty in conceiving anyway. Five will probably never be able to conceive for various reasons, including previous infections with sexually-transmitted diseases.

After four months of trying to conceive, only about half of an average group of women will succeed in becoming pregnant. If they used a perfectly safe method two out of three times that they had intercourse, it would take a year for half to become pregnant. If they used the method for ten out of twelve months of the year, then twenty-five out of a hundred could be expected to get pregnant in a year. If they had unprotected sex for one month a year and used the method for eleven months, then it could be expected that over twelve would become pregnant in a year.

What this means is that if condoms produce a failure rate of around twelve in a hundred per year, then they must be leaking often. It is about the same thing as having intercourse for a whole month without any protection at all but taking the pill the rest of the year. Somehow or other secretions from a man and a woman are very frequently meeting each other.

This conclusion is confirmed by a study of 2,000 acts of intercourse by eighty heterosexual and seven homosexual couples, with fourteen types of condoms. The overall failure rate from slippage or rupture was 11.3%, even higher than the one in twelve (8.3%) theoretical rate predicted above.[421]

Think about it: a woman can only become pregnant on three days a month—while ovulating and shortly afterwards. After a single accident with a condom there is only a one in ten or so chance of it being a fertile day anyway. Even if it were, pregnancy may not follow. However, it is possible to catch HIV infection every day of the month. The overall risk of pregnancy after one episode of unprotected sex is 2–4%;[422] the risk of HIV from an infected partner after unprotected vaginal sex is probably 0.5%, in the absence of other sexually-transmitted diseases. An increasing number of people have become pregnant recently because they switched from a more reliable contraceptive to the condom because of AIDS.[423] The numbers using condoms are now equal to those using the pill in the UK.[424]

If up to fifteen out of a hundred couples each year are actually managing to conceive despite condom use, there must be frequent accidents—probably one time out of twelve, from the figures above. If you are having sex regularly with an infected person, it is like throwing dice. Every time you throw a twelve is how often the condom has let you down. Would you trust your life to a condom?[425] Remember that one episode of unprotected sex can be enough to infect you. Over the next few years there will be a growing number of angry men and women who have become infected, despite their using a condom, having thought they were safe.[426]

Various reports have been published on couples using condoms where only one partner is positive.[427] In one study, up to a quarter of the partners became infected with HIV in only one to three years, despite use of the condom. Others may say these people were careless. All I am saying is that I agree with the Family Planning Association. If correctly used, the condom can be a reliable contraceptive and will almost certainly reduce enormously your risk of getting AIDS, but the reports show that it is hard to use safely.

Another study of partners using condoms suggests that the risk of catching HIV is reduced by 85%.[428] That sounds excellent, but it is not. If you persist in sleeping regularly with someone who is positive or with numbers of unknown people who are possibly positive, then eventually, condom or no condom, you may get AIDS. Vaginal or anal sex using a condom is not a low-risk or no-risk activity. It carries a medium risk at best.[429] Dr Norman Hearst and Dr Stephen Hulley (Centre for AIDS Prevention Studies in San Francisco) have estimated that even with condom use an uninfected partner had a one in eleven chance of becoming infected after 500 sexual contacts. I think this is rather high.

World Health Organisation: 'The most effective way to prevent sexual transmission of HIV is to abstain, or for two people who are not infected to be faithful to one another. Alternatively, the correct use of a condom will reduce the risk significantly.'

World AIDS Day 1991 and 1992.

A calculation can be as follows. Let us assume the estimate many use is correct that the risk of transmission is roughly one in 200 per episode of unprotected sex with an infected partner. Let us assume 95% protection from the condom for the sake of argument, or a twenty-fold risk reduction. This would give a total risk of one in 4,000 per episode of unprotected sex. Let us assume a couple has sex just under three times a week, or 150 times a year. The risk of the partner becoming infected in one year despite using a condom then becomes 3.7% or almost 20% in five years. If we only rate the condom protection as 90% instead of 95%, then the five-year infection rate could rise to 40% or 7.4% per year.

How do these theoretical estimates fit with experience? An Italian study of almost 400 women with infected partners found the following:

1.2% always using condoms were infected per year overall.

7.3% not using condoms regularly infected per year overall.

12.3% not using condoms regularly with highly-infectious partners became infected per year.

2.6% not using condoms regularly with partners of low infectiousness became infected per year.

Partners were considered highly infectious if their white cell (CD4) counts were low or if they were becoming unwell.[430] Inconsistent condom use increased risk around six times. Anal sex doubled the risk. AIDS in the partner trebled the risk.

In another study, almost 200 women with HIV-infected haemophiliac partners were studied. Between 1985 and 1992, one in ten became infected. The risk of infection increased with time as the men deteriorated.[431] It is very difficult to obtain meaningful figures for these risks because there are a number of variables: stage of infection, sexual practice, presence of other sex diseases, frequency of intercourse, frequency of condom use. For this reason different studies can give varying results.

A combined European study of 563 heterosexuals with infected partners in stable relationships from nine countries was carried out between 1987 and 1991. People were enrolled in the study month by month so some were part of it for only a short time. Altogether, 12% of the men and 20% of the women became infected. Risk increased to men with stage of illness, and intercourse during menstruation. For women the risk increased with her age, stage of the man's infection and anal intercourse. None of twenty-four couples always using condoms became infected.[432]

We do not know what the risk is from a single sexual contact with someone who is positive. It certainly depends on many other factors such as whether either partner also has gonorrhoea or syphilis. Any sores will be full of white cells and virus. Circumcision reduces risk. It seems people are most infectious for the first twelve to fifteen weeks after infection with HIV, and then years later when beginning to feel unwell again. Some individuals may be more susceptible than others genetically. In conclusion, it seems the risk from a single accident with a condom or a single unprotected contact is small, but some have become infected this way.[433]

Condom manufacturers' literature states that condoms are designed for vaginal sex only and are not suitable for protection from HIV transmission by the anal route. Particularly hazardous is the use of oil-based lubricants as these rot the rubber in minutes. Recently, some new 'extra strong' condoms have been marketed with lower failure rates for anal intercourse.[434]

What is safe sex?

So what is the correct health message? It is that condoms do not make sex safe, they simply make it safer. Safe sex is sex between two partners who are not infected. This means a partnership between two people who are uninfected—perhaps they were virgins—and who now remain faithful to each other for life and do not inject drugs. If you are going to have sex in an unsafe situation you are foolish indeed not to use a condom, and you must use it very carefully every single time. But don't kid yourself that you will never get AIDS. (See previous chapter for further background on risks.)

Because condom use also provides a measure of protection against other sexually-transmitted diseases, and because genital ulceration caused by them makes the body so vulnerable to HIV, it may be that a key part of condom protection is reducing the incidence of ulceration. This is so particularly in developing countries.[435]

How to use a condom more safely

A condom is tightly rolled up. Make sure it is the right way around. It will only unroll one way. If you have sex in the dark you may need to turn the light on. The teat at the end is there to collect all semen and fluids from the man. This needs to be squeezed empty of air or the condom may leak. With one hand holding the teat, the other is used to roll the condom gently over the entire length of the erect penis. This needs to happen soon after the man is aroused[436] for two reasons: first a small amount of fluid emerges from the end of the penis during arousal as part of the body's natural lubrication before the man enters the woman. This can be full of virus.[437] Secondly, a woman produces a lot of secretions during arousal for lubrication. These may also contain virus if a woman is infected.[438] The early use of the condom is to keep any genital contact separate from the start.

Wear and tear

A woman usually takes longer than a man to become fully aroused and will usually find things more satisfying if there is continuing caressing before her partner enters her. During this period a condom may unroll partly or fall off altogether. It may also suffer general wear and tear. It can snag on a woman's jewellery or on her fingernails. This can happen if, as advocates of condoms suggest, the woman helps the man put on the condom as part of lovemaking. Damage is usually obvious early on. The real danger time can be when a woman helps her partner come inside her. Fingernails and jewellery can cause a minute tear in the condom which enlarges during intercourse. The result is discovered on withdrawal.

Rapid exit

Withdrawal must be prompt for two reasons: first there is a small risk of semen leakage along the shaft of the penis, especially if the teat was full of air. Secondly, as soon as a man has reached climax, the penis starts to soften and what was a tight fit becomes a very loose fit. Condoms can easily leak or slip off inside a woman. The condom end must be held gently as the man withdraws.

Most people dislike using condoms

A huge international campaign has been carried out to try and make the condom more acceptable. When used carefully as above there is no doubt in many couples' minds that it is disruptive and they dislike it: it is a real turn-off. It is the same in countries like the US or African nations.[439] What's so romantic about a condom?[440] After all, that is one reason why people stopped using condoms when the pill came along. The other was unreliability and constant fear of pregnancy. It was the pill, not the condom, that brought about the so-called sexual revolution of the 1960s.

1. To put it on carefully takes precious seconds out of a continuing experience. Some men find that by the time they have got it on so they are happy it is comfortable (may need a couple of tries), their erection has disappeared. A woman is left hanging around and rapidly loses her momentum. Trying to find where you put one, opening the packet, and getting it on correctly can be a joke, but it is disruptive.

2. Making sure it does not roll off can cause tension in the pre-intercourse stage of lovemaking.

3. Checking it is still intact immediately before entry causes further delay.

4. Many men say that the layer of rubber reduces what they can feel[441] (although some who tend to ejaculate too early may find that an advantage). Some women dislike the thought of a piece of rubber in such a personal area.

5. For many couples a central part of their celebration of oneness is to be lying together, with the man inside, immediately after both are satisfied. Many people enjoy being able to 'cool off' in each other's arms like this. Correct condom use requires the man to withdraw immediately. Some see it as a rather abrupt and savage end to a marvellous experience.

6. Some find disposing of the used condom rather revolting. The best method is to tie it up carefully, wrap it up in toilet paper, and flush it away.

In addition there is another vital factor: the very fact that a condom is being used, other than merely to provide some protection against pregnancy, implies slight anxiety about whether a partner is infected. This can cause tension.

Are people using condoms more?

As we have seen in earlier chapters, homosexual men are using condoms more than they used to. This is not surprising since their chances of sleeping with an infected person may now be up to one in three[442] in the United Kingdom or one in two or greater in parts of the United States. However, most experts agree that there is no condom which reliably withstands the rigours of anal intercourse.

Young heterosexual people of both sexes were interviewed at the height of the UK government campaigns and many said they were now intending to use a condom. When a similar large group was interviewed about four months later it showed that very few had actually started doing so, who were not before. In other words, campaigns can stir lots of good intentions but no action. In fact over the period in question the number of new cases of gonorrhoea rose in heterosexuals although it fell in homosexuals. So the number of partners was just as high as before except in the homosexual group who were panicked into more restrained behaviour.

People are constantly trying to invent new ways to promote condoms. One company even gave condoms away with every pair of jeans.[443] It is extremely difficult for a woman who has no boyfriend at the moment to buy a packet of condoms and keep one in her handbag, because in doing so she is having to admit to herself and a prospective partner that she plans to have sex soon with someone whom perhaps she hardly knows. When she goes out for the evening it can be hard for her to take a condom. In doing so she is admitting that she might have sex with someone tonight.[444] Many women feel carrying a condom makes them look promiscuous, when they feel they are not. A further major problem is when to produce it. A romantic evening is turning rapidly into something more. Are you going to show you don't trust the other person by reaching for a condom? Will the other person take offence at you implying that he or she has been sleeping around? Insisting on a condom may take a lot of self-confidence and courage on the part of the woman.[445] Female condoms may be easier,[446] although pregnancy failure rates can be as high as 12%.[447]

Because there are so many natural social barriers to condom use, a major part of some prevention campaigns has been the message: 'Be confident in presenting your partner with a condom.'

How to minimise the disruption

Be prepared. Talk it through with your partner. Practise! But there is another way: change your lifestyle. So many pamphlets tell us how wonderful 'safe sex' is. They say how fulfilling it is just to rub bodies together and have a cuddle. They describe a vast number of other things people can do to have sex safely together. That is not what most people call sex (see p 318).

The choice is so obvious and clear. Find someone you love and trust—someone who is not infected at the moment and will remain faithful to you for life and to whom you will remain faithful. Then you can enjoy unlimited, anxiety-free sex. (Advice to spouse of infected partner p 176.)

Free love

You may reject this. Your philosophy is that if people want to they can sleep together without any great relationship or strings attached. 'We live in a free world and people should be free to do what they like.' Maybe you feel that ultimately you want to be married but you want to have fun now. Friends of mine are afraid that their relationships will become tame and boring if they get married. 'A piece of paper won't make me love her any more.'

As a doctor and as a church leader, I am constantly seeing

the casualties of this, and they are usually women. Life is unfair. Somehow it is usually the woman who comes off worse: she is the one who becomes pregnant and her risk of catching HIV is twice as great as the man's risk from her. She suffers the chronic pain of pelvic inflammatory disease and cervical cancer. And the woman is often the one who is most devastated when a relationship breaks up.

Free love is fine until your lover leaves you at forty-three years of age, and you still have had no children because he would have walked out. A whole generation of people is growing older. Pensioners of tomorrow with no wives, no husbands, no children, no family—only a few casual relationships and old memories. No wonder many are deciding that enough is enough: the right person has not come along so they are staying single and celibate, yet forming long-lasting, warm, caring friendships.

Someone was saying in a newspaper article once how exciting it was to commit adultery. She was saying there was nothing wrong in it. There were some angry letters. One woman said that adultery was wrong for lots of reasons: for her it had meant an elaborate web of cheating, deceits, small lies and big lies. The total betrayal of the trust of another. No wonder it causes such terrible bitterness and hurt. Adultery wrecks marriages and damages children. Surely this is not the best plan for human relationships.

Women leading the way

On one TV programme[448] a young audience was voting on love, sex, condoms and marriage. Huge differences emerged between the boys and the girls. Some boys wanted to 'score' with as many girls as possible. Their reputations and image depended on sleeping with every girl they went out with. Many girls were disgusted. They wanted commitment, friendship, companionship, security—and then they would give themselves in other ways. Romantic ideals live on.

Marriage remains very popular, and the programme suggested that girls are leading the way. I find similar differences expressed almost every time I go into a school to take an AIDS lesson. Girls are often more worried about consequences of sex than boys. Many boys could not care less. It is the girls who seem to worry most about getting pregnant or being let down. I believe that part of the next education phase needs to be to teenage girls and young women, many of whom need little convincing about the desirability of being in a warm, loving, caring, exclusive relationship. This strategy should be designed to give them moral support when under pressure, not to 'sell themselves cheap'.

It is strange that many men want easy women to have fun with, but deep down prefer by far the thought of marrying a virgin.[449] We need to cultivate a new age where romance is in, self-respect is in, faithfulness is in, marriage is in. I don't think it's clever to sleep around or get divorced.

The people I admire are those who work at relationships, who are good at relationships, who have good happy marriages, who can handle things. What's so smart about walking out on every problem? I respect and admire, too, those people who have made a positive decision—for whatever reason—to remain single and celibate.

Advice to someone married to a 'positive' spouse

You may be afraid you or your spouse are already positive. For many women with partners who have haemophilia it has been a terrible shock to discover that their partner may have been HIV-infected several years before, without either of them realising.

This is an increasingly common and agonising situation, in addition to many others where one or other partner is known to be infected through other routes.

Such knowledge can place a severe strain on even the strongest relationships. One big question is over the future of the sexual relationship. Will it continue? What adjustments need to be made? To what degree does the uninfected person wish to 'take a chance'? There are no right or wrong answers, and each couple will need to find their own way forward, with the help of those experienced in HIV counselling.

The important thing is to realise that many people are still uninfected after several months, or even years. As we have seen, it seems that the risk of infection rises when the person becomes ill. Before then the risk may be much lower. You may want to be tested yourself. If you are positive, neither of you need to take as many precautions. If you are negative, then the following is sensible:

1. Use a thick strong condom carefully—see earlier in the chapter.

2. You may want to reduce the frequency of your lovemaking, but be sensible. Stopping altogether may cause terrible tensions and actually result in a rushed mistake. Arousal may be much stronger after abstinence and then it is not as easy to be careful. Do not make love while a woman is menstruating, if she is positive, as the blood will probably contain virus.

3. Deep kissing, where saliva may pass from one mouth to another, is probably not a good idea. Dry kissing carries a much, much lower risk. Oral sex is not sensible.

4. An infected woman should probably avoid pregnancy as there is a significant chance that any child born may also be infected.[450] So use a second method of contraception as well, eg the pill, or consider sterilisation very seriously.

This is a very difficult and traumatic area.

In this chapter we have looked only at condom effectiveness and risk reduction using them. There are, however, major questions over their promotion in many developing countries. In African nations, for example, condoms may be unaffordable, unacceptable and difficult to obtain. We look in more detail at these issues in Chapter 14.

We have looked at the whole issue of the spread of AIDS and some ways to reduce the risks of getting infected, but we have never been faced with a disease which confronts us with so many conflicting moral choices to do with rights and freedom. Some of these issues threaten to tear society apart. We consider the most important of these in the next chapter.

7

Moral Dilemmas

The reason why AIDS is such a sensitive issue is because it touches on so many different aspects of conscience and morality. Different moral dilemmas present themselves in different cultures and nations. In this chapter I want to look at some important issues faced by many countries like the UK or US. Sexuality and sexual behaviour, freedom of the individual versus protection of society, care for others, euthanasia, treatment or testing by force, suicide, use and abuse of drugs, and age of consent are just a few of these dilemmas. Some issues are cross-cultural and are also relevant to developing countries. (For fuller discussion of special issues in poorer nations, see Chapters 13 and 14.)

An indication of how complex these issues are can be seen by the proliferation of HIV-related laws in many countries. In the US alone some 500 new statutes have been passed, with the spawning of large numbers of specialist centres on AIDS law, journals, courses and a new breed of expert lawyers.[451] In order to have a view on regulations and legislation, we need to take a closer look at what is already happening.

Euthanasia—a word to those who care for others

I remember going to see a man dying at home. He asked me to kill him as an act of mercy. Euthanasia literally means 'mercy death'. In some countries it is legal, but in the United

Kingdom it is illegal. Why did he ask? He was in no pain because of the proper use of painkillers, nor was he feeling sick. He had a very slight cough but was eating quite well. His mind was superbly clear but he was confined to bed and unable to walk. He knew he was dying and talked about it freely without fear. He had a faith and felt he knew where he was going.

He felt his life had lost its meaning. He felt he would rather be dead than continue like this. Some doctors in some countries would have killed him, and a third of family doctors in the United Kingdom might have, but for the law.[452] He would have been in a coffin by the following morning. But look at the situation more closely: many different emotions are tied up together and need separating. He felt a terrible burden on his wife. They had a happy marriage and this was destroying it. He had always led the way and now felt helpless.

It is rare for someone to ask for euthanasia without 'burden on other people' being a major factor. If we give way and agree, we are then killing people because they feel they are too much trouble to family or friends. This is a hazardous course. We are then killing people because, say, a friend, partner, or child is getting fed up and resentful. When do you agree that the patient is too much of a burden on others, or disagree and say that others are coping fine?

Sometimes I am asked to 'put someone away'—admit them into a hospital or hospice. Tensions are rising at home or there is no love lost in a relationship—it has been non-existent for years. The carer takes me to one side: 'I want him put away somewhere.' My first priority is that if someone wants to die at home, that person should be able to do so.

Therefore it is vital to provide care and support for relatives and friends to enable that to happen. There are times when we have to admit someone to a hospital for 'social reasons' which usually means the collapse of support at home. You cannot force people to care, nor are they always physically able to. However, one tries if at all possible to create a situation where the sick person's wishes are observed. An atmosphere of resentment, hostility or tension produces unimaginable, unbearable pressures for someone who is dying. They often feel compelled to agree to going back to a hospital or even to ask for euthanasia.

The second major reason why people make this request is because of depression. I am not talking about natural sadness. To feel overwhelmed by sadness because of leaving loved ones, losing strength, and because of dashed hopes for the future is normal. It is abnormal to be spectacularly cheerful in such circumstances. Natural sadness is not depression. Depression is where feelings of sadness are out of all proportion to the situation.

This exaggeration of natural emotion can be caused by all kinds of things including hormonal changes or chemicals in the body, and needs urgent treatment. Occasionally it is because lots of minor or major sad events have been brushed under the carpet for years without tears or low spirits. Behind the mask of ecstatic happiness there has been a growing mountain of grief for losses of various kinds. Eventually something happens and the mask cracks. The person cannot hold back the flood any longer. An exam is failed or the car is written off and the person has a major breakdown. People think they are 'off balance', crying all the time for no obvious reason because they fail to look deeper to the root of major hurts and losses over a longer period of time. Many have breakdowns in adult life because of childhood sexual abuse by a parent, for example—a deadly secret that has never been shared.

When someone is depressed, he or she always loses a sense of self-worth. Everything is useless and hopeless. Everything is an effort and may result in self-centredness or a feeling of being a burden. Suicide is becoming increasingly common in the United Kingdom.[453] If a person is very ill, that person will be unable to commit suicide without help. Would you sit and watch a friend who was depressed, but not physically ill, swallow a hundred tablets without trying to stop him or her? No. Nor would you give the person a bottle of pills if he were unable to walk. You see, depression is quite common when you are unwell. When the body is physically low it can affect the brain so that you feel an exaggerated sadness. Sometimes this is due to chemical imbalances in the blood caused by the illness.

Someone who approves of euthanasia must be absolutely sure that the person is only naturally sad, and not depressed. Even psychiatrists find it hard to distinguish the two.[454] Depression always lifts given time, with or without treatment, although treatment may shorten its course.[455] Are you really going to kill someone who is emotionally ill, who may feel differently in a few weeks? Are you going to kill someone who is feeling a burden, when he may be under pressures you do not understand from others? Yes, you may say, because you feel his quality of life is awful. But who are you to judge?

Many people find being with someone who is ill or disabled, emotionally traumatic and disturbing. Many panic phone calls come from people—even professional carers—who cannot cope with their own anxieties.[456] You may be in danger of killing someone because you have a problem coping and this colours your reaction to the person's request. With your own reaction, the patient's mood, and subtle pressures from others, you are on dangerous ground to do an irreversible, eternal act.

If you are still unconvinced, consider this if you are a doctor or a nurse—especially if you are regularly caring for people who are dying. A nurse visiting dying patients may get a reputation as an 'angel of death'. You know death is never far away when she visits someone in the next bed to you or a neighbour on your street.

Often people are too weak to swallow medicines shortly before they die and the last dose or two has to be given by injection.[457] Sometimes a nurse draws the curtains, injects someone near death, and five minutes later the person is dead. The drug is still largely sitting in the muscle where it was injected. Very little has reached the blood. The injection did not kill the person—he was just much, much closer to death than anyone realised. But it looks awful.

'That lovely doctor came into our house, took one look, and gave him an injection to put him out of his misery. He died two hours after. You wouldn't even let a dog suffer like that. It was the injection that put him to sleep.' Nothing will persuade the person otherwise. She is convinced euthanasia was committed.

Doctors and nurses are in a vulnerable position. If ever there was the faintest suspicion, grounded in fact, that foul play had been committed, we would lose all trust from patients and other colleagues. I cannot warn you more strongly. If you practise euthanasia as part of care of the dying you will cut your own throat, bring into disrepute yourself and the whole of terminal care, an area which scares many people anyway.

From my own perspective, to harm a patient is to break part of the ancient Hippocratic oath. As a doctor I understand how we are made. There is more to life than life. There is a mystery here. No one can create life, and life is to be respected. Abortion and other things have cheapened human life. I believe human life needs to be treated with the highest regard. I will never commit euthanasia and I believe the man I mentioned at the beginning of the chapter was actually relieved when I told him so. I took away an unbearable pressure.[458] It was not an option. If I had said that I was willing to do it, he would then have been faced with a ghastly sense of obligation. This man was unusual in any case. Most people who ask for euthanasia do so because of inadequate relief of pain and other symptoms. With proper control of symptoms and accurate information, the terrible fears about what will happen as they get worse melt away.[459]

Fortunately those attempting euthanasia often fail—even doctors. I remember coming onto a ward one day to see a patient, looking at the drug chart and being amazed to see that three vast overdoses of a particular drug had been given only hours apart to this person without her consent or knowledge. Not even a cry for euthanasia. She survived and died peacefully in her own time a week or two later. The staff had been unable to cope with their own distress. Let's stop playing God in secret, behind closed doors, and start giving back to people control over their own lives, with dignity, self-respect and respect for human life.

Withholding treatment

We need to make a careful distinction between withholding treatment and euthanasia. Making a carefully planned decision not to start a particular treatment, or to stop one that may be artificially prolonging life or directly causing distress in someone who is near death and for whom the possibility of recovery is extremely remote, is not euthanasia. Relatives, friends, the patient himself and staff can be involved in the decision, although responsibility for it must always rest firmly with the treating doctor.

Examples include the decision of an AIDS patient not to continue with radiotherapy or chemotherapy for extensive Kaposi's sarcoma, or not to be mechanically ventilated.[460] An AIDS patient may decide that he cannot bear the thought of another long struggle with many tests and special treatments for his next pneumonia, and decides to stay at home to die.[461] Radical, mutilating surgery may be declined by a cancer patient. Most people with cancer or AIDS die of chest infections. Pneumonia used to be called the 'old man's friend' because it allowed a stricken body finally to die peacefully. It may not always be appropriate to leap in with aggressive treatments. It is not appropriate to give cardiac massage and mouth-to-mouth assistance to an eighty-four-year-old woman who is extremely ill from a wide variety of other illnesses if she has a heart attack and her heart stops. Most attempts to resuscitate such people fail anyway. Of those who are 'brought back to life' many die before ever leaving the hospital. With the elderly the success rate is even lower. What are we playing at? A terrible way to die. There is a time and place for resuscitation and for just letting someone go.

People who have problems with this are usually scared of death. Death is seen as failure. They may be too emotionally attached to allow the person to go. Failure to use common sense in this area, failure to see death as a natural conclusion to the process of living, drives many doctors—especially surgeons—to absurd lengths, ridiculous operations, and ever more exotic procedures designed to fight to the end whatever the costs. Doctors are treating their own problems. Doctors often feel guilty because they raise hopes too high in the first place, the person gets worse and is justifiably puzzled, upset and angry. The doctor feels under pressure to do something (see p 396).

The result is often catastrophic. Terminal care teams pick up the pieces every week of such inappropriate behaviour. We must learn to allow the body to die. Every year new medical methods make death more elusive. We can now keep someone's body warm and healthy for many years without any brain. This is not medicine. This is inhuman science gone mad. (See p 267 for a different approach: hospice.)

Living Wills

As a reaction to what some people see as bad medical care, they are now writing down in advance what they want to happen towards the end of their lives, and they want it to be legally binding. Communication is always a good thing and anything that helps a doctor to understand his or her patient's wishes is to be encouraged. Many treatment decisions are difficult and a strongly expressed view can be very helpful—even if written in advance.[462]

It can be hard to be allowed to die—and I am not talking about euthanasia which is a deliberate act designed to kill. If I was dying of very advanced cancer with many complications,

I would make it absolutely clear to my doctor that my next pneumonia should be my last. There is no need to 'strive officiously to keep alive' when the end is in sight, so why pump me full of antibiotics?[463]

However, once a written directive is backed by law, then doctors risk prosecution if the exact wording is not followed regardless of circumstances—medicine by lawyers. But how could you agree if you thought the person might have been depressed, under pressure or feeling a burden? How could you be sure that every medical option had been fully explained and understood? There is also doubt over our ability to get the diagnosis or prognosis right. These issues also affect the euthanasia debate. Many legal experts say an Act of Parliament for 'Living Wills' or 'Advance Directives' could be a back-door route for legalised euthanasia.

Involving police, magistrates, judges, jury and prisons is no way to care for the dying—much better to encourage good communication, compassionate common sense and expert appropriate treatment, taking into account the expressed wishes of the individual.

Suicide

Suicide is a common terminal event in people with AIDS—usually early in the illness[464]—but also tragically in people who have had a positive test result, especially if counselling afterwards was poor. This is why the new over-the-counter home testing kits which could be available soon are so dangerous. A small but growing number are also committing suicide because they fear they have AIDS. Once, a patient on an AIDS ward went home suddenly for the weekend and gassed himself using the exhaust of his car and a piece of tubing.[465]

When someone has lost his job, been thrown out of his home, been rejected by family and deserted by friends, it is not surprising he feels suicidal. Glances in the street and people muttering in the shops are easily imagined but may be quite real. News of AIDS spreads only too fast. We need to show that we really care and go out of our way to make infected people feel accepted, loved and welcome. If someone is depressed it may be wise to ask them if they have ever thought of harming themselves. You may be afraid of putting a wrong idea into the person's head. You won't, but the answer is vitally important.

If the person says no, then suicide is much less likely. If the person says yes, then ask if they have thought out how they would do it. Most people have not. Someone who can describe to you with clinical detachment and in great detail exactly how he would kill himself is probably at great risk.

The doctor should be told, and the individual should be persuaded to seek medical help. Tablets and other parts of the plan should be destroyed. Often someone who is suicidal has secret supplies.

Threats of suicide can be a most powerful means of blackmail, however: 'If you leave me I shall throw myself under a train,' or, 'If you go on holiday for two weeks I shall probably drown myself. I won't be here when you get back.' But like euthanasia, suicide is harder than people think, and the after-effects of an attempt can be horrible.

Suicide is often attempted as a cry for help. Particularly tragic is the person who takes twenty paracetamol tablets expecting to go off to sleep. After most of a day has passed, the person walks into casualty looking sheepish. The psychiatrist is asked to help. It was a cry, not a serious attempt, but the liver is now permanently damaged. Within a few days the person begins to die an awful death and is dead in a week. Many over-the-counter preparations contain paracetemol.[466]

HIV testing without consent, or mandatory testing

At the time of writing, a doctor in the UK who tests someone's blood without prior agreement could be struck off the medical register or prosecuted. However, at a meeting of the British Medical Association most doctors present voted to do so under special circumstances—usually where they believe the patient's life may be at risk through not knowing that he or she has HIV or AIDS.[467] (See pp 121–124 for testing methods.)

The reason for these rules is to protect people who are infected. People with the infection need protection because although they may be free of any signs of illness for years, it is a hard secret to keep and the knowledge that you are positive can be totally devastating. People lose jobs, houses, friends and partners as a result. They cannot get a mortgage, a car loan, or life insurance.[468] Life insurance companies are worried. American actuaries have reckoned that AIDS claims could cost United States companies $50 billion by the year 2000.

The other reason for the regulations is, strangely, the ultimate protection of society. Control of sexually-transmitted diseases has always been hard because people are reluctant to seek help so the disease is untreated and more people are infected. They are afraid of being judged by doctors and nurses. The whole ethos of a clinic is to go overboard in providing a non-judgemental, tolerant, relaxed, attractive atmosphere with easy access and long opening hours. The aim is to entice people who may be infected so they can be tested, and infections cured. A clinic in West London prides itself in being busy with people coming from large distances because of its pleasant atmosphere. Judgemental, condescending behaviour puts people off and they continue to infect other people. It drives the problem underground, endangering the health of a whole community. And all this was before AIDS.

If people were afraid that while attending a hospital clinic for an unrelated reason or while in a hospital being prepared for an operation, a sample of blood would routinely be tested for HIV, there would be one result: they would be too scared to seek medical help at all. People would die at home of appendicitis or even from treatable chest infections as a result of developing AIDS. The entire problem would go underground. (See p 342 for issues in poorer nations.)

In one respect, however, the problem of AIDS is unlike syphilis. If you can make a diagnosis of syphilis you can treat it, cure it and protect the whole community. With AIDS there is no cure and the person always remains a risk to sexual partners. Driving the problem underground will certainly deny infected people access to normal medical care. If the person attends for his hernia operation and is not routinely tested, he will go away none the wiser. Spread is then stopped only when full-spread AIDS is diagnosed from a strange infection or tumour, or the person is HIV-tested for another reason, counselled and changes behaviour. These are complex issues.

While the arguments *against* testing without consent are very strong indeed, the situation is not clear cut and the opposite views are going to grow in strength.[469] Protecting those who are infected is praiseworthy, but it may put others at risk. For this reason there are various Acts of Parliament in England that allow a person to be detained against his will if, in the opinion of a doctor, he is likely to endanger the health of others.[470] In the United States, these matters are being debated, state by state. In Illinois, it is legal for any physician to test patients undergoing treatment for HIV and to disclose the result to sexual partners or others thought to be at risk. Colorado and Missouri are very likely to implement similar measures.

Take the plight of a surgeon: should he not know when to take special care not to cut or scratch himself? It would be wrong to refuse to operate on someone who was ill and needed surgery, but what about someone wanting cosmetic surgery or even a sex change operation?[471] Is it right for someone who may know he is positive to ask a surgeon to take that risk when the patient's own life is not at stake.[472]

Most emergency rooms now use paper strips to close minor wounds instead of stitches. In most cases with small wounds the results are just as good, if not better, than with stitches because stitches can get infected and cause a body reaction. A stitch or two may reduce the risk of a slight scar, especially in a young girl, if the cut is deep or the patient is particular. But if someone has the virus, is the risk of stitching acceptable? Metal surgical clips can be used to close wounds after surgery. It has been suggested that they should be used with all high-risk patients.[473] Just how many people will need medical care for AIDS over the next twenty years? More than 20 million. Even if the risk from an individual patient is small, the risk can multiply millions of times.

The fact is that a large number of doctors and nurses world-wide are going to die of AIDS over the next decade or two unless there is a cure or a vaccine. In the US alone, estimates have been made that over 100 health care workers will become infected through patient care each year, although some say this is too high a figure.[474] Only thirty-two documented cases with sixty-nine other possible cases had been detected up until 1992 in the US. By September 1993 there were sixty-four definite and 118 possible cases worldwide.[475]

Accidents with needles and during operations happen in every hospital every day—most too minor to report but still capable of transmitting infection.[476] Years ago such people often died in the course of duty, from tuberculosis, for example. But today it is incredibly rare. A fireman occasionally dies fighting a fire or a policeman in trying to save a man from drowning. Doctors and nurses rarely die from their patients' infections. This will not be so in the future. Britain's Trades Union Congress (TUC) has suggested routinely screening everyone who is admitted to a hospital to protect health care workers[477] although at the moment the risks are much higher from private lifestyles of members of staff.[478]

The fears of health care workers are real and may be affecting recruitment in high-incidence countries. In the US, applicants for medical school places fell in 1988 to the lowest

Health care workers with documented and possible occupationally acquired HIV infection, by occupation (United States) to September 1992[479]

Occupation	Documented	Possible
Dental worker, including dentist	0	6
Embalmer/mortuary technician	0	3
Ambulanceman or woman	0	7
Care assistant	1	5
Cleaner/maintenance worker	1	5
Laboratory technician, clinical	11	12
Laboratory technician, non-clinical	1	1
Nurse	12	14
Doctor, non-surgical	4	7
Surgeon	0	2
Respiratory therapist	1	1
Surgical technician	1	1
Technician/therapist, other than those listed above	0	3
Other health care occupations	0	2
Total	32	69

level since 1970, attributed among other things to a fear of occupational HIV infection.[480] It is worth considering the total lifetime risk to a medical student beginning to train as a doctor in a country like Malawi where up to half the patients on hospital wards are infected. (See pp 347–351 for further discussion of risks to surgeons in developing countries.)

The argument in favour of selective testing without consent is that the alternative is to assume that everyone is positive and take incredibly elaborate precautions. Time may be wasted and lives lost.

A certain man is known to have been a drug addict up to a year ago and needs open heart surgery. Treating him as 'presumed HIV infected' adds enormously to the operation cost. The theatre has to be closed for cleaning afterwards.[481] A twenty-minute operation took two and a half hours of theatre time when all the procedures were followed.[482]

A simple test could save all that, nine times out of ten.

Some countries are now preparing to force certain groups of people to be tested. Military recruits in the United States army have all been tested routinely for some time. Iraq is testing all long-term visitors to the country. Bavaria in West Germany has tested groups as a matter of law. I think many people are going to disappear rather than be tested.

However, I am convinced that unless a cure is found quickly, HIV testing will become part of the routine work-up before any operation in a number of countries. I think it will be justified by surgeons as in the patient's interests on the grounds that fevers and chest infections after the operation may be mistaken for normal consequences of anaesthetic and surgery, correct treatment will not be given and the patient could suffer. At least one surgeon in the United Kingdom is regularly testing people for HIV regardless of whether they are in a risk group or not. This is without consent and without the approval of the British Medical Association which voted overwhelmingly against such an approach.[483]

The public climate is shifting rapidly in many countries. For example, in the US a jury decided that a woman had committed fraud by not disclosing her AIDS illness to a surgical team before having a breast reduction operation. One of the team accidentally cut herself with a scalpel and became infected. She was awarded compensation of over $100,000.[484]

I also think HIV testing will be done on many patients in hospital wards with unusual symptoms of almost any kind. AIDS is such a complex disease because it opens the body up to so many other kinds of illnesses. It must therefore be on a physician's list of possibilities in an enormous number of people who are ill these days. Without the test the diagnosis will have to be made by excluding every other possibility, by which time the patient may be dead. This becomes vitally important as soon as we have any anti-HIV drugs that might be effective if given early (p 70). Once this happens, testing without consent will become widespread and justified on the grounds that prompt treatment could prolong or save life— although the real motive may be different.

It may seem shocking to test people for a disease without their knowledge, but we have been doing it for years: blood testing for syphilis is common for similar reasons. It mimics such an enormous number of diseases. People are not always confronted with their result. In fact the vast majority of blood tests are done with what is called 'implied consent'. By agreeing to come into a hospital the person is accepting treatment. By agreeing to allow a blood sample to be taken 'for various things—like to see if you are anaemic' a person can often be tested for twenty or more different things. A diabetic woman develops severe thrush, a symptom of AIDS that can also be caused by badly controlled diabetes. The doctors think AIDS is highly unlikely and do not want to make her anxious by asking her permission to do a test and then leave her in suspense until the test result is back. So they may decide to test her anyway and only tell her the result if it is positive.

However, the great problem is keeping the result strictly confidential. Medical teams must improve at this, especially family doctors and occupational physicians in work places.[485]

Counselling following a positive test is vitally important. As we have seen, it is not uncommon for someone to commit suicide following the discovery of a positive result.

So far we have looked only at testing of a person without consent in order to influence either the treatment given, precautions taken or that person's behaviour. However, there is another moral dilemma: the testing of unmarked blood samples as part of an anonymous fact-finding exercise.

We have been in a crazy situation in the United Kingdom where we have not really had any idea at all how many people were infected. We knew only the majority of those who developed AIDS. Nor did we really know how the epidemic was spreading.

However, there is a simple way to find out, which is cheap, breaks no confidence and affects no individuals in any way at all. This way is to instruct various laboratories in certain hospitals not to throw their old blood bottles away—many keep them anyway for a week or so—but to remove all identifying markers on them and send them to the public health laboratory for AIDS testing. The results are quick and helpful: maybe showing that over a year the number of women infected at a London teaching hospital increased, whereas in East Anglia the number was constant.

Some say it is immoral to test someone for HIV and not tell them if the result is positive. Therefore no one should be tested unless the intention is to give the result. But this is a different situation where a group of people are being sampled anonymously. Anyone can ask for a test to be done at any time if he or she wants. No extra blood is taken and only existing blood samples are used so there is no discomfort or inconvenience.

In the first edition of this book in 1987, I urged the government to carry out such a programme. I am pleased to say that by the time the second edition had come out, the process had started and the initial phase of testing is now complete. As a result, for the very first time we have a more precise, up-to-date picture of HIV infection across the UK.

The other problem area is mandatory testing, for example of engaged couples in Illinois. Mandatory testing is hard to enforce, whatever your opinion may be. In Illinois, marriage applications in 1988 dropped by 67% as couples went to other states to get married.[486]

Revenge sex and other situations

What do you do if someone you know is positive and has decided to get revenge on society by having sex with as many other people as possible? A man visiting New York woke up after a date to find 'Welcome to the AIDS club' written on his mirror. He is now infected.[487] A man was recently murdered in New York after announcing to the man he had just had sex with that he was positive. The murdered man had made the mistake of laughing.

A newspaper in the UK reported that a boy prostitute in London was taken out of circulation and into custody because he was determined to infect others.[488] This report was hotly denied by social services.[489] More recently, reports appeared of a man in Birmingham with haemophilia, who might have had sex with several women while knowing he had HIV. Most became infected.[490]

A drug addict in Norway 'infected fifty people after he discovered he had the disease'.[491] This opens up the broader issues of confidentiality: a businessman is positive and has no intention of telling his wife, who is wanting to have a baby. If she is positive, pregnancy could mean death for her and her child. Do you just sit back and wait for the inevitable? This whole area of law is confused: there are no test cases yet in the United Kingdom. The Public Health (Infectious Disease) Regulations of 1985 and 1988 and the Act of 1984 could be interpreted as giving a hospital the authority via a magistrate to compulsorily detain such a person for treatment for a limited period only.[492]

Human rights are always complex. You cannot have rights without responsibilities. You have a right to bring up your own children, but you must not abuse that right by abusing your children. The businessman has a right to confidentiality, but his wife has rights too. She has the right to live to seventy or more and not catch HIV. She has the right to be told and to choose about having a baby. Whose right is greatest? An expert on medical law, Professor Ian Kennedy, believes that doctors could be sued if they fail to inform an uninfected husband or wife, even if forbidden to do so by the patient.[493] If someone is raped, should that person have the right to insist that the rapist is tested?[494]

I think many doctors are going to recognise that a small minority may be using their rights to confidentiality as a passport to injure and destroy others. Practice varies among 'contact tracers' in sex disease clinics in the UK. Some will contact partners without the person's consent as a last resort if the person will not co-operate despite many hours of counselling.

Partner notification guidelines have recently been issued by the UK government to help find a way through the moral maze.[495]

It is incredibly worrying that a number of people who know they are positive have returned to clinics only a few weeks later with a new infection of gonorrhoea.[496] Some have contracted this from promiscuous behaviour without a condom. In one UK study, nearly a quarter of gay men who knew they had HIV returned with a new acute sexually-transmitted infection.[497] They are wilfully putting others at risk. These are questions that doctors and governments are going to be faced with sooner than they realise.[498]

If someone knows he or she is positive, and sleeps with someone who is not without warning them of the situation first, and that person becomes positive, it has been suggested that the man or woman concerned could be prosecuted for grievous bodily harm.[499]

The Solicitor General for Scotland, Mr Peter Frazer, announced that people who maliciously or recklessly infect someone with the virus may be prosecuted for assault under existing Scottish laws. A drug addict was jailed for three years for spitting in a policeman's eyes 'to give him AIDS'.[500]

A New York judge has ruled that damages can be claimed from a sexual partner if you can prove that he or she infected you and that the partner knew he or she was infectious and did not tell you. A lawsuit for a case of herpes involved a claim for over $1 million.[501] One man in Arizona faces two charges of assault and sodomy. This will change to a charge of murder if either victim dies.[502] In West Germany such an offender can be charged with manslaughter.[503]

In 1993 a Swedish injecting drug user was found guilty of rape and deliberate transmission of HIV in a Stockholm court. Strains of virus from both parties were analysed genetically and found to be very similar. The chances of such similarity in such a rapidly-mutating virus were considered so low that it was concluded that he was the source of infection—upheld by the Court of Appeal. At least 200 lawsuits are pending in the US by infected people wanting to sue previous sexual partners.[504] The lesson is that gene technology can now be used to prove who infected you. A leading laboratory in Edinburgh with the right facilities to do the work is now concerned that its work may be overwhelmed by the need to verify court evidence.[505] The social consequences of HIV gene typing could be enormous, with violent threats of revenge. In the UK, prosecution allows people infected as a result of crime to put in a claim to the criminal injuries compensation board.

For the sake of the community, prostitutes should not be allowed to practise if they are positive. How many men do you think each prostitute services each year? According to a UK report, up to 200 per week or 10,000 a year! A study of fifty London prostitutes showed that nine out of ten thought there should be compulsory testing, and eight out of ten thought that a prostitute should be prosecuted if she worked knowing she was infected.[506]

However, what happens after prosecution? I have visited a women's prison in the UK where there are a number of HIV-infected prostitutes, jailed for soliciting and not paying fines. They know they are infected, but have no other way to survive financially following release. Their friendships, accommodation and supply of drugs are linked with selling sex. Making certain behaviour illegal does not make a problem go away.

There are other issues: alternative employment, new life, drug rehabilitation (assuming the person wants these things).

Another problem is that control measures can backfire and make the situation worse. For example, a crack-down on the Thai sex industry by police resulted in people being reluctant to come forward if they thought they might have HIV. As a result, doctors had great difficulty monitoring spread.[507]

Yet another case of rape by someone knowing he was infected occurred recently in France,[508] while a woman in the UK has been accused of knowingly infecting her boyfriend during a three-year relationship.[509] In Switzerland, an HIV-infected man was jailed for two years for knowingly passing on infection.[510] In the US, a man was convicted of attempted murder for the same reason.[511]

It has been suggested that all people who are infected should be issued with identity cards. Such a proposal has been roundly condemned because of experiences of retaliation and discrimination in the community.[512]

Infected doctors, nurses and dentists

While health care workers may be anxious at times about the risk of being infected by their patients, there is also enormous public concern about the far smaller risks of being infected by an HIV-carrying doctor, nurse or dentist. We know the risk is small because despite the growing number of infected care workers, very few cases of care-worker transmission to patient have been seen. In the US, almost 16,000 have been tested so far following treatment by thirty-two infected care workers. Apart from five patients from a Florida dentist, and possibly two others in the US prison service (unproven connection), no other cases have been identified.[513]

There have been several cases recently in the UK where infection of a surgeon only came to light after the person had treated a very large number of people. In one example of a senior gynaecologist, the person was estimated to have treated up to 17,000 women and been involved in over 6,000 operations.[514] Hospital authorities have often been unsure what to do. Where do you begin? How do you trace such a large number of people, many of whom may have moved more than once over the last ten years? Even if you have a complete list of addresses and phone numbers, how long would it take to contact them all? You might need more than 100 trained team members.

It is not surprising that information has sometimes leaked out in an uncontrolled manner before helplines were ready, or before a proper public announcement. Often the individual has been quickly identified in media coverage, making the person's life a misery, affecting family, violating privacy and confidentiality, and making it less likely others will come forward promptly if they think they too could be infected.

The risk of someone being infected by a health worker is very low.[515] For this to happen, the surgeon would need to be cut badly without realising; so badly in fact that he or she cuts right through the glove into the pulp of a finger, carrying on so blood contaminates a patient's wound. This is hardly likely. Nevertheless, we have to face the fact that in a tragic series of events a number of different people became infected by the same dentist, and we have seen the more infectious hepatitis B virus transmitted from a surgeon to patients.[516]

The 'dentist' cases happened in Florida a few years ago. We know he was the source because as we have seen we can now type the tens of thousands of minor strains of HIV. The strains were all closely related indicating the same infection source.[517] Unfortunately you do not need many stories like that to keep the tabloid press busy for years.

It seems clear to me that care workers who think they may be infected and are or have been involved in invasive procedures have a public duty to arrange to have an HIV test, and to inform their employers promptly if the result is positive. In the case of the surgeon, the issue is not just transmission of infection, but also possibly manual dexterity, given that late HIV infection can sometimes affect someone's ability to perform complex tasks (see pp 86–88).

The British Medical Association, The Royal College of Surgeons and the UK government agreed together in 1993 that those involved in invasive procedures (operations, injections and other procedures where wound contamination could occur) should cease if they are carrying HIV. They should receive practical help and support in switching to non-invasive medical jobs. In practice, this can often be quite difficult and a terrible blow to an experienced surgeon for example.[518] The General Medical Council has gone further and said that doctors failing to disclose they have HIV to a senior colleague could be struck off the medical register.[519]

Relative risks to patients[520]

HIV from infected surgeon (HIV)	1 in 42,000 to 420,000
Hepatitis B death from infected surgeon (HepB)	1 in 76,000 to 1.4 million
Death after transfusion HIV neg blood	1 in 60,000/unit transfused (USA)
Death from a general anaesthetic	1 in 10,000 operations

In other words, even if your surgeon is infected, some would say the greater risk is still from the anaesthetic— not to mention the risks from a major operation itself, which can be as high as 1 in 10 of serious complication or death.

Employers in turn clearly have a duty to do all they can to protect the confidentiality of the individual, and to provide appropriate help. This is also in the public interest. It is surely *against* the public interest to broadcast the name of an infected surgeon to 56 million people on primetime news if it means another ten infected surgeons vow to take their secret to the grave.

Employers also clearly have a duty to recall patients where there has been a risk of infection, however small. Those operated on, for example, need to be recalled. Failure to do so can have terrible consequences, as we have seen in the past. It is essential to retain public trust, and if people feel there has been a cover-up, the result can be a backlash against the very people we are trying to protect. People do not need to be told the identity of the member of the health care team who is infected. It is true that many will guess, but it is better for a few hundred to guess than for it to become national knowledge.

There should be an agreement with national media to abide by a code of practice so that if, say, an infected individual is named in the local press, that name is not then regarded as national information in the public domain. The hounding of individuals in the UK has been truly disgraceful. Where do you go? Where do you live? What about your children? Once photographs are printed the end of normal private life has arrived. This is a bitter reward for someone who has had the courage to be honest and open.

Ideally patients need to be contacted by letter or telephone before they hear in the press. They should be offered access to telephone advice, or a personal interview, and a test if they wish. In the case referred to above there were over 4,000 callers, so hospitals need to have a plan prepared. The UK government has now issued guidelines which do not go far enough in protecting identity.[521]

Unless doctors and other care workers can be assured they will be well treated, they will delay coming forward, if necessary until days before death. If this continues to happen, pressure may become irresistible to test, say, all surgeons on an annual basis. This would be much cheaper and more straightforward than supervising recall of up to 30,000 patients a year, many of whom are severely stressed by the experience.

It is true that annual testing would miss a few infected in the last few months. However, it would ensure that no surgeon is able to expose patients to infection for more than a year, so greatly limiting the numbers to be recalled.

I think that compulsory testing would be a great step backwards, since once you start with surgeons, where do you stop? Airline pilots are already routinely tested by some airlines, as we have seen, because of worries about mental performance. Before we know where we are, a great number of different groups could end up being tested on a regular basis, with resultant loss of freedoms, breaches of confidentiality, oppression and fear. Nevertheless, I see its introduction for some health care workers as inevitable, unless surgeons agree to testing on a voluntary basis. Such a measure may even have been implemented by the time you read this book.

Procedures and laws vary greatly from country to country. In the US, for example, a surgeon could face ten years in prison for operating without revealing he has HIV or AIDS.[522]

Legalisation of brothels

Recently there was an outcry from some in the UK after the Mothers' Union appeared to support the legalisation of brothels in the fight against AIDS. Although it later voted against the suggestion,[523] the debate was significant—similar to debates over legalisation of drugs.

Some say that legalising organised brothels means that prostitution can be regulated, and the health of prostitutes can be checked. The argument goes that this protects prostitutes not only from untreated sexually-transmitted diseases, but also from the ever-present risk of a violent death in an alleyway, in the back of a car, or in the home of a customer.

However, having official brothels means in many nations brightly signposted and advertised sex houses with official backing. This seems a very odd approach to HIV prevention at a time when governments need to be encouraging young people to be restrained and faithful in relationships. What kind of messages are we giving young people? Many also feel that it is degrading for a woman to have her body sold for sex by others.

In the UK, it is no longer an offence for a woman to accept money for sex on a personal basis—an enlightened measure which means that prostitutes are no longer forced into a kind of slavery through vice rings. It is, however, an offence for other people to publicly solicit for clients, run a business even as two women, or to live off the earnings of prostitutes.[524] A representative of the English Collective of prostitutes said that 'legalisation would lead to sex ghettos, and an assembly line of sex with high taxes and few benefits for the women',[525] particularly as anyone found to have HIV would be likely to be thrown out on the streets. In Sweden, where prostitution has always been legal, there are now growing pressures for anti-prostitution laws, because the numbers of prostitutes are growing fast amid fears of AIDS.[526]

Sex education in schools

While HIV infection raises many issues, so does prevention, most of all among young people in schools. What is an appropriate message? What is the right age? Should people be allowed to opt out?

Many have feared that certain groups will use AIDS as a platform, either aggressively promoting gay lifestyles as normal to young teenagers, or aggressively promoting a right-wing moral crusade.

Young people clearly need to know the facts about HIV, and also need room to think through for themselves how they are going to respond.

In the UK, the Christian-based AIDS organisation ACET has been very successful in developing a national schools programme, presenting the facts in a context encouraging people to see sex in terms of health, relationships, choices and their long-term future.

As we will see later on, most schools reject a simplistic message based on using condoms, and also reject a moralistic approach. However, they do want values to be communicated in a way which gives a positive view of waiting for the right person and of being faithful.

The US Vice-President said recently: 'When eighth-graders are squandering the gift of youthful innocence in premarital sex, the solution is not to give them a condom. The solution is to give them a value-based education.'[527]

In New York City, the Board of Education has insisted that all new teachers agree to 'stress that abstinence is the most appropriate premarital protection against AIDS' and to 'devote substantially more time and attention to abstinence than to other methods of protection'.[528] With half a million New Yorkers HIV-infected, a third of boys and a fifth of girls sexually active by the age of fifteen, there is unease about just giving out condoms.

See Chapter 12 for fuller discussion (p 292 onwards) .

Age of consent

One traditional way to discourage sexual activity in the young is through a legal minimum 'age of consent' below which sexual activity becomes a crime.

Age of consent varies widely from one country to another, even in Europe (see table), and from one kind of sexual activity to another. In many countries there are campaigns to lower the age of consent, particularly where it is much higher for homosexual acts. The law is a blunt instrument with which to regulate private behaviour between consenting individuals. Prosecutions are rarely brought except where there is evidence of exploitation. Pressures are likely to grow for a unified age for both heterosexual and homosexual sex. Pressure was great in the UK which had the highest age of consent for homosexual men in Western Europe until March 1994.

Some argue on the basis of their own views on morality that all homosexual acts should be illegal, and therefore an age of consent of twenty-one is already too low. However, there is inconsistency in the argument since the same people may regard adultery or heterosexual sex before marriage as morally wrong, but would not make these things illegal.

The basic question is this: Do you want to see people put in prison with criminal records for violating an age of consent as it stands? If the answer is no, then the age of consent needs review, or it could make a mockery of the law.

Age of consent[529]

	Heterosexual	Gay	Lesbian
Austria	14	18	14
Belgium	16	16	16
Cyprus	16	Illegal	16
Denmark	15	15	15
Finland	16	18	18
France	15	15	15
Germany (W)	14	18	14
Germany (E)	14	14	14
Greece	15	15	15
Ireland	17	17	17
Italy	14	14	14
Luxembourg	16	16	16
Netherlands	12	12	12
Norway	16	16	16
Portugal	12	12	12
Spain	12	12	12
Sweden	15	15	15
Switzerland	16	16	16
UK	16	18*	16

* 21, changed to 18 in 1994—further reduction?

Telling the truth?

I will never forget the day I went to visit a particular person who was dying at home. I was accosted in the hallway by an anxious relative who was convinced that the only reason I was there was to tell the patient his diagnosis and that he was dying. Nothing I could say would convince this relative otherwise. She was terrified. In fact we found as a team that working with this family became impossible. The sticking point was that I said that although I would never mention his probable death unless he himself asked, I was not prepared to lie to him. I might give an indirect answer such as, 'Why do you ask?' or, 'You don't seem to be getting any better, do you?' but I was not prepared to say, 'Of course not, don't be stupid!'

The reason is very simple: trust. One day he would have realised I was lying. Actually, as far as I could see from what he said, he knew he was dying anyway—most people do. Most people with cancer or AIDS have guessed what is happening long before they are told, although there can sometimes be denial, associated with fear or guilt. Having established myself as a liar whenever it suits me to save embarrassment or calm fear, what happens when the person asks if they will die in terrible pain? This time I answer truthfully—but will I be believed? Often when people are first referred to us, they are convinced they are going to 'suffocate to death'. They may have terrible nightmares and be consumed with fears. Every time they get a cough we get a telephone call—the reason is overwhelming fear of what may be around the corner.

The truth is that no one suffocates to death these days. Hospices have advanced our care of those with lung disease enormously over the last twenty years. That is the truth—but will the public believe it? Fear of death can be worse than the dying itself.

Trust is the most powerful tool a doctor has. It is the reason why support teams and hospices are so successful. They inspire trust because they do not engage in the same frauds, cover-ups and webs of petty deceit that are practised daily on the wards of every hospital. If only doctors realised that people see through it all!

The reason for dishonesty by doctors and dishonesty by families and friends is simply this: we live in a society which likes to pretend that death does not exist. AIDS then hits us like a thunderbolt straight between the eyes, because it brings us face to face with death and all our deepest fears. But before we take a look at the whole life/death issue, I want to turn to just one more moral dilemma which I get faced with every day as a church leader. The question people ask is this: Do you agree with those who say that AIDS is the wrath or judgement of God?

8

Wrath or Reaping?

Wrath of God?

Is AIDS the wrath of God? I am asked what I think about this issue almost every day, because I am a church leader as well as a doctor and often find myself talking to churches and other church leaders about AIDS. It is one of those areas where you know that any phrase or sentence you say or write could be turned into a banner headline of whatever kind the editor thinks will sell the most papers or media time. I am also aware that you may be one of the thousands of readers of this book who will judge it by whether you agree with what I say. You will either be pleased you bought it or want to burn it. You will either say I am judgemental or a heretic or a liberal. What follows is a personal view from a church leader who takes seriously what the Bible says.

It is also a view consistent, as far as I can see, with the historic teachings of the church on sexual behaviour over 2,000 years, whether Orthodox, Catholic, Anglican, Episcopalian, Baptist, Methodist, Lutheran, Presbyterian, Independent Evangelical, Pentecostal, New Church charismatic, or whatever. In fact Christian teaching on sexual behaviour and morality has been remarkably consistent and united, as it is today outside certain groups within particular denominations. The big issue is how a traditional Christian view on morality can be equated with God's call to love.

In the mid-1980s medical advice filtering through the media was that AIDS was spread only by anal sex. Anal sex was described by many in the press as an unnatural act that caused bleeding and infection of the partner. The public impression was that unless you were gay you could not get AIDS. A number of clergymen and church leaders then grabbed their Bibles and began a series of private and public pronouncements in the United States, the United Kingdom and other countries denouncing homosexuality, listing plagues described in the Old and New Testaments, and declaring that this was obviously God's plague on homosexuals[530]—obviously as it only appeared to affect them.

A Catholic Professor of Philosophy in the US said at an international conference recently: 'The gay community was the originator of the AIDS troubles in America,' and went on to suggest that gay men should accept AIDS as 'just punishment for their disgusting sins'.[531]

This attitude is not confined to Western nations. In Uganda it was reported on state radio that a goat, speaking in a loud voice, had prophesied that the AIDS epidemic was a divine punishment for mankind's wickedness in not obeying the Ten Commandments, and predicted a terrible famine. It terrified local villagers and died shortly afterwards.[532]

Such reactions are fuelled by a distorted perception of sexual sin which is part of our culture and not part of Jesus' own sayings. Before you reject this out of hand, you who are churchgoers, read on. Incidentally, I find it is usually men who are so vehement in condemning the homosexual man. Women are usually far more tolerant. Yet the same men are more tolerant of two lesbians. Why? Does God find sex between two men more offensive than between two women or an adulterous relationship? AIDS is almost unknown in lesbians.

First, I expect those church leaders are now acutely embarrassed. They are on record as declaring that this is God's judgement on homosexuals, although there are now known to be many more women and babies infected than there ever were homosexual men. They fire salvoes at the visible tip of the iceberg, ignoring the millions of women, children and heterosexual men beneath the surface. As we saw in Chapter 1, 90% of new HIV infections worldwide are now among heterosexuals. The 'wrath' theology is then adjusted to include all who are promiscuous—again acutely mistaken.[533] What do you say to those millions of children who may die in Africa or elsewhere as a result of medical treatments (blood and injections)? Children are also dying in the United Kingdom, in America, Romania, Russia and many other countries.

When coupled with the public image of the church as 'anti-condom', the comments about AIDS being the 'wrath of God' have been seen as doubly negative. The Catholic Church in particular has been extremely uncomfortable with AIDS campaigns promoting condom use, while strongly advocating compassionate care and understanding.[534] Protestant churches tend to be more relaxed, as long as condom use is placed alongside the options of celibacy and faithfulness.

It is hard to generalise, and responses vary with country and area, but the Pope restated the official Catholic position on AIDS by encouraging compassionate unconditional care, with self-control, chastity and faithfulness. Many were dismayed at Vatican suggestions that even married couples where one is infected should not be allowed to use condoms. With 92 million members in Africa alone, the Catholic Church has great influence.[535]

Nothing new

'Wrath of God' theories are nothing new. Several centuries ago a plague for which there was no cure swept the known world. Signs of infection were absent sometimes for many years and controversies raged over which country it had all started in. It was spread by sexual intercourse. I am referring to syphilis which, as we have seen, only became curable with the advent of penicillin in 1944.

At the time, many saw syphilis as the judgement of God on

the sexually immoral. This had two effects: search for a cure was inhibited or actively discouraged—after all, you were interfering with the natural course of judgement. Also, those with syphilis were treated in a less sympathetic way: 'It is their own fault and they put society at risk.'

A friend of mine spent some months in a certain developing country in 1974. Many men came into the hospital clinic where he was working because they had difficulty passing water. Gonorrhoea infection had caused scarring and narrowing of the delicate tube (urethra) inside the penis. Sometimes these people would have full bladders and be in great discomfort. The way to treat this is by pushing a series of rods into the penis, each one larger than the one before, to dilate the stricture. This causes excruciating, unbearable pain unless you use local anaesthetic cream. It is so painful that most surgeons in the United Kingdom do this under a general anaesthetic. The cream was stacked on the shelves and men were screaming out in agony.

Greatly shocked by this my friend asked why the pain-killing cream or a full anaesthetic was not being used. The answer was that this was an immoral disease and the person must be punished. I wish it were not so, but these people had been influenced by atmosphere and culture imported by church missionaries. What has that appalling attitude got in common with the way of Jesus?

You may recoil from this, but you must realise that in the United States, the United Kingdom and some other countries, parts of the church are still fostering the very same attitudes to the very same kind of epidemic. The words are not the same, but the same atmosphere of rejection of the person is there.

Be consistent

Be consistent: if AIDS is the wrath of God, then syphilis was too. I cannot see any real difference between AIDS and any other disease from the medical point of view. The cause and mechanism of illness are different, but people still need care. The agent of the wrath of God is often recorded as being an angel in the Old and New Testaments. It is portrayed as a supernatural intervention that is selective. Contrast this with AIDS, caused by a virus which has probably existed in some shape or form for thousands of years. It has existed in animals for a long time, and maybe also in humans. The explosive spread—as with syphilis—has been along the lines of international travel and sexual relationships. It behaves according to the rules of every other infection with its own particular preferences and effects.

As I said at the beginning of the book—what is so special about AIDS? In one sense, nothing at all. You have been misinformed. The reaction of extreme fear associated with AIDS is unusual. But fear, lack of signs and high death rate from a viral disease are not the same thing as God's judgement. For me, the key to the whole thing is the attitude of Jesus.

Caught in the act

At the crack of dawn Jesus was at the temple teaching a huge crowd. Sitting and standing, leaning against the walls, they listened quietly as Jesus sat down. It was still cold under the stark sunlight and the vast stones were damp with dew. Jesus' voice quietly rose and fell. There was silence apart from an occasional cough or the bleat of an animal outside.

Suddenly all heads turned at the sound of a great commotion. Twenty or thirty people burst in shouting and screaming. Jesus stopped. He was used to such interruptions. They happened almost every day—either by friends bringing someone wanting to be healed or by the authorities hoping to provoke a confrontation and arrest him.

A woman was thrown down at his feet. She and Jesus stood up together. She had been discovered in bed half an hour ago with another woman's husband. Caught in the act. The men who brought her were furious, seething with anger. They demanded a response from Jesus: 'The law says we must drag her away, pick up rocks and boulders, and stone her to death. What do you say?'

It was yet another trap and Jesus knew it. If he had agreed with the law they would have dragged him away and stoned him for being judgemental and severe. If he had not agreed they would have arrested him for being too liberal.

Who's perfect?

Jesus did nothing at all. He said nothing at all. The mob were pressing in, repeating their question over and over again, pushing and shoving aggressively. All the while the people in the court were watching and waiting. Tension was rising. Someone was going to get hurt—either Jesus or the woman was likely to be lynched. The very forces who could have prevented it were standing right there in the temple.

Jesus knelt down on the ground under the harsh glare and threats of the men and was silent. He wrote on the ground with his finger. The shouting and abuse got louder.

Jesus stood up and looked at them. Instantly there was quiet. Jesus looked into the eyes of each man standing there. 'You who are so perfect, you who have never cheated anyone, lied, or been selfish, you who are always so perfectly loving and kind, you who never lose your temper, you who are so generous, you who have never had a lustful thought . . . Yes, you come forward now, come and take a stone, come and throw it at this woman. Be the first to throw.'[536]

Jesus looked at each man in turn, but they shrank away, uncomfortable under his gaze. He knelt down again and stared at the ground as he wrote with his finger in the dust. The older men began to peel off from the crowd and disappeared down the temple steps. One at a time they left in silence. Gone were the shouts, the threats, and the abuse. Eventually none was left—only those who had come to hear Jesus teach.

No condemnation

Jesus stood up. The woman was still standing there, her head hung in shame, humiliation and embarrassment. She stood afraid, unable to move, afraid of the men waiting outside, afraid of what Jesus was thinking.

Jesus looked at her. Spies in the crowd were about to slip out and report that Jesus had been trapped: he had given himself away as a liberal by letting an adulterer off free.

Jesus said to the woman, 'Where are they? Has no one condemned you?'

'No one, sir,' she replied. Jesus then said two vitally important things: 'Then neither do I condemn you,' and then he added: 'Do not sin again.'[537]

Men had caught a man and a woman making love. One of them was married to someone else. They let off the man and judged the woman. Double standards: their own they excused, the other they condemned. As far as they were concerned, they were just expressing the natural wrath and displeasure of God, but Jesus rejected their whole attitude. Jesus was concerned not just with actions but also with attitude. As far as he was concerned, to have an adulterous fantasy could be as bad as committing adultery.[538] One person may be no worse than the other—just one had the opportunity and the guts to actually do it, the other no opportunity or was too afraid.

The man who is angry with his brother could be as bad as someone who kills. Read what Jesus said for yourself.[539] Actions are not everything. What goes on in the secret places of your heart and imagination is also vitally important.[540]

Never do it again

Jesus did not distinguish between the subtleties of wrong. We are all wrong. We have all done wrong or thought wrong. None of us is perfect.[541] As the only perfect man, he was the only person who had the perfect right to condemn the woman, but he did not. Why not?

Because he loved her and understood himself what it was like to be tempted.[542]

Did he excuse her? Not at all. Did he encourage her? Not at all. Did he allow her to get off free? Not at all. He rebuked her. He told her she had been wrong. He told her never to do it again. He told her never to do anything else wrong again. 'Go and learn from your lesson' was his message.

They were *all* wrong: the men were hypocrites. When Jesus said that, every single one realised it was true. Every single one of them had had lustful thoughts and fantasies about other people's wives at some time or other. Every single one of them, if they were really honest, knew that deep down inside they were not as nice as they tried to appear on the outside. Only they and their families knew what they were really like at home with the door closed. Only they knew how selfish and mean they could be sometimes. Their own consciences convicted them, and they backed away. In some ways they were no better and no worse than the woman. If she deserved stoning, so did they.

The trouble is that in every town, in every village, in every church, in every country—and maybe in your home, maybe in yourself—there are attitudes just as revolting to Jesus as the attitudes of that crowd: judgemental, harsh, intolerant, vicious, cruel and bitter. 'No!' you may say. 'I'm not like that, nor is anyone I know.' Consider this then:

Banner headlines

What is your attitude to a clergyman who is prosecuted for sexually abusing children? Banner headlines continue to hit us over church leaders who have been charged with sexually assaulting children.

So much for vicars assaulting small boys. What is your attitude to a married priest who is discovered in bed with a parishioner's wife, or in a public toilet with his trousers and pants down, having anal intercourse with another man?

In most circles inside and outside the church, the reaction to all these things is shock and outrage. You say it is despicable because of his position. That person has undoubtedly lost his ability to lead a congregation. He has been living a charade, a façade behind which lies a guilt-ridden twilight world or else he has rewritten the rule book to make his conduct compatible with his faith. But in your sweeping anger you have condemned him. Your outrage is identical to that angry crowd confronting the woman.

Double standards

Clergy do not have some super gift of God that keeps them perfect. In fact the Bible does not distinguish between clergy and laity at this point. We are all a royal priesthood.[543] All who claim to be Christians are called to live up to our calling.[544] None of us is exempt. There are no double standards. As you would expect, there are minimum standards for life and conduct laid down for those appointed to positions of leadership in the church and certainly such responsibility brings special accountability. However, these minimum standards such as managing the household well, being sober and self-controlled, are no more or less than those expected of all of us. It is interesting that the lists of qualifications are all to do with character, not gift or experience.[545]

Individuals who behave in the ways listed above need to be accepted as people, while we may not necessarily accept everything they do or say. As people we find this almost impossible—we either accept the person and what he or she does, or land up rejecting the behaviour and the person. It is not what you say, but the way you say it that can be most important. Some people say they care about drug addicts but give out an atmosphere of coldness. Some people say that as Jesus loved all people, they too accept all people, but still display deep-rooted prejudices at every turn. You who are perfect—you cast the first stone.

God calls us to accept all people and to extend his love to them regardless of whether or not we agree with what they do.

'Impossible!' you say. 'How can this be reconciled with God's absolute standards?' Jesus came for all men. Not for the perfect but to invite 'sinners to repentance'.[546] Did Jesus come to bring forgiveness and peace to the repentant murderer? Of course he did. God's love and mercy is so unbelievably great that if even Hitler had genuinely repented and given his life to God in that bunker in 1945, the Bible tells us he would be in heaven now. Some Christians find this hard to accept. They cannot understand the true reality of God's mercy and forgiveness. Death-bed conversion is real. The thief crucified next to Jesus was told that within a few hours he would be with Jesus 'in paradise'.[547]

Judgement without tears is obscene

You may reject all this; you may go through the Bible quoting texts about God's wrath and anger. It is possible to be correct but horribly wrong. It is possible to be correct about God's displeasure but lack love. A well-known Christian leader once said that 'to speak of judgement without tears is obscene'. Where are your tears? Go and find your tears of grief for those who are suffering, dying and, you say, in line for judgement. When you have found your tears, then talk to me of judgement—but start with yourself.

Reaping natural consequences?

It is a fact of life that everything has consequences. If you drink and drive you may injure or kill yourself and others. If you sniff cocaine you may get a hole inside your nose—the nose was not designed for cocaine. If you line your lungs with tobacco tar you can get a chronic irritation which may result in coughs and cancer. If you eat badly-cooked chicken you can get food poisoning. If you sleep with someone who is not a virgin, you could catch a number of illnesses which he or she may have caught from a previous partner.

These things are so obvious. Cause and effect is also a

central theme in the teaching of Jesus. The Bible teaches that we are creatures of choice. We are not automatons. We are free to choose God's way or our way. If that were not so there would be no point in telling us how to live because we would be unable to respond in any other way at all. But with freedom comes responsibility. The Bible teaches that each of us will have to give account one day for everything we have said, thought, done, should have done and did not do.

The Christian position is that within the Bible our loving Father has recorded guidelines for healthy, stress-free, fulfilled living: 'How to be healthy and whole.' So what is the Christian view of sex? Here is a personal view.

Unlimited sex

Sex was invented by God to be enjoyed. It is one of the most amazing and intensely enjoyable experiences God gave mankind. In God's plan, he intended a man and a woman to marry and in the context of that promise of commitment, care, love and understanding, to explore together the kaleidoscope pleasures of physical love. God intended husband and wife to have unlimited sex: as often as they both would like and enjoy. Out of that beautiful loving relationship were to come children who would grow up feeling loved and secure, with a mum and a dad, grandparents, aunts, uncles and cousins. God loves families. He created human beings to belong to each other, and those whose families had died or were far away to be cared for if they wanted by other families or communities.

Our bodies were not designed for multiple sexual encounters. Such a lifestyle has consequences. It is physically unhealthy. Before AIDS, promiscuity was already becoming more and more unhealthy. It was fairly risky until the advent of antibiotics dealt with gonorrhoea and syphilis. Then some penicillin-resistant strains of gonorrhoea emerged, along with various other infections such as herpes and chlamydia (Pelvic Inflammatory Disease). Now we know that early sex and multiple partners can also cause cervical cancer. This was all before AIDS. Promiscuity has always been unhealthy. Now it can be fatal.

Emotionally, sleeping around has always been hazardous. The result is usually destabilisation of any semi-permanent or permanent relationship. Although polygamy was practised in the Old Testament, the track record of its success and happiness is disastrous. Read the story of Abraham.[548] Adultery usually has catastrophic consequences for one person at least. I have yet to come across a case where it did not. Divorce, too, is nearly always a traumatic disaster leaving lifelong scars. Sleeping around fractures relationships and will always be emotionally risky, unless there are no relationships. If there are no relationships then nothing is at risk. A prostitute has no emotional investment in her client— nor her client with her—so there is no loss or trauma. However, there may develop a more sinister and deeper damage to the ability to form lasting loyal commitments. The risk is a lonely bankruptcy of friendship and support after middle life has sapped physical drives and taken its toll on attractiveness and vitality.

Sleeping with multiple partners can have permanent spiritual effects too. The Bible teaches clearly that sex is a wonderful experience and one of the deepest mysteries known to human beings. When a man and a woman sleep together, the Bible says they become 'one flesh'.[549] We see the physical expression of this spiritual event when a 'half cell' (sperm) from a man fuses with a 'half cell' (egg) from a woman and the two become literally 'one flesh'. In that moment of history a new being is formed; life is created.

When two people have sexual intercourse, the Bible teaches that irrespective of whether conception occurs, something has taken place which can never be undone.

Sex was designed as the ultimate expression of exclusive covenant love between a man and a woman. Devoid of relationship it is robbed of its quality and enjoyment and becomes a mere mechanical sensation. No wonder many unmarried people reject sleeping around and choose celibacy. They see through the glamorous veneer to the emptiness beneath. Those who are promiscuous are often driven into further and further searches for the ultimate in sexual satisfaction. Once you have divorced the physical act from the whole-person experience you have no hope at all of true fulfilment. Women usually realise this more than men. None of these things will satisfy your heart. You have been cruelly deceived and there may be consequences.

The Christian position is that when we break any of God's designs for living we create tension in our relationship with him. God is perfect and cannot tolerate sin. Nor can he reward us with the warmth of his love and approval when we have turned our backs on his best for us. Sin affects your nearness to God if you are a Christian and prevents your finding God if you are not. There is nothing especially wrong in sexual sin, although its effects can be very destructive of relationships and communities. As we have seen, there is one sense in which it is no more displeasing to God than any other sins against others.

I feel I must say again that often we fall into absurd double standards. People reject homosexual acts or adultery as more wrong in some way than lying or cheating or stealing or being cruel or hating someone. There is no such distinction in the Bible when it comes to separation from God.[550] Sin is sin— the other differences are merely cultural values and must be rejected. The Bible teaches that we are all imperfect. We all think wrong, feel wrong and do wrong. We all fall far short of God's standards. None of us deserves any reward or favours from God, and there is nothing we can do to earn his pleasure. That is why I believe no one has the right to turn and point the finger at someone with AIDS.

Impossible barrier

You can never be good enough. Human imperfections always remain an impossible barrier between us and God. Without

Jesus Christ, you can no more put human beings and God together than olive oil and water: they always separate.

That is why Jesus said, 'I am the way and the truth and the life. No one comes to the Father except through me.'[551] There are, we are told, hundreds of ways to God. Maybe, but none of them leads you to a personal relationship with a God who is almighty, omnipotent, unknowable, unreachable and untouchable. Other religions may promise some kind of ethereal consciousness, but that is no substitute for a personal relationship. The reason is obvious. Other religions say that closely following a certain formula for holiness will deal with your imperfection. If only it could. The best formulas in the world and the most ardent efforts might possibly get you a mile or two nearer God. The trouble is that our imperfections distance us from God by several light years! But even after a lifetime of devoted holiness, you would have a chasm of several million miles to cross.[552]

No wonder Jesus himself said he was the only way to oneness with God the Father. Christians believe the good news that God himself provided a rescue plan for mankind because significant movement by us in his direction was impossible. So God himself moved towards us and entered our time-space world. He came in human form as Jesus.

When Jesus died, that whole issue of separation was dealt with for all time. Every single thing that separated us—all the consequences of our wrong doing and wrong attitudes—were lumped on Jesus' shoulders. As a sacrifice for all time he, the perfect God-man, allowed himself to die for us so that we might be forgiven and released from the consequences of what we have done. The result is now a doorway—a narrow one—to union with God our Father. You enter the door not by justifying to God what a wonderful person you are, but by believing and accepting all Jesus came to do—and by making a decision to give your life to him in obedience.

Unless you really understand the way the Bible portrays this separation and how Jesus overcame it, you will never fully grasp what Jesus said to the woman and the accusing crowd that morning; they were all finished. None of them had the remotest hope of peace with God. The men and women in the crowd, the adulteress herself, they were hopelessly blocked from a relationship with their Father. That is, outside of following, believing and trusting in Jesus, the only way, the truth about God and the means of finding the life of God.

Changed lives

To all those who accept Jesus as Lord and turn away from everything wrong (repent means to turn around), he has given a brand new life.[553] That is why Jesus told a would-be follower that he had to be 'born again'.[554]

When I became a Christian, in one sense I died.[555] Baptism is a symbol of my burial. When I rose out of the water it was a symbol of my new birth.[556] The Bible says I am now a new creation: 'The life I now have is not my life, but the life which Christ lives in me.'[557] This is another mystery.

When someone becomes a Christian, the results are often dramatic.

Parents or children become easier to live with. Marriages begin a new start. Friendships are transformed. A friend of mine who became a Christian invited all his friends to his baptism (we use a local swimming pool). They all turned up with their heavy metal leather jackets and boots. Two were so amazed at what had happened to their friend that when they saw it wasn't just a passing fad, they became Christians as well.[558] When you've seen the real thing, who wants a substitute? Ordinary people changed by something outside themselves.

A friend from the United States told me that he became a Christian partly through his mother's conversion. She was dying of severe kidney disease. The poisons were steadily accumulating in her body. She was not a believer but went to a healing meeting. She was prayed with for healing and felt she had been instantly healed. She went back to the clinic as usual.

The doctors were amazed. All the results of medical tests on her kidneys had returned to normal. Life was never the same for her. She became a Christian, and so did her son some time later.

I met someone recently after an AIDS talk. He told me he had been a heroin addict until three or four years ago when he became a Christian. He broke the habit immediately and is now a leader in his church. This is not unusual. Jesus gives people power by the Holy Spirit when they become Christians.[559]

You can be free to choose God's way even though chained to all kinds of things—addiction, childhood memories, or parts of your own human nature. Jesus came to set you free. You choose to follow him and he does the rest. You exercise your will and he will give you all the resources you need.[560]

Father's love

After a meeting at a London medical school, I overheard a conversation between a medical student and a member of the hospital Christian Union. She was basically asking herself why she couldn't believe in God. 'I admire you people. I wish I could believe. You have it all together. You know where you are going. It's all right for you.'

I joined in. I asked her if she really wanted an answer to that question because I believed God wanted to answer it for her. I told her that God loved her whether she believed it or not. I told her the story of Jesus and the woman at the well.[561] Jesus broke the taboos by asking her for a drink. He then told her to go and fetch her husband. She replied that she didn't have one. Jesus agreed with her: 'You have been married five times and the man you are now living with is not your husband.' She was shocked. How did he know? She rushed to the village to tell them about this man who knew everything about her.

Such insights can be a part of Christian life today. I prayed for a moment and then said that I felt that part of the reason this girl could not believe was because of her family. She had never known what it was to feel loved, especially by her father, and so could not accept that God could care about her, love her as his child.

She sat down and started to cry. Tears poured down her face as she started to talk about her childhood, not a particularly unhappy one, but one devoid of open affection. She was hurting, bruised and wounded. I asked if she wanted me to pray for her emotions and her past. She did. Even before I prayed her eyes seemed to open and she found she believed deep down. But it is hard to trust a heavenly Father's love if you have never experienced an earthly father's love. After we had prayed she made it clear she wanted to give her whole life to God. She realised she had been living life her way and now wanted to live life God's way. She wanted to turn her back on the past and begin again. She gave her life to God in a very moving prayer. There were tears in my eyes and in her friend's when we had finished.

About a year later I found myself sitting next to her at a conference. Friends had told me previously how much she had changed, how much happier and fulfilled she was, and how her student friends had all been along to various things with her to try and puzzle it out.

Father's discipline

People who have never known love find it hard to accept love—whether from a friend, a spouse, or from God. Likewise, people who have never known the balanced firmness and discipline of a loving father and mother can find it hard to understand the discipline, firmness and standards of God.

Jesus loves all people, but not necessarily what people do. He got angry and violent with traders using the temple area to make money out of pilgrims. He walked through the stalls, tipping up the trestle tables and throwing their goods on the ground.[562] There was chaos: their best wares and coins were flying everywhere. Then Jesus came at them again, this time with a whip of cords to drive them right out of the temple.[563] 'Gentle Jesus meek and mild' is not the whole Jesus of the Bible. And yet he loved them.

Many of Jesus' words to religious leaders were aggressive and cutting with biting sarcasm and savage wit. Wherever he went he slaughtered hypocrisy, double standards, false religion and disregard for God's holiness. Today we shrink from preaching on many of the things Jesus said because they are so strong.

The thing on which Jesus was strongest of all was love. 'Love your neighbour' is hard enough—particularly when the story of the Good Samaritan shows us that your neighbour is whoever you come into contact with, regardless of nationality, background, circumstances, or personal risk.[564]

Loving your neighbour is not enough

Jesus then made one of the most devastating commands that has ever been made. Loving our neighbour is totally inadequate. We are also called to love our enemies, to express God's perfect love to those who hate us, despise us, want to hurt us, and beat us up.[565] Jesus calls us to love those who rape us, cheat us, and those who twist and distort things we say. He commands us to pray for people who persecute us or spitefully use us.

This is not a command to mere forgiveness—though that itself is painfully costly and hard at times. This is a command to actively, positively seek to express warmth, compassion, kindness and understanding to those we humanly would hate and regard as our worst enemies. We are told to pray for their happiness. This was not idle talk: Jesus lived out his message all the way to his crucifixion.

This may seem objectionable, impossible and bizarre—but it is what Jesus said. After all, even the most horrible people tend to be nice to their friends. What is so special about being nice to your friends? What is so remarkable about loving those who love you? Nothing at all. We are called to be a visual aid, an active demonstration, a living temple of God's supreme love. Even more amazing is that God's love for us is incalculably greater than our love for others—because God is infinite and perfect.

Just as we are commanded to love, regardless of response, in a way which is totally without conditions or strings attached, so God our Father loves all people regardless of their response to him.

Now you can see that God does not hate or reject people because he does not like what they do. He weeps over our slowness, our obstinacy, our self-centredness, our stupidity.

When it all goes wrong

When God made creation, he designed man and woman to be physically united in a marriage covenant, to be perfectly loving and perfectly faithful. What happens when it all goes wrong? When people make each other's lives hell in a desperately unhappy marriage, when people cheat each other in adultery, when people sleep around without the covenant commitment of marriage, when people express their sexuality by torturing their partners for pleasure, when children are sexually seduced by adults . . . ? When it all goes wrong, what is the response of our Maker?

Sadness and dismay are his response. Where others are being hurt or emotionally damaged the response is anger. Where people choose to ignore a relationship with him, the result is no relationship with him. A living death, a living hell. An eternal disaster of constant separation. It is not that God's will is for any to be separated from him,[566] but that God is holy. Outside Christ—which is our choice—there can be no reconciliation.[567]

So does God condemn the adulterer? Not at all. He is sad at separation from the one he loves that may result. Does God condemn the practising homosexual? Not at all. He is sad at the distance the sin creates. Does God condemn the hypocrite, the liar, or the person who is mean with money? No, he is sad that the person has missed the way. Does God condemn the person whose rages spill over into violence? No, he is sad that the person is driven by these things.

However, the Bible teaches us that God's sadness and God's anger are closely linked. God is furious at some of the things we do. God's anger is the result of his perfect holiness and justice expressed through creation. God, although our loving heavenly Father, can never compromise. Anger and judgement are the discipline sides of love, to those who refuse to turn away from what is wrong, and refuse to follow him.[568]

At the end of the day the tension between God's love and God's anger is difficult to understand. God is himself a mystery to the human brain limited in time and space to a four-dimensional world.

You reap what you sow.[569] If you sow a certain way of life, you will reap the consequences of it. This is not God's wrath or judgement. This is a normal part of living. God is a loving Father whose wish it is to see the whole of creation united with him again as was the original plan.[570]

It is not his desire to see anyone perish, but for all to come into their full inheritance:[571] life outside the limitations of space and time, a wonderful life for ever free from anguish, pain and suffering.

However, we are created in freedom, and with that come guidelines and responsibilities. With choices come consequences—some of which are, we are told, unpleasant. We are warned that we cannot always undo what we have done and the biggest consequence of all is having to face our Maker after death with our track record.[572] That may not be such a pleasant experience. It may be a terrible shock to those who thought God didn't even exist. But at that time there will be no further opportunities to undo what has been done. The result will be separation from God with all the time-space world stripped away. A continuation of a relationship—or a lack of it. There are people right now who are separated from God and know it. They need to be reconciled to him and experience the warmth of his love.

People think finding God as a Father is very complicated. Becoming a Christian is as simple as apologising to God in your own words for living life your way and agreeing to live life his way, turning your back on the past, acknowledging Jesus as Lord to be worshipped and obeyed, and trusting him for everything. That is the way to experience the love of God as your Father. That is the way to find forgiveness and cleansing for all you have ever done wrong, and that is the way to receive the help, comfort and power of the Holy Spirit.

There are others who are separated who have no idea at all. So consumed are they with earning money, building a business, or making a nice home that they pay no attention to the empty spaces inside. Many of these people finally start being real about themselves when confronted by their own imminent death.

If only I had known what I know now

People who become Christians in later life often say, 'If only I had known what I know now. I would not have got divorced. I would still know my kids. I wasted so much of my life. Why didn't anyone tell me before?' They probably did, it just took a sudden jolt to shake them out of their complacency. Death of a friend, adultery by a wife or husband, death of a child, diagnosis of AIDS. With AIDS there is an added dimension. Maybe if the person had become a believer a decade ago, he would not be infected. He could still have been alive in twenty years' time.

Quite often people have not heard before. The UK is in a post-Christian era with various outward trappings of Christian life left, often devoid of content. In the church we tend to think everyone knows what Christianity is—but in fact very few do. Saying a prayer or two when in trouble and going to church do not make you a Christian. Being a follower of Jesus is what makes you a Christian. Jesus said that even the devil believes.

It is the desire above all else to do God's will that makes the difference. 'Whoever cares for his own safety is lost; but if a man will let himself be lost for my sake, that man is safe.'[573] In businesses we often talk of the cost benefit analysis. Is a project likely to be worthwhile? In the church we major on benefits, but when did you last hear a sermon about the cost? Jesus majored on the cost, just as he majored on choice, responsibility, accountability and consequences.

Strong stuff

It was Jesus himself who said that if my right eye caused me to go wrong then I should pluck it out (figuratively speaking) and throw it away rather than 'be thrown into hell where the devouring worm never dies and the fire is not quenched'.[574] Strong words from the strongest man the world has ever seen. You may not like them and I may not like talking about this whole area, but it is part of the truth. To say otherwise is to make God out to be some amoral, ethereal substance, neither able to feel nor think. Some indescribable, unknowable something-or-other as vague as energy or cosmos. My God is more than that: Author, Originator, Prime Mover, who created a conscious, moral, decision-making, spiritually-aware creature capable of relationships. Man was made in God's own image, a creature to have a relationship with his Maker, who is revealed to him in terms of an ultimate relationship: that of Father to son or daughter.[575]

How do we respond?

So how do we respond in a practical way? Even those who passionately defend their promiscuity or homosexual sex on moral grounds concede that if I found a friend of mine, a leader of a church, was having an affair with another man's wife, I should tell him to stop. In fact I usually find people outside the church are even fiercer in speaking out against such behaviour than many in the church. Those in the church are expected to behave! If I ask why, they say that a clergyman must act in a moral fashion. I agree.

The Bible is quite clear that those who call themselves Christians are called to be loving, kind, generous, honest and either faithful to their spouses or celibate.[576] To remain single, following the example of Jesus, is shown to be a positive, releasing decision, because it frees the person enormously to be mobile, able to go wherever God wants.[577] The Bible is exceptionally clear in outlawing sex between unmarried people and sex with other people's spouses. Sex between two men or two women is considered in just the same way as sex between unmarried people. For those in the church it is forbidden. Sex between a son and his mother or a father and his daughter or with animals is also outlawed. In fact any form of sexual intercourse outside of marriage is utterly forbidden.[578]

Sex is not unique in this regard. To bear a grudge is also forbidden.[579] To be moody and feel sorry for myself all the time is forbidden. To get drunk is forbidden.[580] The way of Jesus is the way of perfect love.[581]

This feels very negative—boundaries always feel negative. If I tell my four-year-old son he can cycle around the park but must keep within sight of me, he will feel I am negative. Boundaries are essential. Any child psychologist will tell you what happens when children don't know their boundaries. They are always testing to find the limits of what is acceptable. When there are no limits—or worse, the limits always vary— the child becomes insecure and can grow up immature. He may also be constantly at risk through lack of supervision.

Boundaries for healthy living

Out-of-bounds areas are marked for protection and safety. The Falklands War left hundreds of square miles of deserted land surrounded by barbed-wire. The reason is that hundreds of thousands of tiny plastic explosive charges lie inches beneath the soil. Treading on one can cost you a leg or a foot. They cannot be detected because they contain no metal and they cannot be destroyed. Those areas have been out-of-bounds for a decade and will probably remain so for several decades to come.

It would be strange if there were no fences, no barbed-wire, no warning signs. You can climb over if you like. No one will stop you, although they may shout at you not to be so stupid. You have been warned by people who care and by people who knew that your instincts would be to run over the beautiful inviting fields and meadows.

The out-of-bounds areas laid down for us are not some great negative moralistic statement, but warning signs: 'Enter here at your peril, it could cost you.' It will cost you. It may cost you emotionally, physically, psychologically, and will certainly cost you spiritually. When we flout what God has given us as guidelines for life, whether by being selfish, dishonest, gossiping, being unkind, or by being unfaithful or uncontrolled in our sexual lives, there are spiritual consequences. It creates tension in our walk or communion with him. It creates a barrier that can only be removed by confessing to God that we have been wrong and have disobeyed. This is the only route to forgiveness, cleansing, wholeness and inner healing.[582]

In conclusion

In conclusion, then, my own view based on a thorough reading of the Bible, together with the historic teachings of the church, is that AIDS is not an expression of the wrath or judgement of God, but is a part of the world of cause and effect in which we live. When it comes to the practicalities of healthy living, the Bible confirms what common sense tells us: that we are not designed for multiple sexual encounters and there is another way to live. However, all with AIDS need our unconditional care. Such basic Christian principles are timeless and cultureless, transcending all people groups.

A Christian response to AIDS

We need a vision to meet the challenge: demonstrating the love of God and teaching people how to live healthy lives. Part of this will be seeking to challenge and fight oppression, stigmatisation and prejudice wherever we find them, and also challenging our society to reconsider its values. The church in every age is called to be salt and light transforming the whole of society by its witness and work, not just the lives of believers.

We need to recognise that as the church we have also contributed to the AIDS situation today by failing in previous decades to give a clear lead, to challenge behaviour, to model an alternative lifestyle and to proclaim the gospel. Many of those finding faith today are finding faith when the HIV damage has already been done.

So having considered some of the questions about sexuality and moral codes, we need to look at one other big issue before we look in detail at how we can respond practically. First, then, the issue of death. It's an issue I face as a terminal care doctor every week of my life.

Death and dying are no strangers to me in cancer work, yet walking onto an AIDS ward for the first time was quite a shock. This was an acute hospital ward of mainly young men, many of whom would be going home. What kind of care people ill with AIDS receive will depend to a large extent on whether the rest of us have sorted out our own death and mortality, or whether we are going to pretend death doesn't exist. Medicine is not known for its honesty—least of all over life and death issues—and the church is also struggling. Why?

9

Some Life and Death Issues

Just one person

I will never forget the first person I met with AIDS: a young student desperately ill in a side-room of a busy hospital ward. He was anxious, sweaty and panting for breath. His hands gripped the sides of the bed with fear. His thin face was covered with an oxygen mask, his chest was covered in wires and tubing. He was alone and about to die.

From that moment on I found I was involved. Here was a human being, made in God's image and in great need. How could I respond other than to care and help, laying aside any personal feelings I might have had about lifestyles, and the means by which he had become infected?

Dying without family, friends or dignity

I asked about his family and his medication. I was told his parents lived some distance away, knew nothing and thought he was fit and well at university. He did not want them to be contacted because he feared a terrible reaction when they found out what was wrong. He had hidden his illness from them completely.

I was told the simple medication I suggested could not be given because there was a chance he might pull through.[583] In my view the team would be phoning his mum or dad just a few hours from then, to inform them of the death and of the

233

diagnosis. By the time they arrived his body would be in the mortuary, sealed in an opaque body bag following an agonising death. What kind of care was that?[584]

I came off the ward feeling angry, upset, frustrated at the lack of response to suggested medication changes, and realising that life would never be quite the same again. I later found out that almost three-quarters of those with AIDS in the UK lived within ten miles of my home and place of work. I quickly discovered that many others were dying badly, in pain, alone, afraid, separated from those they loved, and often trapped in a hospital ward because no one could care for them at home. At the time, many services available for other illnesses would not get involved. There was a massive gap.

In the prime of their lives

The most shocking thing of all was that unlike a cancer ward where people tended to be retirement age or older, here was an entire ward of young people in the prime of their lives, every one of whom was going to die from a totally preventable rapidly spreading infection. As a care-of-the-dying specialist I could not turn away, whatever the reasons for the illness, or the lifestyles of those who were ill.

I had had mixed feelings about even visiting the ward. Some of my colleagues had refused to get involved and I had felt less than keen. After all, so they told me, AIDS was basically a sex disease of gay men. Was this really an illness I wanted to become heavily involved in?

Correct but horribly wrong

My Christian background told me that most of those infected were ill because they had rejected God's ways.[585] It was easy to feel detached or even critical. It was also easy to react when confronted by a whole ward of young gay men, many of whom were openly expressing physical affection and intimacy.

As we have seen, so often as Christians we do nothing or find ourselves rushing to open our Bibles, to declare to ourselves and to others that something is wrong. Yet in our sudden reaction we can lose sight of God's mercy, love and forgiveness.

Just one more statistic?

I went back to the ward a few days later to find the young man had died the day before. They had taken my advice. They found as I predicted that medication to relax and help remove fear and feelings of breathlessness had improved his condition. The level of oxygen in his blood went up, not down. Far from killing him, the medication had allowed the inevitable to take place with comfort, dignity and peace. He saw his family before he died.

As a result of this experience I began with others to set up hospice-style home care teams for people with AIDS. Many with AIDS reacted, telling me that the emphasis should be on 'living with AIDS', not on dying. My reply was that such an approach was fine so long as you were well, but many were dying badly. Doctors also reacted, telling me there was no 'terminal phase', that AIDS was totally unlike cancer, and that the emphasis should be on active treatment. A part of these two reactions was undoubtedly fear of death or death denial, since those dying so obviously needed help, and there is often a stage of chronic illness and gradual deterioration when palliative care is needed.

Death denial

Since 1945, those in industrial nations have been living in an escapist, death-denying society. Before then the two main killers of young people were war and pneumonia. Now Europe has been at peace for over a generation (apart from civil wars), memories of Vietnam are fading, and we have penicillin and other antibiotics. These days most people assume they will live to a ripe old age. Any discussion of sickness or death is considered morbid. And now comes AIDS.

As part of a lecture on attitudes to dying I needed a photograph of a coffin. I found the mortuary attendant and an undertaker inside the hospital gates preparing to take a body outside. I asked to take a photograph of the coffin—a fibreglass box for transport to the undertakers—and they got very aggressive. They said I was sick and it was against the rules. Even though I was a doctor and the photograph was for teaching professional carers they refused. In fact I took it on the pavement outside as they were loading it into a white unmarked Ford transit van.[586] I still use the slide today.

Why the fuss? The person was unidentifiable. What is so peculiar about dying? It is just as much a part of the cycle of life as birth. The reason is that we are afraid of death. Death is the terrible unknown which robs and destroys. This fear spills over into panic, fear of illness, operations, flying, or many other things. As we will see later in this chapter, this has a profound effect on doctors and what they do.

So where are all the people who know where they are going, who have no fear of death?

In countries like the UK, you might have expected to find them in the church, but the church tends to absorb the culture of its country. The church in the West is full of the same death-denying mentality. This can lead to a watered-down gospel promising good things now (peace, security, happiness, prosperity) because all the future rewards (heaven, eternal joy and peace with God) have lost their meaning. People who are always talking about heaven can be regarded as needing a psychiatrist—and yet that is the hope that drove the earliest Christians towards their goal. The prize St Paul was absolutely determined to win was God's call to the life above in Christ Jesus.[587] He was perfectly content to continue this life as long as God wanted because to 'live is Christ' but 'to die is gain'.[588] So what has gone wrong? If even Christians are afraid, what hope is there of dealing with the fears in the rest of our society?

The church's reaction to death

Look at the reactions of many churches to someone in their congregation who has just been told he will be dead by Christmas. The younger the congregation, the more extreme the reaction, which is why many of the rapidly growing churches are in difficulties over this whole area.

Horror

The person or his family or the church recoils with horror at the prospect of death. Having carefully put aside all thoughts about getting old, the body wearing out, and having ignored the absolute inevitability of death, the news comes as an inexplicable, unexpected disaster. The deaths of friends, colleagues and relatives at similar ages and stages have always been written off with the philosophy of 'it will never happen to me'. The shock now produces devastation.

Frantic search for cure

Every avenue is pursued and every door pushed. Second opinions are asked for. Ever more mutilating procedures are discussed. The treating doctors often drive this madness along themselves, as a part of their own feelings of inadequacy and failure. 'Cure at all costs.'

Desperate prayers

Fear of death is perhaps what lies behind some of the tremendous drive towards supernatural healing in the church. Books on healing are bestsellers.[589] Healing conferences are packed. Healing meetings have been standing-room only unless you arrive very early.

Within a congregation there is a drive to desperate prayers—and maybe fasting. Not the balanced prayers of faith, but the desperate prayers of fear. Gripping, overwhelming, paralysing fear of a terrible disaster. I have seen people reacting out of fear and their own emotional problems. The person they are so strenuously praying for may be totally at peace about 'going home' but others are utterly opposed to allowing events to take their natural course.

Please do not misunderstand this. I believe God heals supernaturally. Major healings of conditions doctors are unable to cure may happen every day and I say this as a doctor. I regularly pray for people to be healed and sometimes things happen. This recent growing experience of God's healing power has gone hand in hand with a renewed emphasis on the Holy Spirit who had become a mere nebulous, ethereal 'thing' in the life and teaching of the church. The Holy Spirit is described by Jesus as the agent of his power. I am sure we are going to see far more evidence of that power over the next few years in countries like the UK, where the rationalistic mindset seems to mean supernatural intervention is more unusual, compared to many developing countries. God has given gifts and resources to the church and expects them to be used.

Miraculous healing

People often ask me if I know of any cases of miraculous healing of those with AIDS. The answer is that a number of reports are circulating, many from developing countries, but none yet that I know of relating to people in the UK, or of cases I have been able to verify.[590]

If we believe God made the universe in an outpouring of almighty cosmic power, then it follows that the same God must have power and authority over every aspect of what he has made. He can boil a kettle of water at his command, turn water into wine, turn your home into rubble, move a huge tree twenty feet, quieten a storm, create a second moon to go round the earth, or remove a virus from someone's body.

God's kingdom now yet still to come

Scripture teaches us that God in his infinite wisdom and mercy has chosen to constrain much of his own power at this stage in the earth's history until the second coming of Jesus.[591] In the meantime we have been given a foretaste of the coming kingdom.

There is a sense in which the kingdom of God is already here.[592] We are encouraged to pray. When we pray according to God's will, we are told that God hears us and desires to act in response.[593]

The truth is that in all things God is sovereign. Who is healed and why remains a mystery. Far fewer people are healed at the moment than think they have been healed. Unless we get our fears of death sorted out we will never have a true perspective on healing.

John Wimber, well known for his work in Christian healing, before praying for a dying person will always ask: 'Is this their appointed time to die?' Wimber has no fear of death and does not necessarily see death as failure.

Confusion

Let's be honest. Usually the person is not healed. Unless you are some especially gifted person, your success rate is low with people who are terminally ill. This often leads to confusion—especially if people have been convinced that healing will take place or has occurred.

There is a lot of unreality in the church over this which is the result of fears of death and teaching by some that God wants to heal all who are sick. Unless there is honesty, openness and integrity, the healing ministry will be brought into disrepute. If you have been healed, then just as Jesus told the lepers to get their cure certified by the priests (medical experts at the time), get it checked out. Why are you so afraid of an X-ray? If God is God and he has healed you, the X-ray of your arthritis-ridden hips will be normal. If you have been healed of high blood pressure, it will be normal and remain so when (under medical supervision) the drugs are stopped.

Some conditions flare up and die down, so it is hard for a doctor to certify a cure until a long time has gone by without any further episodes.

Examples are asthma, ear infections, sinusitis, epilepsy, arthritis and AIDS. Because of the so-called placebo effect (see p 77) many symptoms such as pain may disappear for minutes, hours or weeks simply as a result of suggestion. Yet the disease may remain.

Questioning

The person or family may be angry: 'Why hasn't God healed me if he healed someone else in our church? Why me?' This can try the faith of the ill person, their family and their friends.

Isolation

All too often separation occurs between those who have faith that healing has already occurred or is about to be completed, and those who are being faced with the daily reality of subtle changes in health, growing weakness, steady loss of weight, depressing blood tests, increasing pain, or shortness of breath. One group can be praying and fasting while the other is also praying but is tied up with the important process of preparing for death. This is a tragedy, especially if the latter group is tiny or non-existent apart from the ill person. If both groups are substantial, the result can be a split congregation.

Dying people tend to be marginalised anyway. We kid ourselves that we are caring but we are in fact rejecting. This has always been so of cancer—and has been part of the reason for hospices—and is especially so of AIDS. Apart from all the terrible fears and fantasies about touching a person who is

dying with cancer (many deep down fear they can catch
cancer even though they know this is irrational), there are all
the intense fears of catching a plague related to AIDS.

When you don't know what to say, the result may be either
ludicrous conversation or oppressive awkward silence.
Because both are uncomfortable, many people shy away
from visiting someone who is near death or has been bereaved.
If they do visit, the conversation is stilted and often
meaningless to the ill person who finds entertaining visitors
exhausting. Visiting times can become nightmares: the most
vulnerable part of the day when literally anyone can burst onto
the ward into your bedside chair and be unmovable for an
hour—unless a large number of others arrive.[594] For further
discussion of grief and loss, see Chapter 10.

So what is the answer to it all? The answer I believe lies in
understanding the mystery of life and of death. Because nearly
all my medical work is to do with those who are dying, dead or
bereaved, I am continually confronted by this issue.

'He had just left his body behind'

The first dead person I ever saw as a medical student was a
huge, bloated, blue-faced man who had been pounded and
punctured during a cardiac arrest. Doctors had jumped on his
chest and jabbed him with needles. He came around, groaned,
vomited and died. They shocked him again, pounded him
some more, sucked out the vomit and eventually gave up. I
waited and watched. Everyone drifted away. The curtains
were abruptly closed off. Who was he? Who were his family?
What about his wife?

I remember holding his hand and praying for him silently as
he lay there, his brain gradually dying. A junior doctor came
in armed with huge needles and began practising entering a
vein in the neck. I asked him to stop, but he refused. He
carried on until he got bored and wandered out. That doctor
was in charge of the patient, but couldn't be bothered to find

out if his wife was waiting outside. His whole attitude was cynical, as though the man was merely an object, a piece of meat.[595]

I was angry and upset. How could people who had been trained to care react like this? I vowed no one I was with would ever die in such indignity.

As a Christian I believe I understood something the doctor had completely missed: a profound mystery had just taken place and I had been privileged to be present when it happened. Here was a man, a person, an individual with personality and energy, who in a moment had left this world bounded by space and time. While I watched he had just left his body behind.

Going into the dissecting room for the first time as a medical student is a strange experience. Here are people laid out on slabs; people of all shapes and sizes, distorted by long lying in formalin. Hard skin and fixed muscles. Empty shells: no one there, all long since departed. This is a mystery, the key to understanding life itself and our Creator.

That is why I count it such a privilege to look after people who are nearing the end of their lives. It is a spiritual event. Some would say that the nearest an atheist gets to a religious experience is his own death, and approaching death heightens spiritual awareness in every way.

That is why deathbed conversion is so common. As we saw in an earlier chapter, Jesus welcomed the dying thief into his kingdom.[596] It seems strange that a patient who becomes a Christian in the last week of life should be loved by God in the same way as a faithful believer who has served God for decades. Jesus said that the first shall be last and the last shall be first.[597] Those who care need to look out for clues to where the person is: a newly-opened Gideon's Bible on the bedside locker, a crucifix which appears one day above the bed, a rosary in the patient's hand. These are all ways in which people tell us that things are changing inside. Sometimes conversion takes place without a word being said. A man I admitted to St Joseph's Hospice announced he was an atheist. Two weeks later he asked to see a priest. The man had undergone a radical turn-around as he approached the end.[598]

Without faith, death is the ultimate enemy; death is the robber and the destroyer. With faith in Christ, death is merely a doorway to eternity. Faith confronts us with an issue: will I enjoy eternity when I get there? Will eternity with God be heaven—or will I find eternity an unpleasant hell?

Because I have found forgiveness, inner peace and reconciliation with God through turning to Jesus, I am looking forward to dying. While I am alive I am delighted to be allowed time here to spend with my family, building up the church, serving the community, worshipping and praising God—which is one of the most enjoyable things in my life— and telling people the good news, extending God's kingdom. However, I am just a visitor, passing through. There is nothing here which compares to what is to come. The next life is the true reality—because it is unchangeable. The earth we live on, the solar system, galaxies, space, the whole cosmos as we know it today has a very limited existence. You and I can outlive it all.

When we begin to find God's perspective on this time-space world, then death truly loses its sting. AIDS has lost its power. As doctors, the death of a patient is no longer failure but the natural transition from one existence to another. Death is not taboo any longer. We can talk about it and face up to our own mortality.

When we are with a patient who asks us if he is going to die, he can sense that we are at peace and not afraid. We can stay with him and not run away. We don't avoid spending time but are able to share experiences with him. We will not abandon him because hope of cure has abandoned us.

As a student I spent a four-week residential elective at St Christopher's Hospice. Someone said that you didn't have to have a faith to work there, but those who had no faith didn't tend to last very long.

If you are a Christian I believe you have the answer. For you the mystery is understood. You know the meaning of life and the meaning of death. You understand what is happening when someone is dying. You can give meaning and hope to a person who is reaching out to God. Because Christ himself lives within you, you bring Christ to each person you meet. Every time you speak, smile, or take someone's hand, that person comes into touch with some aspect of Christ himself.

In summary we have seen how AIDS is sweeping across the globe, leaving a terrible trail of human destruction, why the only solution in the foreseeable future is a radical change of values and human behaviour, and how failure to deal with fundamental issues like death and dying now compounds the problem of providing good care. AIDS makes us think through again our views on sexuality and life itself. It confronts us at the very root of our being and at the end of the day leaves us with choices about how we respond, not just to AIDS and those who are dying from it, but also to the ultimate issue: What is the meaning of life? What is the meaning of *my* life? Am I really just a collection of molecules, or is there another dimension?

There is another question: What is the church going to do about AIDS? What Christian response can be made and how do we make a start?

IO

When Church Members Need Help

Having looked at many of the issues raised by AIDS I now want to ask some practical questions of church leaders and members of congregations. What are you going to do the first time someone with AIDS walks into the vestry or church office? For many, despite reading this book and listening to people speak, their first direct experience of AIDS is still going to come as a shock. How are you going to care for people with HIV in your church, especially when people in churches may still be worried about things like the communion cup? How are you going to look after a church member dying at home?

Exploding myths

Priority number one must be to get educated. Church leaders need to be up to date and well informed. Books, conferences and visiting speakers are all ways to achieve this. Even a ten-minute presentation as part of a Sunday service can be long enough to bring home the impact of AIDS, if done by someone with personal experience of the illness, possibly from an organisation like ACET, working in the field as a Christian agency. Remember that AIDS is a new area and whatever you knew three years ago may be out of date.

Church congregations need clear information about risks, the communion cup and about social contact. They also need clear teaching on some of the ethical issues involved. Teaching needs to be given about God's accepting love, as well as his standards, emphasising the need to care unconditionally, challenging prejudice and judgementalism (see Chapter 8).

Caring for church members

Your chances of being confronted by someone with HIV or AIDS over the next few months or years will of course depend on many factors of which the greatest perhaps is where you live, closely followed by the previous lifestyles of people in the church. However, it is usually a great shock when it happens and can hit churches sooner than they expect. Churches sending workers to developing countries are often immediately faced by the huge challenges of AIDS in the letters and other communications from such places.

Your first involvement may be caring for others in the community rather than for your own members. We tend to think of AIDS as something out there rather than a problem within, yet AIDS is also marching into the church. Any growing church which is seeing people come into faith, with lifestyles changing and lives transformed, is likely to find imported HIV sooner or later.

Infection usually survives conversion

It is sobering to think how many of your congregation have come into faith in the last ten years. If many have done so, then HIV may be nearer than you think. Conversion or a rediscovery of faith can happen gradually or suddenly, but infection always remains, barring God's intervention in a miracle of healing.[599]

AIDS time bomb in the church

As we have seen, someone who joined a church in 1988 may have been unknowingly infected in the early 1980s. The person may still be perfectly fit and well today. In a few years' time the person may be a recognised leader with many responsibilities. One day the person may come to you looking obviously unwell after having been afflicted with various medical problems for some time. Now he's tested positive for HIV.

This scenario has already become reality for a number of churches in the UK and is a very common scenario in other countries, particularly in African nations. The pastoral implications are huge when you have a congregation which has mushroomed from maybe 500 to 5,000 in five years and you realise that up to a fifth of your adult members could be carrying the virus.

AIDS in the church office

It is a huge step for someone to tell you they have HIV or AIDS. In many cases it means revealing intensely personal things about the past; things which have been prayed over and forgotten years ago. This is in addition to the shock of coming to terms with a future death from AIDS. It often seems particularly tragic when someone who has made a fresh start has to pay such a very personal and public price for what happened so long ago.

Such tragedies can tear churches apart, with people asking over and over again why God has not chosen to heal the person after the greater miracle of life-changing conversion.

Can you keep a secret?

Once someone in your church has told you they have HIV or AIDS, a journey has started which will probably have a profound effect on you and the church over many years. Confidentiality is important. As we have seen already, we live in harsh times when it comes to AIDS. Violence, discrimination, verbal abuse and hostility are common reactions in many nations from an intolerant minority; common enough to create an atmosphere of tension and fear if the diagnosis becomes known.

A diagnosis of AIDS or HIV infection is sensitive information which may need to be kept strictly confidential for a long time. You may be able to create a supportive environment in the church. However, churches are by their nature public groups meeting in public places. Anyone can turn up to meetings and new people join. You cannot be certain how one or two on the edge of things might react, especially those who perhaps have not been Christians very long or who have deep personal problems of their own.

People with AIDS may leave your church

I remember talking recently to a mother with a young child. She told me that she had moved 100 miles away from her church after the news that she had HIV gradually spread. She said the church had been caring. She had felt accepted and cared for by the leaders and supported by her home group which met in someone's house during the week.

Unfortunately, once her situation became widely known in the church, she began to notice a change. She felt people were avoiding her. No one wanted to have her child to play any more. No one wanted to share the communion cup with her. She felt isolated, insecure, rejected and afraid. After a few weeks she left. I am pleased to say she is now happily settled elsewhere.

Her story made me think. The same could so easily have happened in my own church. Much of the supposed rejection could have been her own hypersensitivity and insecurity, but it is quite likely that one or two may have made inappropriate comments, or behaved in a hurtful and unkind way.

For these reasons we need to address the issue of who is told before the event, rather than working out a policy an hour after realising someone has HIV. Do all the leaders need to know at this stage? What about their spouses? If one person in the church knows, will others be told—'just for prayer, of course'?

Big leaks can start slowly

News may leak gradually before an explosion occurs. Take the situation of four senior leaders who know, each confiding in one other person over the next six months. Each of the new four also confide in one other, while the four leaders also tell two or three others. The result is that in just twelve months at least fourteen to sixteen people already know. After the second year the number knowing has grown to twenty, and by the third year to twenty-five.

One day a conversation is overheard by someone else who very likely tells another ten in as many days. By the end of the month people at work have found out and are saying they will refuse to co-operate unless the person is laid off. The result could be loss of job, loss of income, public humiliation and a big question mark: Does every other person in the church know?

Now is the time to prepare

We need to prepare before someone turns out to have HIV. Perhaps someone in your church is already infected, but he or she—or you—has yet to find out. Sometimes I am asked to speak to a church because the leaders are now aware of someone with HIV who is becoming unwell. They realise people are going to guess soon and they want help now, so when people find out there will not be any panic. It would have been better to have visited the year before.

It can be hard to know when to widen the network of those who are aware of the situation. The timing and occasion are best determined by the person with HIV. The process becomes easier if one or two new people are told at a time, before involving larger groups. Often the person with HIV feels anxious about possible reactions. As each person is found to be accepting, warm and encouraging, it helps to overcome the big lie which says that people will reject once they know.

This fear of being known is a curse because it robs and destroys friendship. Whenever someone lives under the shadow of discovery, there will always be deep insecurity. It is only as we find people still love us despite our failings that we begin to see and feel what the love of God is like.

Openness can bring release

The more open we can be, the more AIDS becomes normalised as a part of our suffering world, and in turn the easier it is for others to be open in the future. More importantly, the more open we are, the easier it is to organise help.

One rule of thumb is to operate on a need-to-know basis. And as illness develops, the need to know becomes gradually greater for a larger circle of people.

Practical care at home

The needs of those with AIDS are in many ways exactly the same as the needs of those with other kinds of illness. There is always the need for friendship, but often the greatest needs are practical. It is easy for barriers to form and for people to feel a burden, unable to ask for help. On the other hand, wanting to help can make us feel awkward and embarrassed, not knowing what to say or do.

Here is a brief outline of ten practical steps that any church can take to support a church member, most of which also apply in many ways to caring for others in the community. This is not a definitive guide, and it is written particularly with an industrialised country like the UK in mind. Many of the basic principles of care are valid in different cultural and economic situations, but other aspects require adaptation.

Before getting involved in looking after someone at home, you will do well to contact an agency like ACET, or to get hold of some of the other resources listed at the back of this book.

1. Show you still care

Someone with HIV is likely to feel especially vulnerable after telling you the news, or just after knowing someone else has told you. What will the next meeting be like? Will there be a smile, a hug or an awkward turning away? People may say it does not make any difference, but is that really true, or are they just pretending? Surely I am a liability, an embarrassment, a burden on the church? Go out of your way to express appreciation, acceptance, love, care and support in those first critical days.

Learn about the illness so you are well informed and can help others later on who may be struggling with ignorance. There is a list of further resources at the back of this book.

2. Maintain friendship

Try to maintain as much normal life as possible. The person who has HIV will probably want to carry on as usual rather than be dragged down by thinking about the illness all day long. Be sensitive to changing physical needs, moods and feelings about the future. It is perfectly normal for people to swing from optimism to pessimism, from grand plans to the depths of despair, from acceptance of the situation to denial.

This is just part of the process of adjustment to grief and loss. Often we think of grief as an emotion triggered by the death of someone we love. However, grief is a process of adjustment triggered by losses of any kind. As we have seen in earlier chapters, the losses for someone dying with AIDS are numerous and often devastating. Loss of health; loss of memory, sight, physical comfort, sleep, control over one's body; loss of future plans, ambitions, hopes and dreams; loss of friends, family, job, physical attractiveness, energy; loss of independence and freedom; loss of future; loss of life on earth. It is no surprise, then, to find people oscillating between denial, anger, sadness and acceptance, or with mixtures of all four. AIDS can be a heavy burden to carry.

3. Listen to the questions

The Psalms are full of heart cries towards God. Why is this happening to me? What is God doing? This seems so unfair. Questions and statements like these are cries of pain and anguish which need a listening ear rather than a trite reply. The person may just want you to sit and listen while feelings are expressed. There are no simple answers to human suffering, as Job's friends discovered.

Anger can often be directed at others such as members of the family, neighbours, friends, doctors, nurses, volunteers and members of the church. Anger and sadness are closely linked. They can both be a part of the process of grieving for a life that has been unexpectedly shortened. The anger may be directed at you too. It is important not to take such rejection too personally, and to continue to offer friendship.

Sometimes anger can become a test of friendship. You may be on trial yourself. Is your love great enough to keep coming back? In the meantime, while offering continued support, there may be another who is better placed to maintain the closest links.

4. Open your home

Be ready to offer a meal, a sofa, a bed, a place to stay for the weekend, or a place to sit quietly during the day. Often a

change of environment can help not only the person who is
unwell, but also the other carers. Many with AIDS have no
real homes or families. Many have been effectively orphaned
by their condition, or by previous circumstances. Many are
living on their own, or with friends, in situations where dying
at home may be difficult, or impossible. As we open up a
network of homes and relationships, we are offering new
choices to people who may feel they have none.

5. Draw others in

In our desire to preserve confidentiality, to care and to protect,
it is easy for intense relationships to develop, and to reach a
situation where 'lock up' occurs. It is easy as a carer to
convince yourself that no one understands the person better
than you, and that you alone have an 'inside track' on the
situation. You want to be involved in all decisions; to be
present at every discussion. It is easy to have mixed feelings
about others becoming involved. Yet that very intensity can
become more than the relationship can bear when illness
develops.

As the situation unfolds, it is wise to draw others in. As a
church leader myself, I feel it is vitally important that at least
one member of the church leadership is closely involved,
providing pastoral support to the person and to the carers,
spotting signs of pressure or difficulty and helping to find
ways through.

At every stage you will need the backing of the person
concerned to involve others in this. If this is constantly
blocked at every turn, you may have some hard talking to do. I
have seen many situations break down at home, with people
landing up in hospital simply because no one was willing to
think seriously about the future.

6. Seek expert help

At some stage or other you are going to need expert help. It is
all very well providing emotional support as a friend, but

when events unfold you may need extra professional advice and support at home. It may be that there is no local service available.

In the UK you can find out by telephoning the local Town Hall, the Health Authority, the nearest AIDS ward or clinic, the nearest clinic for sexually-transmitted diseases (GUM clinics), or by telephoning the National AIDS Helpline. You can also find out if ACET Home Care is available in your area by telephoning the head office—numbers on pages 415–418. Even if there are no volunteers or team members in your part of the country, you can still benefit from advice from your nearest ACET office. In every part of the UK there should be an NHS doctor available to visit even at nights and weekends, a community nurse, a social worker, an occupational therapist, a physiotherapist and a home help. Sometimes people are scared about confidentiality, preferring to use specialist agencies like ACET combined with hospital support. However, no specialist agency can be a full substitute for the integrated network of community care available in most areas. If the person is unhappy about his family doctor's approach, it is now very easy to register with a different practice.

Community care varies from country to country, but the trend in many places is towards caring for people in the community. Neither the richest nor the poorest nations can afford to keep people with AIDS in hospital when they do not need acute medical care. In almost every country there are now government departments or local government offices which can supply information on general care resources available, and on AIDS specific resources.

As we have seen in Chapter 1, anxiety can produce many of the symptoms of early HIV illness, and as in other areas of medicine it is possible for people to convince themselves and others that they have HIV when there is no evidence of this. Because medical confidentiality is so strict in many nations, it is only possible for health care professionals to obtain confirmation of diagnosis after written permission from the person concerned, and even then it can be difficult. However, such confirmation is important (see p 381).

7. *Be ready for the long haul*

Both those with HIV and those who care for them can be bewildered by rapid changes in the illness. One week there may be such a marked deterioration that they assume the end must be near, while the next week things may be back to their usual state. AIDS is a disease of ups and downs. People can be close to death, yet recover with prompt treatment, and be home again. People with AIDS are living longer in many countries with improved treatment, as we have already seen. Therefore it is wise to plan for a level of support that may need to be sustained for a long time.

People often ask me when the end will come. The answer is that no one knows, although we can often be certain about one thing: death is not here yet. With onset of new symptoms it is natural for everyone to become anxious. I often say to people that although it is true they are going to die of this illness, barring a miracle or a sudden new discovery, it is also true that they are not dying at this moment. We can often look back and see that maybe over the last few days things have actually improved a little.

One of my greatest joys has been seeing people begin to make realistic plans again: a last holiday, a project to complete, a book to write, friends to see, a place to visit. Our aim is to redeem time; to give back dignity, freedom and choice. That is why expert care is so important. When it comes to practical care, nothing is more rewarding to me than something as simple and important as being able to give someone their first good night's sleep in months, so that the following day can be enjoyed.

8. Fear of death can be worse than death itself

Remember that the process of dying can be far more worrying to people than death itself, particularly if the person is sustained by the hope of eternal life. Common worries can include losing control over bowels or bladder, becoming mentally feeble with loss of memory, becoming disabled and confined to a wheelchair, losing hair as a result of chemotherapy for cancers, having to be washed and dressed by another.

Other worries can include the fear of uncontrolled symptoms of pain, breathlessness or other kinds. Finally, there is also the fear of losing control, of others marching in as strength fades, and of the wrong decisions being made.

The way to deal with these fears is to address them, and to try to discover what lies behind them. I remember someone asking me one day whether he would suffocate to death. There was real fear in his eyes as he gripped my arm waiting for the reply. Before answering, it occurred to me to ask why he was asking the question and, even more importantly, why he asked today when I was visiting so regularly.

The answer tumbled out that he had woken in a terrible fright the previous night in the middle of a nightmare. He had seen himself lowered into the ground in a coffin while still alive. Despite his shouts and his hammering on the sides of the box, they had covered him with earth. He had suffocated to death.

We were then able to talk about the dream, and I was also able to promise him first that he would not suffer from feelings of suffocation if he developed a pneumonia, and secondly that death when it did come would be certain. No one would suddenly whisk him away. He could remain in the house for some time. As a result of the conversation he felt at peace and the fear never returned. It is an important principle to find out what lies behind a question before wading in with an insensitive and immediate response.

9. Support the carers too

Sometimes all the attention can naturally fall on the one who is ill, ignoring those giving most of the support. Sometimes partners, family and friends can unexpectedly run out of steam. Things can become too much, juggling job, children, other responsibilities and the needs of someone with AIDS. An effective early warning system is vitally important.

Those doing all the work need to know they too have someone who is special to them, watching out for their own needs, stepping in with practical help, sharing the load, providing a shoulder to cry on, and being a friend in times of trouble. The greatest help is often practical. You could spend an hour a day counselling a carer who is near breaking point when the time would be better spent sitting in the home for a morning or an afternoon so the carer can go out. Perhaps you can take the person who is unwell out for the day, or have the person to stay for a night or two, possibly longer.

Do not wait for people to shout for help, as they will often tell you much too late. Keep in touch regularly, even when things seem to be going very well. Time can fly by. Write a note to yourself in the diary when you are going to telephone next or drop round again.

Be honest about your own needs, to yourself and to others. You are a special person too in God's eyes. He loves you too. Allow yourself to be vulnerable. Let the right people see when you too are feeling the strain and are hurting inside—obviously you need to be careful not to share too widely, nor to dump your own emotional needs on someone who is ill, or on the main carer. Maybe you will encourage someone when they see that you are human too. Be ready to say no, to draw the line, to have recovery time of your own. That is why it is a good idea to involve a few others. You never know just when you will need their support.

10. *Be ready to help around the clock at the end*

You will need to be well-organised if the person wishes to die
at home. It is likely that the last day or two, or even longer,
will be quite harrowing. There may be a need for a continuous
presence in the home, in addition to professionals coming in
and out. If you are in an area served by ACET Home Care or a
similar service, you may find volunteers are available to help.
If not, you may need to identify a few sensible friends who
would be willing to help on a rota basis, and who are
acceptable to the person who is ill. The main need is likely to
be for the sort of help that a caring relative would provide, to
help in various practical ways (see Appendix B).

On the whole, the care approach is the same as would be
taken locally for any illness, whether you are living in
London, Washington, Kampala or Bangkok. The only thing
you need to take extra care about is exposure of skin to body
secretions. Spillages of blood or other secretions should be
wiped up wearing a pair of gloves. The easiest thing to do is
mop up using disposable paper towels, and then to soak the
area for two or three minutes with a freshly-made solution of
one part bleach to nine parts water. The area can then be
cleaned in the normal way (see Chapter 5).

Gloves are not needed at other times. As we have seen,
intact skin is an excellent barrier to HIV. Even if there is some
skin contact with secretions, infection is most unlikely to
occur unless the skin is damaged. It is wise to cover cuts with
a waterproof plaster before going into the home.

Although this may all seem rather daunting, it is most
unlikely that you will be managing on your own. In many
countries you will find community nurses and other health
care workers are also providing support and advice. In other
places, churches have found themselves having to develop
their own community services because there is nothing
available in their area.

When the moment of death comes, those in the home can

feel uncertain as to what to do. There is no need for great activity when someone dies. The normal cultural rituals can be observed, remembering that secretions from the body will still be infectious. There may be one or two who need to be contacted, and would like to be able to say goodbye before the person is taken out of the home.

I want to look now at extending our care from our own church to the wider community. Should we? Can we?

11

Others Need Help Too

Caring for church members is one thing, but what about those with AIDS who are part of the wider community? They may be dying in the most terrible conditions. Are we able to sit back and ignore their plight?

As soon as you talk about social action in some churches you can sense a problem. For some people, social action is associated with a liberal gospel where anything goes so long as you are kind. Some say it is far more important to deal with the root of the problem by preaching the gospel and seeing lives changed. However, the teaching of Jesus makes it clear that both need to go together.[600] Evangelical churches emphasise the need to preach the gospel. However, it could be said that evangelism without love is an obscenity to God, because a gospel message without love is a gross denial of what God is like. Love will always go further than words to meet practical needs. As Christians, we are called to love people as an expression of God's love—not as a means of manipulating them into joining the church. We love because people are worth it, made in the image of God.

The church in the United Kingdom and the United States pioneered many aspects of medical care that we take for granted today. Almost all of the first hospitals and associated caring agencies were started by Christians. Medical care was spread all over the world by a small army of dedicated men and women who often died abroad of the very illnesses they went out to fight. Their living conditions were dire and primitive in Africa, Asia, South America or China.

A missionary tradition

These men and women were driven by an overwhelming compassion for those in other nations, many of whom they felt were often without care and without hope. For them, bringing treatment for leprosy, malaria, tuberculosis or smallpox was bringing the practical love of God. As a result of that work, churches in South America, Africa and Asia are the fastest growing in the world, at a rate enormously faster than the birth rate. These countries are now sending missionaries to Europe, the United Kingdom and the United States.

I cannot find a closer parallel to leprosy a century ago than AIDS today. Now is the time for the church to climb off the fence, to stop taking pot-shots at the tip of the iceberg—the bit they see (erroneously) in the West as consisting entirely of promiscuous homosexual men and drug addicts—and to start considering the whole picture: the millions of men and women dying worldwide, and those dying on our doorstep. God calls us to accept all people and extend his love to them, regardless of whether or not we agree with what they do.

Public involvement

Church leaders and their congregations need to be visibly involved; not just seen to be caring for their own. They need to be quoted in the local press, on local radio, and down on record in the national media as declaring a commitment to get involved. The message is that we care about what is happening and want to make a difference.

Leaders especially need to come forward and to be examples—filmed talking to people with AIDS, holding their hands, receiving communion with them, or giving them a hug. At the end of the day, actions like these are things that really encourage others. Fears are not dispelled by words alone, but by seeing that people are not afraid. If church leaders cannot do this, our efforts to mobilise a congregation will become hollow.

Community support

Is it practical to set up a small community support group to help those outside the 'family' of the church? How could we go about it? What about those who cannot be cared for at home? Could we use a church building to provide some sort of residential care or hospice for those who cannot manage at home?

Experience has shown that these things are possible in a wide variety of community settings, whether in a country like the UK or one like Uganda. The approach may vary greatly according to the local situation, but the overriding principles of compassionate care remain the same.

Everyone cares for their friends

Jesus said that caring for our friends, or members of our own social networks, is something that everybody does: it is *not* a great sign of his kingdom.[601] He said that true love is to care for those who are not members of our own family; people we would not associate with; people we do not like and might not be naturally drawn to. In fact Jesus went even further and told us that we were to love our enemies, those who want to stab us in the back, those who run us down, those who hate us, those who undermine us, those who attack us, those who are against us.[602]

If this is the test of true love, then we can never be content to care just for our own. The test of true love will be our willingness to care for others in our community and for children left behind, without any hidden agenda or additional motive other than that which drove the Good Samaritan.[603]

Jesus wants us to care as the natural response of our nature to the need of those around us. He wants us to care because he

cares and we are channels of that care. As people come into
contact with us, and feel our touch, our love, our compassion,
they are coming into contact with something of Jesus
himself.[604]

As we have seen in a previous chapter, this is a mystery. As
we enter a room we carry his presence into the place. I
remember as a junior doctor, working in a busy hospital, I
came into contact with a great number of staff. Once or twice I
came home and talked to Sheila my wife about a particular
nurse on one of the wards who seemed to radiate something I
had come to recognise in the past.

She had never said anything, neither did she wear some kind
of badge or symbol. I remember after some months, with
slight embarrassment, I asked her if by any chance she was a
Christian. Of course the answer was that she loved the Lord
very much. It showed. She carried the aroma of Christ with
her.[605] You can smell believers as they walk into the room!

So our calling then is not to shut up the love of God in some
kind of Christian ghetto just caring for each other, but to allow
that love to be expressed through caring for others.

Isn't care the responsibility of the government?

Some say that it is the responsibility of the government to
care, not the church. I believe it is the responsibility of both.
One of the primary responsibilities of government is to spread
wealth and resources by collecting taxes and providing
services and benefits, whether in education, health care, road
building or other ways.

The balance between individual, group and government
responsibility is a political question, but one thing is clear. As
Christians we are called to be a nation's conscience,
responding to need ourselves, and also encouraging a
compassionate government response.

Where possible, I believe it is entirely right and proper that
the government contributes to or provides some or all of the

running costs of church-based care and prevention programmes, so long as the running of those programmes
remains within the church and there is not a loss of control.
We need to be careful that Christian initiatives do not become
mere extensions of government or international agencies. That
is why we need such a clear vision about what God is calling
us to do. Without that we will be rapidly swept off course by
someone else's vision, politics or priorities.

The issue is care for people, closely linked to social justice
and basic human rights. If I am healthy, well fed and have a
high standard of living, then the teaching of Jesus is that my
'neighbour' has an expectation perhaps that he or she will not
starve or be deprived of the basic necessities of life. The
church is one vehicle for provision; voluntary agencies and
government departments are others. All can work together to
get the job done.

Partnership between church and funding agencies can
impose useful disciplines. It can help us think through what
we are doing, as well as encourage us to measure our
effectiveness and to plan strategically.

In many developing countries, the government depends on
international aid, often channelled through Christian agencies,
with projects overseen jointly by the donor and national
government. These arrangements are often very successful,
because governments are able to tap into an established
network of Christian medical missions that have been
providing first-class care and prevention programmes in the
country for decades.

The test of unconditional love

The test of unconditional love is twofold when it comes to
AIDS. First, does it matter to you how someone came to be
infected, or why someone's parents have died? Will that
knowledge alter the way you see that person or the way that
person is treated? Many people feel it is easier to care for an

orphan or a dying baby than for an adult who is ill. That is certainly the situation in Romania. Everyone wants to help AIDS babies, and the care of adults or prevention can almost be ignored. But is that the way of Jesus?

I remember doing some research into the needs of men, women and children with AIDS in the UK and how those needs were changing. It was a very moving experience to go through ACET's home care records and be reminded of so many we had cared for who had died—a number of whom I had visited at home or spoken to.

I wanted to discover if the needs people had, such as the need for rehousing, symptom control, nursing care and other things, were related in any way to the age of the person, the main medical problems and the route of infection. If so, it could help us plan better care for others in the future.

When I tried to collect the information, I found that many of the records were incomplete. There was often no indication of how the person had become infected. In many cases the route was known, but the nurses had hesitated to record it. The reason was that part of our whole approach to care is that the route by which someone became infected is irrelevant unless the person wants to tell us. Our love is unconditional because it is the same expressed to all, regardless of how they have come to be ill.

Is our love always the same?

The second practical test of unconditional love is perhaps even more important and is this: two people are dying with AIDS, and one has indicated he or she would like to become a Christian. Does this person get better care than the other? If so, then our care has become conditional. This is a real challenge to us and should cause us to consider how we think and respond to a variety of situations in the church.

Some may react here by pointing out that there is a sense in which God's love is full of conditions—this is the basis of

God's judgement. Perhaps Chapter 8 needs reading again to see the whole thing in balance.

Community care or caring for our own?

What we are talking about here is a church or Christian organisation which feels a particular call to provide care for those who are ill with AIDS as part of the general call to care for others. If the care has become conditional in subtle ways on whether the person shows signs of wanting to join our church, then the programme needs redefining. It is not really community care at all, but just an extension of church life. That may be fine to you, but other agencies may be extremely reluctant to ask you to help, unless it is to care for those who already have a strong Christian faith.

Building on what we have

In many different countries, members of churches or Christian organisations have begun to set up AIDS care initiatives. Some have been very successful in providing practical, emotional or spiritual support. Others have found it more difficult. In the UK, many churches have linked together to provide care at home through ACET.

The advantage of home care is that you do not need a building, or even a formal office, in order to begin. You can start by resourcing the work from within the existing structures and facilities of the church. Indeed, it is possible to provide very effective AIDS care through general care programmes, so long as people are adequately trained, and those with AIDS locally are willing to receive help from a non-specialist agency. Examples might include a cancer hospice opening its doors to those with AIDS, or a bereavement support group or a project caring for families in need or for orphans.

As we have seen, in most countries of the world the church has a huge established caring network, and a long track record of delivering high-quality care. There may be other care programmes running already which can be extended or adapted to help those with AIDS.

There are no blueprints for success. You will need expert advice if you want to go ahead, and will need to adapt lessons others have learned to your own situation. (See Appendices B and C for an outline of some principles which have been found useful in the UK.)

Care at home is fine as far as it goes, but what do you do when care at home is impossible? What about hospices?

Caring in a hospice

Even if we set up a community programme, there may be people we are caring for who cannot manage at home. For a variety of reasons they may need to be cared for in a hospital or a hospice. Many churches have access to buildings, or may consider buying one. How can we tell if this is a sensible way forward, and how can we make sure the project will be successful?

Why hospices are setting the pace

Over the years, I have talked to a number of people who were set on starting some kind of hospice or in-patient unit for those with AIDS, whether in a country like Uganda or in the UK. What exactly is a hospice? The hospice movement has grown enormously over the last twenty-five years, having had its origins in the UK earlier this century.

It is aimed at providing a place where those with terminal illnesses can find peace and security in a specialist environment with a particular expertise in symptom control. Hospices are usually separate from hospitals, are often independently funded, and seek to provide emotional and spiritual support, as well as practical care.

The hospice philosophy spread fast from the 1970s onwards in the UK at first and then elsewhere because traditional medicine seemed obsessed with cure and had little time for the incurable. At the same time, those with symptoms such as pain were often very badly treated. Hi-tech medicine has sometimes lost touch with the needs of people. Thus the drive to build these hospices often came from relatives of loved ones who had died badly.

When AIDS became more and more evident, most of those who were ill in many countries were treated at first by specialists in either sexually-transmitted diseases or chest problems, neither of whom had much experience of looking after the dying.

The aim is to help people die well by caring for them as whole people, physically, emotionally, socially and spiritually. The unit of care is not just the person who is dying, but also the family, or the group of people around that person.

Cure at all costs?

Eventually, many of those with AIDS themselves began to want to opt out of an aggressive fight to the death, robbing them so often of time and dignity. It was also realised that the reason people with AIDS often ended up in hospital was because the carers at home had become exhausted. Therefore, there was also a growing need for short-term respite care in an environment more friendly and relaxed than a busy hospital ward.

As we have seen, improving treatments have meant people with AIDS have been surviving longer, but with more chronic disabilities such as memory loss, partial blindness or loss of mobility, so the need for hospices is growing.

Mildmay Mission Hospital: a model for many

The Mildmay Mission Hospital in the East End of London was set up in 1892, but closed in the early 1980s. After much prayer and a lot of fund-raising it opened again, becoming Europe's first AIDS hospice at a time when very few cancer hospices would accept those with AIDS. Although some other hospices in the UK do now take small numbers of those with AIDS, the need has grown. The London Lighthouse opened soon after, while the Mildmay has since opened two more wards. The Mildmay has a long history of overseas links, continued today through training courses in the UK and in Africa, particularly aimed at equipping doctors and nurses to care for those with AIDS in developing countries.

Some people cannot die at home for various reasons, even if that is their wish. This may be because they live on their own and they do not live in an area served by home-care teams. It may be that they live in a part of the world where organised care is almost non-existent for any illness, let alone AIDS. It may be that they have become so disabled and forgetful that others at home are unwilling or unable to look after them. It may be that particular medical problems have emerged which are very difficult to manage at home. Or it may be that there are strong cultural objections in the neighbourhood to looking after someone with AIDS. For example, in certain areas of Africa, the disease may be thought to be a result of a curse from a witch doctor.

Others do not wish to die at home. Perhaps they feel safer in a hospice. Perhaps they do not want others in the household to have memories of them dying at home. Perhaps they feel they do not want the pressure of placing a burden on people they do not feel particularly close to—an ex-partner, for example, who is still sharing the same accommodation.

The provision of hospice care can be a wonderful thing, and the Mildmay is a great example of Christian witness in such provision—indeed the hospice movement has been largely shaped by the work of many Christian pioneers in the field. Therefore hospice provision is often the first thought of many groups. But often also the last project to get started. This is because providing a hospice is a major undertaking and many groups quite wisely have second thoughts once they have taken expert advice.

One example of the pitfalls awaiting hospice builders is a miscalculation of real need. Just as there is a need to research the need for home care, there is an even greater need to research the need for hospice beds. I remember talking to a missionary organisation recently, just in time to stop them going ahead spending thousands of pounds on building an AIDS hospice in Romania. The town they had chosen had almost no HIV infection at all and would not have been able to fill the hospice for ten to twenty years. Meanwhile, other cities elsewhere were overwhelmed by sick and dying children.

There is a real need for expert advice. For example, you may have access to a property, but after all the costs of conversion you may still not have the building which is practical. It may be better to build something from scratch.

Forming a ten-year vision

You will need a steering group or committee prepared to see the vision through and sustain it. You need long-range plans and vision—for at least ten years. It may take you three of those years to get from agreeing the plan to being able to welcome your first patient.

It is all too easy to go bankrupt with a beautiful building. Many cancer hospices in the UK have failed to open on the day the building finished, or have only partially opened, because all the fund-raising effort went into the building and not enough thought was given to running costs. Most people like to see something for their money, so they give to capital projects and are less happy to support staff salaries.

It is easy to sit back expecting the government automatically to pick up the bill for running your project, but it may turn round and ask why it should when it was not consulted in the first place and perhaps feels that people can be cared for adequately elsewhere. (See Appendix A—size of need.)

Other approaches can be considered. For example, there may be a need for something more like a halfway house between what you would expect in a hospice and what could be provided at home. In Dundee, Scotland, ACET has been providing care at home for some years. But what do you do for people who have no home? ACET has now set up two small housing units for the homeless, into which we can bring home care.

Home care and hospices, however, still leave a massive gap for up to 10 million children left behind by the year 2000 (WHO).

AIDS orphans—how have churches responded?

Whenever we care for young people who are dying, we find children swept up in the process. Churches have responded in many creative ways, depending on the local situation. Many adults ACET cares for in the UK have young children. Sometimes the youngest children have been infected at or shortly after birth. As we have seen, the risk may vary from around 15–30%. The uninfected children are going to lose one or both parents. What are we going to do? In the US there were already 14,500 uninfected children by 1991 whose mothers had died, with a further 4,500 alive with HIV.[606] In Uganda alone there may already be 50,000 children who have lost one or both parents from AIDS.

I remember visiting a Ugandan village where many adults had died. At first there were just a few orphans, but numbers had grown rapidly. In Africa, a child who has lost even one parent is likely to be in big trouble, because the family may already have been living at a subsistence level. To lose both parents is usually a disaster, especially if the family is large with maybe six or more dependants.

There were 400 orphans in the village, so what should be done? Many grandparents were spending their time trying to help bring the children up. The children had no source of income, no one to pay their modest school fees, so they had dropped out of school. Nearby was a village that had been closed by the government. The generation of parents had been wiped out. Only grandparents and children were left, and the village could not survive.

It is easy to march in and build orphanages as residential institutions providing love, education and care, but this may not be the best answer. There may be a simpler approach. Attending to one area of need may release the community to provide the rest.

If school fees can be found, the problem can be greatly eased. It is a tragedy that the local schools, which may offer an excellent education, may be half-empty because AIDS orphans are dropping out. It is a mistake then to educate them separately as this reinforces the separation and stigma. It can also be a mistake to house them separately. Isolation from village community life may make integration more difficult later on as adults. They may have difficulty finding husbands or wives as they do not belong. Institutions can never provide the same experience of home as a family.

Sponsorship in families

For these reasons, an effective way to help in a country like Uganda can be to provide school fees. Often this is all that is needed. The children are then back in class with their friends. They are supervised and may even be fed in the middle of the day. Sleeping accommodation at home is often far less of a problem and in some countries in Africa the food supply may be adequate and inexpensive. Families usually grow most of their own.

Sponsorship in homes means that hundreds of orphans can be cared for individually in as normal an environment as possible. It is low cost with few extra staff needed. The staff role becomes that of a community visitor, advising, monitoring, supporting and encouraging. Sponsorship schemes are funded by a number of different relief and development agencies, such as TEAR Fund, in partnership with local churches and national agencies (see Appendix G).

Orphanages may be needed

Although we have seen that community placements can offer good provision at low cost in some countries, it may not always be possible. If the network of extended families and village resources is totally overwhelmed, then institutional help may be the only alternative. The principles of running such places are the same as for any other orphanage project. It is good not to separate those who are orphans because of AIDS from those orphaned by other events such as war, tuberculosis, accidents or malaria.

The scale of the problem defies comprehension. In many areas at the moment, nine- or ten-year-old children are acting as Mum and Dad to younger brothers and sisters, often after nursing their own parents until they died. The children have to collect firewood and water, cook their own food—and grow it—supervise young ones and repair their homes. They have nothing.

Just a very little help can make all the difference. One project in Eastern Uganda has been helping children rebuild their huts, so at least they have somewhere safe and dry to sleep at night.[607] The workers also give out food and other essential items.

Income-generation projects

There are often situations in developing countries where a small amount of capital and training can equip people to become self-sufficient. While one example may be orphans who are growing up and need to provide for themselves, another important example can be women who have no means of survival, shelter or subsistence except through sex. In some countries the women may be seen as prostitutes; in others they may be seen as bar girls, or 'kept women'.

In Uganda there are thousands of women without family support or jobs. Many survive through the gifts of a number of men who stay with them regularly when in town. AIDS campaigns are useless to those who will starve without providing sex. A small cottage industry can enable a number of women to find a new life, with new freedom, dignity and control over their own lives—lives free from the constant fear of exposure to HIV. For example, in one area a group of women were given pigs and other livestock to breed and sell, as well as to feed themselves and their families. These issues are also important in countries like Thailand. One project has set up a needlework industry for former prostitutes (see p 329).

As in every area of this terrible epidemic, it is easy to feel totally overwhelmed. Where do you start? How do you begin to tackle such a vast, global, growing problem? The answer is to start somewhere. As has often been said, you cannot change the whole world, but you can change someone's world somewhere.

If as a result of your help an adult with AIDS is able to die at home, free of pain and at peace; if a family recently orphaned are taken into a home and cared for together until they grow up; if as a result of an AIDS lesson five young people are still alive in ten years' time who would otherwise have died of AIDS, then you have indeed made a big difference. Just think what 100, 1,000 or 10,000 people could do together. Even more so, the whole church across your country, across the continent, across the world.

Jesus did not heal all the sickness in the world. He came and touched the lives of those around him, giving hope and purpose to a suffering world. As we ask God to show us who our neighbour is, his answer could involve us in the lives of those in another continent, or in the lives of those who live next door.

Some are called to give care in practical ways. Others are neither called nor gifted to set up or be involved in projects, build hospices or start agencies. However, there are so many other ways to be supportive: prayer, financial help, encouragement—to name but a few.

Whenever we begin caring for those with AIDS, we are faced with a terrible thought. Here are a growing number of people dying of a very unpleasant and incurable disease, yet every day many more are becoming infected, becoming ill, dying or becoming orphans. If we cannot cure it and the virus is spreading so fast, then we must urgently do all we can to prevent further tragedy and destruction.

We need to decide what to tell our children, since they are in the frontline of danger, and we need to tell them in a way that is most likely to help them see the risks and change their behaviour. School is an ideal place to start, but what do we tell the children?

12

Saving Lives

Why prevention is often swamped by care

What do you do if you are walking along the road one day and two cars spin off the road in quick succession as they reach a dangerous bend? Do you run to help the victims? Do you run up the road to yell a warning to traffic? Do you go into a house and phone for an ambulance and the police?

Most of us respond to the immediate, which is why in many countries care for those with AIDS is eating up most of the AIDS budget. Prevention is usually an afterthought in spending terms, which is madness considering that infection is lethal and incurable, yet almost totally preventable. Infection is also very expensive.

In the UK, for example, out of a total AIDS budget of over £200 million, less than 10% is spent on prevention among 53 million people, while 90% is spent on services for a few thousand who are unwell. Even more disturbing is that the UK spends more on this tiny number than the World Health Organisation spends on the entire Global AIDS Programme,[608] most of which is for prevention.

Economics of prevention

Effective prevention campaigns could halve new HIV infections, according to the World Health Organisation.[609] A

276

global programme in all developing countries would cost $1.5 to $2.9 billion a year—less than the cost of the Desert Storm campaign in the Gulf War, and less than the cost of a can of Coke for each person in the world. The saving in direct and indirect costs by the year 2000 could be as great as $90 billion.[610]

Prevention saves huge care costs

The economics in favour of prevention are staggering, yet little action is taken. Every person who develops AIDS costs the UK government between £25,000 and £40,000 from diagnosis to death. Each life saved through education saves the same amount. In the US, the equivalent costs per person are $66,000 to $100,000.

Worldwide the care of those with AIDS is already costing £5 billion each year. The indirect costs of lost productivity, lost markets and the training of new workers are said to be up to £50 billion annually. By the year 2000, in Thailand alone the cumulative total cost of AIDS could reach £9 billion.[611]

How much does it cost to save a life? The figure is harder to come by, but let us argue from common-sense principles. Let us suppose that a schools worker with experience of working in home care spends a whole year taking classes in schools and talking to young people. The person sees up to 8,000 pupils in the year, as well as talking to a large number of staff, parents and others.

Let us suppose that only one individual changes behaviour so that infection is avoided. The educator would still have saved the government between £10,000 and £25,000 even after deducting salary costs.

Health education is free

How many lives do you think a good educator could save? Ten? Twenty? Thirty? Fifty? If the educator saves just ten lives per year, the government saves up to £250,000 each year; if twenty, then £500,000. What a big earner! How many people in sales and marketing do you know who earn their employers £250–500,000 in extra profits each year?

High impact AIDS prevention is quite simply one of the most cost-effective things a government can possibly spend money on. The reason for this extraordinary fact in industrialised nations is that AIDS is such a difficult and expensive illness to treat. The drugs used are some of the most complex and costly ever produced. One of the drugs, AZT, is so expensive that a doctor in Uganda would have to save every penny he earned for ten years to pay for one year's treatment of just one person.[612]

The cost of AIDS

The cost of treating one person with AIDS in the UK is the same as the Ugandan government spends on the entire health budget for almost 25,000 people for a year.[613] Education is cost effective in Uganda too. I am excluding here, of course, any other measure of cost apart from economic. How can you place a cost on human life?

Incidentally, I have sometimes been asked by people in developing countries to help provide supplies of 'wonder' drugs. The trouble is that as we have seen drugs like AZT just delay death and they are toxic, so complex laboratory monitoring is needed. Other cheaper medicines will have a far greater impact for the same price.

For example, many people with AIDS will be helped by receiving antibiotics to treat chest infections, antifungals to treat thrush in the mouth, antidiarrhoeal drugs and painkillers. None of these may be available to those in rural areas on a regular basis. A year's supply of AZT could be exchanged for medicines to prolong life and control symptoms in up to 200 people with AIDS.

Swapping third world debts for programmes

Developing countries are often crippled by interest payments
to Western banks, financing previous loans. One creative
solution to debt and HIV prevention is 'debt swaps' which
convert a release from debt into AIDS programmes.

The debt crisis was triggered by huge oil price rises in 1973
and 1980 which led to oil-producing (OPEC) nations
depositing massive amounts of currency in Western banks.
These were lent via the World Bank and the International
Monetary Fund to developing countries at low rates of interest
to help modernisation. However, much was spent on arms.
The average expenditure on arms per person is $38 compared
to $12 on health. Some went on prestige projects like nuclear
power stations or luxury items. Some was reinvested back into
Western banks. It has been suggested that one African head of
state had a personal fortune that exceeded his country's entire
national debt.

However, these countries have also been crippled by rising
interest rates and a fall in prices of their exports. Starting with
Mexico in 1982, many countries began to default on
payments. Between 1982 and 1987 the total foreign debt of
developing countries almost doubled from $650,000,000,000
to $1,190,000,000,000, while Africa's debt rose from
$212,000,000,000 in 1986 to $272,000,000,000 in 1990.[614]

Today many countries pay up to a third of their entire gross
national product in debt service. In 1990 every man, woman
and child in the developing world paid an average equivalent
of £17.40 to Western banks. In the same year, the UK took
back £2,493,000,000 *more* from developing countries than
they gave in grants, aid and new loans. Not surprisingly, these
countries are suffering. Health spending has fallen by half in
the world's poorest thirty-seven nations over the last few
years.[615]

This is how debt swaps work. Let us suppose that a country
owes £1 million to a British bank, with interest due of £50,000

a year. The country cannot afford even to pay the interest, let alone repay the money. The bank's shareholders know they are unlikely to get much of the money back in the near future. Along comes an agency offering to 'buy' the debt off the bank for, say, £400,000. Any interest will now be payable to the agency. The bank is delighted to cut its losses and recover some of its capital, so it agrees.

The agency then goes to the country to negotiate. Paying interest is very difficult because it has to be paid in foreign currency which can only be obtained by exporting goods. In some countries, much of the trade revenue goes straight back to Western banks. The agency agrees to cancel the debt completely if the country will agree to spend the equivalent of £800,000 in local currency on employing local people in AIDS programmes.

The country agrees. The debt is wiped, thousands of local people are given educator jobs, no foreign currency is used and the agency has funded an £800,000 programme with only £400,000. Although progress is slow, debt swaps are becoming a reality.[616] It is sometimes difficult, however, to be sure that funds released are used entirely as intended.

When deaths damage the economy

Indirect costs of AIDS are the biggest problem in many developing countries. When a young person dies who is well educated, highly skilled and a key person in some part of your country's economy, a part of that economy dies. For example, if a factory in Malawi loses four out of six of its directors from AIDS in a year, you can be sure that production will fall, and so will the export orders, further damaging the economy.

If key designers, sales and marketing executives, engineers or people with mechanical skills die in the UK, then there is a cost to the government. The economy shrinks. Although this is hard to measure, and you may not think it matters when unemployment is high, in the longer term the loss is significant. We see it most noticeably in the entertainment world: there was only one Rudolph Nureyev, only one Rock Hudson, only one Freddie Mercury (see p 83).

But this talk of finances is to reduce humans to items for sale or purchase. People are worth more than a few thousand pounds. Whether they are famous or unknown, people are people and have value for who they are as individuals. Yet as we have seen, many governments spend practically nothing on prevention in comparison to care.

Ten years before health savings

Unfortunately, as with anti-smoking campaigns, prevention costs money up front, while government spending will have to continue for at least another decade because HIV, like tobacco, has a very slow effect. The 120,000 who will die this year because of tobacco (UK figs) are more than likely dying because of smoke inhaled ten years or more ago. Although it is true there is some improvement to health if people stop, much of the damage is permanent and progressive.

With HIV prevention, health services will probably see no real reduction in illness from prevention campaigns today until well into the next century.

World sexual activity[617]
Every day there are at least:
100 million acts of sexual intercourse
910,000 conceptions
965,000 cases of sexually-transmitted diseases
150,000 abortions

Do health campaigns work?

Does health prevention work anyway? How do we know if any of the millions spent so far have had any effect at all? All health promotion tries to show people cause and effect, persuading them that the effects are so terrible that it is worth paying a big personal price to stop doing something they like doing very much.

An example is drinking and driving. People need convincing that they are likely to have an accident if they have drunk too much. People also need to feel afraid that they stand a big risk of losing their licence, even if they are good drivers.

If they are rammed by another car and the police turn up, they could be breathalysed, and if there are random checks on the road . . .

The evidence shows that some behaviour does change while media campaigns are running, but once they stop, then behaviour tends to return to previous patterns. However, when adverts are backed by intensive breathalyser campaigns, including randomly stopping cars, then behaviour changes dramatically. There has to be a personal 'me' factor.

The same applies to the new speed trap cameras in London. These have been set up along busy roads to take photographs automatically of any car that goes more than a certain margin over the speed limit. The effect on the roads where they are placed has been dramatic—although it is wearing off a bit now that many motorists have worked out where they are positioned.

The health campaign against smoking has been something of a slow starter in comparison. Although we discovered the link between cancer and smoking forty years ago, smoking habits have only begun to change significantly in the last few years.

Advertising has encouraged risks

Perhaps the reason why anti-smoking campaigns have hardly worked is that no government has dared to do the obvious: ban cigarette advertising.[618] It would be very expensive, as huge revenues are earned from taxes on tobacco. If someone tried to get a licence for nicotine as a new drug today, it would never be approved.

Nicotine is strongly addictive. Just watch the agony of someone trying to give up. Nicotine addiction can break the will of some of the strongest characters. Nicotine and tar are highly dangerous, and kill more people each year than heroin. Yet despite all this, no British government has grasped the nettle. As a result, smoking continues at a high level. Everywhere they turn, those trying to escape the habit are reminded of what they are desperate to forget.

We have the same problem with AIDS: on the one hand the UK government spends £12–15 million each year trying to persuade the nation to use condoms, and to reduce the number of partner changes. At the same time, the television and film industry spends larger sums making just one film which has the effect of promoting the opposite. It has been estimated that 90% of all sex scenes on TV or the big screen are shown as taking place outside marriage, mostly in new or relatively short-term relationships.

The safer sex message is drowned out by a massive industry feeding images of rubber-free sex, yet with partners who could well be infected. When did a character on screen last produce a condom or ask about previous partners or offer to have an HIV test so they could forget about condoms? It does happen, but not that often. It is true that condom use has almost doubled in the UK from 1984 to 1992, but perhaps the response could have been far greater. There is also a big difference between occasional use and regular use over a long period.

Behaviour can change

Studies have shown that behaviour does change, and can do so quite quickly. We have seen huge changes in the sexual behaviour of gay men, for example, in many countries. This has usually happened as people have been hit by the deaths of close friends from AIDS. We see the impact not only in survey results asking people about sexual practice, but more importantly in the fall of new cases of rectal gonorrhoea. This is a useful marker for exposure to HIV. If people are abstaining, adopting safer practices or using condoms, then gonorrhoea rates fall. Maintaining behaviour change has been more difficult, especially among young gay men.

Condom use and health campaigns

1. Zambia:
Peer educators reached 80% of sex workers in Bulawayo. Over 3 million condoms given out in thirty months. Consistent condom use rose from 5% to 48%.

2. Mexico:
200 peer educators reached sex workers. In twelve months the percentage not using condoms with the previous ten partners fell from 17% to 1%. Those using them on last ten occasions rose from 50% to 80%.

3. Switzerland:
'Stop' campaign—condom sales up from 6.5 million (1986) to 13.8 million (1991). Use by 17–20-year-olds rose from 19% to 73%. No evidence found of increased promiscuity.

4. Zaire:
Condom sales up from 0.5 million (1987) to 18 million.

Little evidence yet exists for any decrease in spread of HIV in large populations as a result of greater use of condoms.[619] It is also hard to prove that extra condoms are used. This needs urgent evaluation.[620]

We have seen huge changes among drug injectors in several countries, many of whom have ceased sharing equipment or injecting as a result of education. We have also seen condom sales increase in many areas following AIDS campaigns targeted at the general population. All these changes have been seen in a very short space of time compared to the slow response to anti-smoking campaigns. This gives us some hope for the future.

Young people take greatest risks

Half of all new HIV infections are in those who are younger than twenty-five years old, so prevention must start young.[621] However, surveys show that those changing behaviour the most as a result of campaigns are those who would be likely anyway to be settling down, changing partners less frequently. For example, in the UK and some other countries, gay men aged thirty-five to forty-five have reduced dramatically their number of partners, while younger men unfortunately seem to be taking bigger risks again. We see this in the rising number of young gay men going to sex disease clinics with new cases of gonorrhoea—a sure sign that they are having unprotected sex.

Those in the firing line are young people. Every year in countries like the UK, the age of puberty falls a little more for reasons which are unclear, although it is related to increasing body weight in girls. At the same time, the age of settling down is being effectively pushed in the other direction, with longer training and apprenticeships and changing social pressures.

Male sex drive is strongest in those who are youngest and it hits boys at a time when they are least able to handle it all emotionally. A twelve-year-old boy and girl may be experiencing strong urges to explore sex at a time when they are incapable of working out a stable adult relationship. These pressures continue to fuel the debate for and against lowering the age of consent (see Chapter Seven).

Sex education needs to start at a younger age

The UK national sex survey[622] shows that the number of partners each person has in a lifetime is increasing fast—currently eight, but expected to rise to twelve for the generation becoming sexually active today.

We know that in many towns and cities in the UK over half of all sixteen-year-olds are sexually active, possibly with an even higher figure in some other nations. In Uganda a survey of teenage mothers found that 70% had their first sexual encounter before their fourteenth birthday. Research in the US has shown that the number of partners people have in their lives can be directly related to the age they first have sex.

Girls becoming sexually active at ten to fourteen years are four times as likely to have more than five partners a year in later life, three times more likely to report sex with bisexual men, and twice as likely to have had a sexually-transmitted disease in the last five years. This is compared to those becoming sexually active after their seventeenth birthday.[623]

Young girls are particularly vulnerable to HIV and other sex diseases because of the immaturity of the female genital tract, particularly in those thirteen years old and younger.[624] This may be part of the reason why one Ugandan study found that there were five times as many fifteen to nineteen-year-old women with AIDS than men of the same age.[625] The other reason may be that young girls in many countries are targeted by older men as less likely to be infected. It is also true that for physiological reasons a woman is twice as likely to get HIV from an infected man than a man is from an infected woman.

As we have seen, it is far easier to prevent risky habits than to change them once established. Parental attitude and religious faith have also been found to be important influences on teenage sexual activity.[626]

Incidentally, we also know there is a big link with smoking. One study in the UK has shown that those who smoke under the age of sixteen are six times as likely to be sexually active as those who do not, possibly because both activities are to do with wanting to take risks, to experiment and to rebel.[627]

For all these reasons it is obvious that we need to start young and that a big part of the national campaigns needs to be directed towards schools, or where youth tend to meet. In some countries, less than half of all teenagers attend full-time education. Those becoming teenagers today are entering a different world. Unless we find a vaccine or cure for HIV, they are going to see some difficult things. With 1 in 250 of the whole global adult population already infected, they are likely to find this has risen to 1 in 100 by the time they leave school or university.

The AIDS generation is growing up

In many countries, or towns and cities in Europe, they will find possibly one in thirty to one in five of those they meet are already infected, depending on the circles they move in. Among some groups of gay men or drug injectors, higher infection rates than these have been found for some time. However, very high rates can be found in some groups of heterosexuals too, particularly where some of a group have had sexual relationships overseas, or have injected drugs.

Consider a situation where a mixed group of twenty teenagers have been swapping partners over a period of two or three years, with each relationship lasting a few months. Such a group can develop a high rate of HIV infection and other sexually-transmitted diseases. Young people today are the AIDS generation.

So then, AIDS is a preventable illness, and very expensive to treat. The cost of prevention is much less than the cost of ignoring prevention. With the epidemic out of control in most of the world, our young people need to be prepared urgently to live in an AIDS world without dying . . . but what do we say and how do we put it across? Clearly the way we present a message will need to change with the audience and the context to be most effective. An approach for committed Christian teenagers may need to be different from that used in a secular school.

At the most basic level there is no point in preaching a sermon about immorality based on Bible verses, when your audience does not even believe in God. They are unlikely to be impressed by your arguments. A more pragmatic approach is needed. Yet for those wanting to base their lives on the teachings of Jesus, a talk explaining what the Bible teaches about sex will be very helpful.

AIDS in the church youth group

Because of the time delays between infection and illness, it is far more likely that you will find the church youth leader coming to you than one of the teenagers. Teenagers developing illness are more likely to have been infected at a much younger age—by treatments for haemophilia, for example. One person ACET has been caring for recently is a fourteen-year-old boy, who has been living with the knowledge he has HIV for more than half of his life and is now dying.

However, the youth of today are the patients of tomorrow. A recent survey of 1,729 teenage members of church youth groups across the denominations was carried out in the UK by Marc Europe.[628] It showed that levels of sexual activity were lower than the national figures, but still significant. Overall, 14% said they had had sex by the age of sixteen, compared to the national average of 26% for people of a similar age. In a number of cases the church respondents said that sexual activity took place before they had made a personal commitment of their own. Faith can have a powerful influence as a motivating factor in HIV prevention.

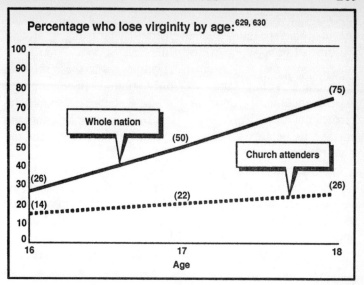

Percentage who lose virginity by age:[629, 630]

Whole nation

Church attenders

(75)

(50)

(26)

(26)

(14)

(22)

Age

16   17   18

Teenagers in church get pregnant

The results show that not only is teenage pregnancy a real
possibility in most churches, but also sexually-transmitted
diseases, including AIDS. Most churches find these things
hard to face. It can be a terrible shock to find that the daughter
of the church leader is three months pregnant, or that 'nice
young lads' have been buying and selling drugs on church
premises.

Unless we think that somehow our church is entirely
separate from and irrelevant to the community in which we
live, we mustn't be surprised to find that the things which go
on in almost every street in the land also go on from time to
time in the lives of those connected in some way with our
churches.

Starting sex education earlier in churches

We need to take sex education and AIDS prevention seriously
with young people in our churches, before they become

sexually active. The survey above shows us this means starting before teenagers reach sixteen years old, probably at around the time of puberty, or even earlier.

Some may feel that insensitive approaches to these subjects at such a young age are only bound to encourage experimentation. I agree, and all sex education should be carried out sensitively in a balanced way, emphasising the positive aspects of marriage and family life, waiting for the right person.

Unfortunately, in a video and satellite age the fact is that whether you are aware of it or not, many thirteen- or fourteen-year-olds are regularly watching 18-rated pornography, either in their own homes with borrowed videos, or in their friends' homes while parents are out or busy.

As most parents know, many nine- or ten-year-olds are now regularly watching 15-rated films in the same way—and older people also need to realise that because ratings have become more relaxed, it means ten-year-olds are now seeing things which would have been X-rated some years ago.

Educating parents is vitally important, encouraging them to take the primary responsibility in these areas which are rightfully theirs.

Sex in the playground

Children are bombarded with images and stories of sex. The playground talk of sex has increased so that parents are now finding their five- to eight-year-olds asking for explanations about sex because of the things they are being told by other boys and girls at school.

In such a sex-obsessed world, the almost complete silence of the church is nothing short of bizarre—especially as the Bible itself is full of stories about sex and sexual imagery, or about sexual standards.

We need to face what is going on and break the sex taboo, bringing our discussions about it into the frame of normal

Christian conversation and experience. We can no longer live in this two-worlds unreality. We are letting our young people down.

'Sex is dirty . . . so save it for someone you love'

We need to be careful about the mixed messages we give in church—for example, 'Sex is dirty . . . so save it for someone you love.' This can be the mixed impression left in the mind of an impressionable child brought up in the church. Another conflicting impression can be: 'Sex is wonderful—but don't tell the children about it.'

We need to communicate that sex is a wonderful gift from God, an amazing experience, as we saw in Chapter 8. We need to teach that *God loves sex—it's the waste of sex outside marriage that causes him grief. Sex was invented by God as a gift to humankind.*[631]

We need to include teaching about sex as part of the overall programme of the church. Possibly a quarter of your congregation may be going home from church to enjoy it with their spouses, their children are obsessed with it, the television and videos from the corner shop are full of it and the Bible is very explicit about it, so why are we still avoiding it?

Role models do matter

We need to make sure youth workers in the church are capable of handling the subject, and more importantly able to set a good example in their own lives. Young people need to see role models worth following; models that are exciting and that work. They need to see marriages in the leaders of the church that are an attractive alternative to the often temporary relationships they see around them. We live in a generation which has almost lost the memory and experience of happy lifelong commitment, yet is searching for it.

The answer is to include sex, sexuality and AIDS as topics

in what the church is already doing, making use of some excellent materials such as Steve Chalke's video *Lessons in Love* (see Appendix H at the end of this book).[632]

Schools programmes

Teaching in church youth groups will only reach a few. What about schools? There can be few lessons which are more controversial. As soon as we think about education on sex or AIDS in schools, we find ourselves caught up in polarised debate. We find strong opinions expressed about general approach, content, methods, context, teacher support, parental opinion and the age it should happen. Millions of words have been written and tens of thousands of hours have been spent in training or in discussions, yet very little is actually happening in many countries.

More attention is now being focussed on this vital area.[633] In the US, a survey of 30,000 high-school pupils shows that an increasing number are now being taught about AIDS and are discussing related topics with their parents. At the same time, there has been a reduction in the numbers reporting sexual risk-taking.[634]

Meanwhile, ACET has developed an education programme in the UK with a simple, practical, low-risk approach which has become immensely popular with teachers, with a take-up rate of our materials in up to 60% of secondary schools.[635] While it can hardly be regarded as a blueprint for success, there are general lessons to be learned, a number of which can be adapted to the situation in different countries.

Instead of getting caught up in discussions of educational theory, it is possible to start from the other end of things; from the point of view of a teacher facing a sceptical class for an AIDS lesson. Teachers in the UK have been facing real difficulties. Educational committees and self-appointed experts can generate a wide variety of materials that may be 'politically correct' and fit with the latest fashions in education, but which turn out to be completely unusable. ACET asked teachers what they needed to do the job. The answers they gave were fed into a new programme.

Here is a summary of twenty lessons ACET has learned, primarily from teachers, parents and governors, drawing from their own experience and wisdom, but also listening to pupils. You may disagree with some of the conclusions, but we ignore the opinions of those in schools at our peril. Later on we consider ten common objections from 'the experts'. Clearly this is a response based on the situation in the UK. A similar process in other nations might produce some differences, but possibly fewer than you might think.

Lesson 1: HIV/AIDS education in schools is sensitive

As we have seen, schools work on AIDS is a sensitive issue because people cannot agree on what should be taught. Staff, parents, governors and national regulations need to be respected.[636]

Be careful to use appropriate language. Recently someone from another AIDS organisation went into a drama school in the UK and began to give a talk on AIDS. The person decided it would be best to communicate using earthy language, so began to be very explicit, using all kinds of crude slang to describe a wide variety of sexual practices. Such an approach is common in many developed countries, promoting 'a more erotic, positive and diverse kind of sexual behaviour'.[637] It is the sex education equivalent of hard-hitting evangelism in the classroom during a lesson on comparative religion. Unnecessary, insensitive and provocative.

After about forty minutes the headmistress intervened, stopped the class, threw the young man out of the school and sent all the pupils home for the rest of the day to recover from the shock.[638] Two weeks later ACET was contacted, and an educator visited, taking a more sensitive approach. We have been invited back. AIDS prevention is difficult because on the one hand we want to hold attention, to be relevant and to have impact, while on the other we must not upset or offend.

AIDS prevention is most effective as an integral part of sex education or education about the risks of addiction. However, in educating about sex or drug abuse, we always have to be careful that we are not just feeding the imagination and encouraging experimentation.

Lesson 2: Facts alone are of limited value

If you go into a classroom and try to give an AIDS talk, you will see that facts alone can be a waste of time. Teenagers are bored rigid with AIDS in low-incidence countries like the UK. The whole subject has been done to death by the media.

People need to see AIDS is real before they are going to listen to you talk about it or seriously consider changing their behaviour.[639] That is one reason why government videos in UK schools have often not been used. Either that, or they were quickly abandoned because the content was felt to be unsuitable.

Lesson 3: Family deaths change behaviour

As we have seen, behaviour often changes dramatically when someone experiences the death of a family member or close friend. The trouble is, by the time many young people in schools today begin to see deaths among their friends, we will have a much higher infection rate.

We do not have to wait at all in countries like Uganda, where in a schools lesson I asked for a show of hands from all those who had been to the AIDS funeral of a family member. Most of the hands shot up. They needed no persuading that AIDS was for real and they were keen to listen.

Lesson 4: We need to make AIDS real to pupils

One way to help make the illness real to pupils is to ask people with AIDS to visit schools. Unfortunately, this can be very difficult to organise and is unlikely to be possible in low-incidence countries, except on a small scale, for several reasons—the commonest given being the risk of anti-heroes.

Many schools do not wish to bring in someone with AIDS who might become something of a role model regarding previous lifestyle. Teachers in the UK recently had a shock over prevention of drug abuse. The government produced striking posters with the slogan 'heroin screws you up'. The picture showed a young man with boils on his face, looking quite ill and sorry for himself.

A number of schools requested these, but found the posters kept disappearing without trace. It seemed that teenage girls were pinning them up on their bedroom walls. The boy had become an anti-hero, the latest pin-up idol.

Many schools may be worried that a gay man might want to promote the view that to have a gay lifestyle is very acceptable and attractive. This would contravene clause 28 of the UK Education Act, which specifically outlaws the promotion of homosexual relationships in schools, although permitting education about orientation to be a part of the school's teaching. You and I may feel this anxiety is unnecessary if those coming in are interviewed first, but for many schools the hesitation remains.

Drug injectors can also become heroes. Many schools are worried that drug users might come across as 'smart', 'streetwise' and 'cool', even if they say they no longer abuse drugs, and warn against it. That leaves only those infected through heterosexual sex or blood products, many of whom are not enthusiastic about being in the public eye in this way.

There is another problem. If we want people to see the reality of the illness, not the fact that you can live perfectly well with HIV for years, then there may not be enough people ill with AIDS to go round in low-incidence countries. Some will be too ill and others may be unwilling. It takes an act of great courage to walk into a school where you are unsure of people's reactions. Another effective way is to use educators who have been involved in the care of those dying at home with AIDS locally. This has been ACET's approach.

A comprehensive review of prevention programmes by the World Health Organisation has shown that person-to-person prevention is especially effective, particularly when 'peer led'. In other words, where the target audience can identify with the educator[640]—for example, similar age, background or experience.

Lesson 5: Professional educators working within a moral framework

Despite all the sensitivities, experience has shown that professionally-based AIDS education is often relatively easy for a church organisation to provide compared to a secular agency.

ACET provides educators to take individual lessons, teams to teach larger groups, and materials and training for school staff. Teaching methods vary from interactive questionnaire, class discussion, role play, dramatic presentations, conferences for large groups and formal teaching assisted by colour slides or video. Every country and situation is unique, but some of the basic principles for effectiveness and wide acceptance are likely to apply.

(a) Care credentials: All ACET educators have helped care for people dying with AIDS locally at home. As the country's largest independent provider of home care for people with AIDS, people know the educators will help pupils develop a positive attitude towards those who are infected. In whatever country education is taking place, it is clear that people with personal experience of care have a big impact—greater than that of educators who have just attended training courses.

(b) Classroom credibility: There is no longer a 'boredom factor' when you are talking about real people dying of a real disease.[641] ACET is also able to bring home the reality of what

is happening in other countries because of its overseas programme.

(c) Proven track record: As it has the country's number one schools programme for AIDS, ACET has a great number of schools willing to act as reference sites. Much of the growth of face-to-face work has been as a result of personal recommendations following presentations to over 135,000 pupils.

In countries like the US, there is debate about whether educators without formal qualifications in health education should be allowed in schools.[642] Experience suggests this is unnecessary so long as individuals are carefully selected for their communication skills with young people, and are properly trained. Extra security is provided by the presence of the class teacher. Paper qualifications do not mean someone will be able to persuasively alter the behaviour of teenagers in school.

(d) Popular approach: AIDS is placed in the whole context of sex education, in the framework of relationships and commitment, empowering people to make their own choices and helping them find their own ways to say no to sex or drug abuse if that is their choice.

Those who know ACET is a church organisation almost always see this as an advantage in the classroom. They realise that no one is going to preach or moralise. It would kill the programme as effectively as crude language killed off one educator's access to the school in the example above.

Lesson 6: Success breeds success

The best advert is personal recommendation based on past experience. A good reputation is essential, and takes time to build. Everything needs to be of the highest standard. Over 600,000 of ACET's full-colour, 16-page booklets have already been requested by schools.[643] They look attractive with illustrations and comic strips, and are designed to survive being dropped in puddles or on the classroom floor. They are given away to each pupil in the knowledge that around 80% are read and kept or passed on to others, such as peers, parents and family.

If we estimate that half of the booklets get taken home, and are read on average at home by two other people, then the 600,000 given out will have reached a total of well over a million people.

This popular resource was test marketed on 30,000 pupils and 100 teachers, and in the process went through three editions until the product was right. Over 95% of teachers said it was the best resource for pupils on AIDS they had ever seen.[644] Success breeds success. The Association of British Insurers saw it and decided to launch it, together with a special teacher pack and a demonstration video, at a press conference in the House of Lords.

It is remarkable that almost all of the initial 350,000 print run was requested by schools in just the first twelve months, together with 10,000 teacher packs (there are only 500,000 pupils in each school year). Many schools reordered before the first year was out. All 250,000 of the second edition were used up in just twenty weeks. In addition, requests have come in from all over the world, while Romanian and Welsh editions have also been produced.

Lesson 7: Compulsory HIV/AIDS education opens new doors

A further impetus has been given to schools work on AIDS in the UK by changes in the national curriculum, first making HIV/AIDS a compulsory subject as part of science, and then moving it to be part of sex education. This caused a great stir. Sex education has been an optional extra from which parents may withdraw their children, and is an area many governing bodies have yet to agree on.

Because the responsibility for sex education in the UK lies entirely with each school's own board of governors, what happens in the classroom varies enormously. If they decided sex education would only be taught to their pupils by parents at home, then there was no formal teaching on sex at all.

Some of the opposition to making AIDS a compulsory subject came from the Christian community. Over 4,000 members of the Exclusive Brethren signed a petition to members of the House of Lords in 1992, asking them to make a conscience clause allowing them to withdraw their children.[645]

They feel that despite the official line that sex education should be within a moral framework, in practice the government materials on sex education and AIDS have been very mechanistic, without adequate balance, and that they should have the right to educate their children on these matters at home.[646]

Although we may debate the rights and wrongs of placing HIV in the science syllabus, the result was a massive new impetus. Schools that had put AIDS to one side as even more controversial than sex education, suddenly had to make new decisions about AIDS and how it should be taught.

We might prefer to see AIDS lessons as part of high-quality sex education in schools, integrated as part of the school's policy for personal, social and health education. The most appropriate teaching methods then include a range of styles and approaches, with pupils actively involved in group work discussion, role play (eg, resisting pressure) and question-naires. At times more formal approaches can also be helpful.

Lesson 8: Help pupils find their own answers

People often ask whether we preach or why we don't, depending on their position. The answer to both camps is the same: sermons only on Sundays. Pupils need to work out their own answers. There is no point at all in trying to back up what you are saying from the Bible when talking to people who have never read it, don't believe in it and don't even believe God exists.

You will merely undermine your message by convincing people that you are giving a biased view of this confusing epidemic. You will be open to the accusation that you are manipulating the facts to get people to accept Christian lifestyles. We are only in the classroom for an hour or two on a couple of occasions, yet the message needs to last a lifetime. Experience has shown that a long-term impact is more likely if pupils take part in the presentation, and come to their own conclusions about changing behaviour or avoiding risk.

A key is a relationship of trust and respect built between the educator and pupils. They need to feel able to talk freely, and to feel that what is being discussed matters and is being covered in a balanced way.

Lesson 9: No need to preach

While it is true that you cannot preach, our experience is that you do not need to. The facts speak very loudly for themselves. It is also true that the kind of person the educator is, and the way the person comes across, can communicate a lot.

When people see someone who is young, single, who enjoys life, has a sense of humour and a normal sex drive, yet is not sleeping around, a new role model is created. These things can emerge in response to pupils' own questions, which can be quite probing. The lesson is designed to help them also talk very frankly and openly.

A survey of a group of HIV-prevention workers in the UK showed that a large number were taking risks and not adopting their own advice. Young people are often very perceptive and can detect double standards, double talk, lack of integrity and hypocrisy. Teaching one thing and doing another undermines the impact you have, and makes it more likely that behaviour will remain unchanged.

The idea of using role models of college age in schools is not new, and has been used successfully in programmes targeting drugs prevention, smoking and sexual behaviour in

the US.[647] However, many studies have shown that if pupils
are presented with an older person who has an overbearing
authoritarian manner telling them to 'be good', they are likely
to react. Some may even be more likely to take risks in the
future as an expression of rebellion against authority.

Teenagers are often far more concerned about their own
health than adults realise. A US study found a high level of
concern about AIDS, schoolwork, making friends, sex,
discrimination and dental problems. Teenage girls were also
worried about violence, rape, menstruation, abuse, pregnancy,
sadness and being overweight. Boys were concerned
additionally about homosexuality, sex, car accidents and low
weight.[648]

Lesson 10: Classes can be large or small

Many theorists say that only small classes are useful. In
practice you are often limited by the timetables and priorities
of the school. If teachers already have booklets or other usable
materials and are teaching the subject themselves, then they
may be very grateful for an outside presentation to a large
group to help reinforce the message.

Drama can be an effective way to communicate to larger
groups, although it is labour intensive and expensive in terms
of pupils reached per hour.[649] Drama has been particularly
helpful in reaching populations in developing countries,
including variations such as the use of puppets in
performances.

The aim is to make the illness real so teachers can teach
about the disease with greater attention from their pupils. The
greatest impact then comes in smaller groups where there is
time for discussion and feedback, and where the educator has
an ongoing presence in the school.

Lesson 11: Teachers need to be closely involved

Most teachers want to be involved, although work pressures
are so great that it can often be very tempting to leave the

302 THE TRUTH ABOUT AIDS

classroom to get on with preparation elsewhere. ACET educators ask the class teacher to be present during sessions. Although some are surprised because they expect pupils will be more inhibited, we have found the advantages more than outweigh the disadvantages.

The aim is to equip and give confidence to class teachers, not to deskill them so they feel the need to leave it all to outside specialists. Watching us at work gives confidence to others. Teachers often feel able to take over much of the work in future years, thus increasing the impact of our work.

If an outsider comes in to talk on a subject like AIDS, the danger is that the message will be entirely disconnected from everything else in school. Even worse is the possibility that there may be conflicting messages.

When teachers sit in, it guarantees that what is said fits in with what they want. It also guards against complaints from parents. There is a witness to exactly what happens in each class. Finally, it ensures that what the school is teaching about HIV is as accurate as possible.

Because every class is not only a pupil presentation, but also a teacher training session, a small number of educators can have a big impact over a year. Between classes there is also the opportunity to talk with staff informally, or to meet the head teacher and advise on syllabus priorities.

Evaluation is essential. Another big advantage of having teachers remain in class during presentations is good feedback. It is essential to evaluate any programme, particularly in schools. ACET encourages teachers to complete evaluation sheets at the end of presentations. They may prefer to wait until after the following week's lesson when they have had feedback from the pupils themselves. From time to time whole classes are asked to complete evaluation forms rating the presentation and booklets.

Lesson 12: Sexual orientation is a separate issue

As we have seen, many schools are very anxious about how gay relationships will be presented in an AIDS talk. There is always a risk that an AIDS lesson by a visiting educator could open up all kinds of sensitive areas in the classroom, including lengthy discussions about sexual orientation, detailed descriptions of anal sex, oral sex, ways to masturbate, demonstrations of putting on condoms and the promotion of gay lifestyles in schools. The teacher may have to spend the next few weeks sorting out the chaos!

Whatever our own views are on these areas, we need to listen carefully to what parents, teachers, governors or community leaders are saying would be most helpful. Schools usually prefer an objective low-key approach using non-emotive language in a matter-of-fact way. They do not want an AIDS lesson to be hijacked by other issues.

It is always best to use plain language where you can, so, for example, I prefer to talk of sex between people of the opposite sex, or sex between men and women, or sex between people of the same sex, instead of 'heterosexual', 'homosexual' or 'gay'.

The latter two terms are very unhelpful and misleading, because many young people are unclear whether you mean someone who has a particular attraction to someone of the same sex or someone who is sexually active.

In the classroom, then, I rarely use the words 'gay' or 'homosexual'. There is another reason. As we have seen, six out of ten men who have homosexual relationships also have sex with women.[650] Some may not think of themselves as gay or bisexual.

When avoiding this kind of language, it is unusual to find problems in the classroom or with parents. We are not there to talk about why or how sexual orientation develops, nor is it part of the job of UK schools to comment on the appropriateness or otherwise of gay or straight sexual activity, except as a health issue.

In my view, it is not usually appropriate to comment on the higher risk of anal intercourse versus vaginal for HIV transmission (two to one), nor that women are twice as likely to get the HIV infection from an infected man, than a man is from an infected woman. Such distinctions are likely to confuse the basic message. All it changes is whether the person would be infected perhaps after four months in the relationship or eight. Nothing more.

Lesson 13: Drug use or misuse must be discussed with integrity

A significant proportion of new infection in many countries is caused by injecting drugs, so it is essential that we tackle this important area. Many are likely to have been offered drugs or to have experimented by the time they are seventeen or eighteen.

A study of 8,000 US teenagers in 1991 showed that almost 3 in 100 had injected illegal drugs—and almost 1 in 100 had shared needles. Those with greater knowledge of HIV were less likely to have experimented.[651]

The first thing we have to recognise is that there is something of a double standard in many countries. Many who are against 'drugs' are in fact addicted themselves. We have already seen how dangerous nicotine addiction is, but the most commonly abused drug in many countries is alcohol. I am ruling out here addiction to substances like caffeine, seen in those who experience terrible headaches and difficulty in concentrating after twenty-four to forty-eight hours of coffee withdrawal.

We need to acknowledge these things before we can talk sensibly with young people about the use of cannabis, ecstasy or crack, or the injection of drugs. It does seem, by the way, that cannabis may turn out to be less physically addictive than tobacco, and perhaps less dangerous to general health.

However, there is certainly a lot of evidence that those using cannabis regularly may be less careful when it comes to thinking about sex. As a relaxant, it removes sexual inhibitions—but then so does alcohol, and alcohol is a very important element in unsafe sex.

There is also some evidence that using cannabis may introduce the user to a circle of friends or a way of life where it becomes part of the norm to try other things. These are usually given freely at first. The charging comes later.

In the middle of the process are some who will need to sell drugs to cover the costs of their own habit. The injector may well be injecting all kinds of things—not just heroin, or what has been sold as heroin. We need to get across the message that sharing needles or syringes is the quickest way to get HIV.

An important part of the approach is to help pupils see how they can avoid situations where they know they will be under pressure to accept drugs. We also need to help them see how they can say no in such a situation, while preserving their self-esteem.

Lesson 14: Condoms need to be discussed in context

The most obvious question facing any educator in schools is how to discuss the condom issue. Christians may have all kinds of objections to the way in which condoms seem to have been promoted as the answer to AIDS. These need to be laid aside when we think about going into schools. We need to take an objective look at the facts, and once again listen to teachers before deciding our approach.

Excellent protection, but not 100% safe. We have looked at the failure rates of condoms for pregnancy and HIV in Chapter 6. A survey of eighteen-year-olds in Glasgow asked for a description of 'safer sex', and 84% mentioned condoms, 68% some aspect of partner selection, but only 2% mentioned abstaining from certain sexual activities as an option.[652] A very one-dimensional message is being given, yet abstinence must increasingly be recognised as a valid—and 100% safe—

option,[653] and is increasingly becoming a central part of thinking on prevention. The New York City Board of Education recently decided that promoting premarital sexual abstinence as an option should be a key part of AIDS education.

Testing is a real alternative. It is hard to think of a more absurd approach than just promoting condoms, particularly in view of the pregnancy failure rates we saw in Chapter Six. If you think through what the campaigns are saying, the conclusion is that all sexually-active adults should use condoms in all relationships for life if either has ever had sex before.

This is a ridiculous message. What happens with couples who have been faithful to each other for years? Are we really expecting them to go on using condoms in addition to the pill for the rest of their fertile lives? What happens when the woman wants to have a baby? Are we seriously expecting women who have gone through the menopause to continue using condoms with their lifelong partners till they die of old age?

As we have seen, the answer is that HIV testing is an excellent alternative to condom use. It costs less to have a test than it does to buy three months' supply of condoms. If both partners are uninfected, they can enjoy anxiety-free, rubber-free sex for the rest of their lives. They will, however, need to be able to trust each other not to have other relationships or to share needles if injecting drugs.

The testing option has hardly been mentioned by the UK government, and has been missing from the poster and TV campaigns because it is not politically correct. Various highly-influential pressure groups have persuaded the government that testing is still too sensitive and controversial, mainly because of discrimination. Many people are still worried that going for a test may affect life insurance. Guidelines have changed (see p 120).

No need to roll condoms on bananas. People often ask whether we give out condoms in the classroom. Our view is that it is almost always unnecessary and inappropriate. Even if we wanted to, most schools would be horrified if we were to roll condoms onto bananas in front of teenagers. We are in the business of giving an all-round message on AIDS, explaining the value and limitations of the condom.

If schools wish to demonstrate the use of condoms, we would expect that to be a part of their overall policy on sex education, after having carefully consulted with parents and governors. In our experience, few schools in the UK feel a demonstration is necessary, desirable or appropriate.

Teaching people to sin safely? While some outside schools want all educators to demonstrate condom use and to teach teenagers that it is good to have fun with sex when you are young, others are horrified, saying that even to mention condoms in class is to invite people to 'sin safely'. Surely, they say, there is a danger that in even talking about sex and condoms we may be encouraging promiscuity?

In the context of a school class we are called to give the facts. We are certainly not wanting to encourage sex outside of marriage, but it would be absurd to avoid any mention of condoms at all. Even if you say condoms should only be used by people who are married, there may be many situations in the future where a couple have got married knowing that one partner is infected from the past. Are their lives also to be placed at risk through a ban on all information about condoms? Young people live in the real world—so do you and I—and we need to demonstrate that in a realistic down-to-earth approach. (See next page for Catholic approach.)

Condom summary. In summary, then, we need to make pupils aware that there are several ways to reduce the risk of HIV or avoid it altogether. As the World Health Organisation says, the most effective way to prevent sexual transmission of

HIV is to abstain, or for two people who are uninfected to remain faithful to each other. Alternatively, the correct use of condoms will reduce the risk significantly. We need to get across that having sex without using a condom could be suicidal with a partner who may be infected. However, condoms may let you down.

Lesson 15: Ethnic minorities often welcome a Christian approach

Over the years, ACET has gained a lot of experience teaching in different kinds of schools in different areas. The same approach to AIDS has found great favour across the spectrum, including schools which are 95% Asian with Muslim, Hindu and Sikh children and parents.

Parents appreciate educators who have a moral framework for their own lives which is similar to their own. Many from ethnic minorities are deeply religious, and find the sexual standards in many Western societies shocking, upsetting and worrying, as they consider the future of their children.

Lesson 16: Catholic schools also welcome sensitive AIDS education

The sensitivities in Catholic schools tend to be greater, although this varies very much from school to school and from country to country. The big issue for Catholics is whether condoms will be mentioned.

Some Catholic schools take the view that it is permissible to talk about how HIV spreads, how it causes illness, and how to help with HIV, but not mention condoms unless pupils ask directly. Others are more relaxed, so long as the lesson is placed firmly in the context of the Christian ideal of sex as part of marriage for life. The range of what is permitted varies from area to area and country to country.

As in every other school context, the best approach is to treat each school and each class as unique, discussing with teachers the approach they want, and any particular sensitivities of the school or of the particular class. This is the only reliable way to avoid misunderstandings, to ensure we serve schools well and to make certain we are operating as part of their team.

In Northern Ireland, the same educator, programme and materials have found warm acceptance in both Catholic and Protestant schools.[654] The problems are therefore often more imagined than real. The key is a strong relationship of trust and respect built with individual educators.

Lesson 17: Lesson content needs to vary with age

Some schools will want to educate pupils who have not yet reached their teenage years. This is perfectly possible without offence or difficulty, but the content will need to be adapted under the guidance of teachers. It is not necessary, for example, to explain about sex in order to teach about Romanian AIDS babies. Some aspects of AIDS can be taught in the context of geography, science, hygiene and other school topics.

Countries vary greatly. In Uganda, for example, elements of sex education and AIDS are often taught to children as young as six. The reason is that in towns or villages where up to a third of the population is HIV-infected, most children will have seen members of their own families die from AIDS. The illness dominates local life, and an explanation has been found to be necessary. In comparison, such topics are very difficult to discuss with young children in a country like Thailand.

Lesson 18: AIDS education needed before some leave school

With many pupils leaving school at the age of sixteen in countries like the UK, AIDS education must start earlier. A recent survey in Dundee showed that those leaving school early are often much less likely to take notice of public health messages later, and this group may take greater risks than those who carry on with general education. School education is therefore particularly important for this group.[655]

Lesson 19: Establishing traditional behaviour patterns as most common can be very effective

Behaviour is often influenced by peer pressure, or by what people think everybody else is doing. Media and peer group conversation tends to exaggerate reality, however. For example, it may give the impression: 'Almost all my friends sleep around,' or, 'Most of my friends use drugs,' or, 'Hardly anyone these days is still a virgin by their eighteenth birthday.' A lot of talk, but little or no performance.

Can these impressions be changed? A US study compared two approaches to prevention of smoking, alcohol abuse and use of marijuana by schoolchildren. The first method taught skills to pupils to help them refuse unwanted offers. The second corrected falsely-high impressions of how many other pupils were experimenting, and of what most others in the school thought of these behaviours.

The second 'normative' approach worked well in altering reported behaviour one year after the programme. The first had fewer measurable effects.[656] It is essential also to reinforce the positive behaviour of the large number of teenagers who do not abuse alcohol or other drugs, or take sexual risks.[657] They may be with the majority.

Lesson 20: Social skills/peer resistance training works

Many studies have shown that classes designed to help pupils develop the ability to say no are effective in behaviour change.[658] Facts are essential to understand the problem, and personal presentation is vital to make the problem real, but pupils may still take risks against their wishes if they feel insecure about themselves with a poor self-image, and are afraid of being looked down on or laughed at.

Schools health programmes may face similar issues in many different countries. A survey of 188 studies in thirty-one countries on health education in schools between 1984 and

1987, has shown that problems and issues faced are remarkably similar from country to country.[659] This is also true in the experience of international agencies like ACET. While cultural sensitivities vary and may require adjustment of content and approach, many basic issues such as motivation, communication and long-term behaviour change remain the same.

The impact of schools programmes is likely to be greatest when mass media campaigns are also part of the overall national picture, as studies on teenage smoking have shown.[660]

Dealing with criticism

In such a sensitive area, whatever one does will be criticised. The test of whether you have the balance about right in schools is probably when you are criticised from several different sides equally, but none too severely.

Constructive criticism must always be taken seriously, especially if it relates to conduct or lesson content. That is why evaluation forms are essential. You want to pick up a slight problem with an educator's approach long before there is a complaint.

We need to understand the background to the criticism. For example, there are hundreds of self-appointed experts in the UK when it comes to AIDS prevention. Hardly any of them have any real experience of teaching about AIDS in schools, or if they do it may be in just one or two schools which are unrepresentative of the country as a whole.

Coping with the 'thought police'

Sometimes comments made from 'non-school' sources can be vitriolic. Valid points may be being made, but I often wonder why they have been allowed into so few schools themselves if they are such experts on getting the message right. Why have their own resources and leaflets found so little favour?

The classroom is a uniquely difficult and sensitive environment and my feeling has always been that it is up to teachers and pupils to tell us what they need.

We must allow teachers to get on with the job. They are the experts, we are the assistants. Failure to recognise this by the HEA and other bodies has been the reason why so little government-sourced material has been used. It is nothing short of a scandal that a modest schools programme like ACET's, intended as no more than a pilot to show what could be done nationally, should turn out to be the largest programme of its kind in the country.

It is sad that after all the millions the UK government has spent, as far as I can see the only quality resource available free in bulk to individual schools has been ACET's own booklet. There appears to be nothing else.

Perhaps there is little new under the sun when it comes to HIV prevention—or criticisms of it. Negative reactions to ACET's schools programme tend to be very repetitive along ten main themes. Similar reactions are likely to be found to other schools programmes run by Christians elsewhere, so ten common objections are listed and discussed below.

Objection 1: 'Large classes are a waste of time'

It is obvious that the more time spent with a group of pupils, and the higher the presenter-to-pupil ratio, the greater the impact is likely to be, but we have already seen that larger classes may be the only ones on offer in a school. A school which opts for a single large presentation one year as an experiment, will often open up more of the timetable the following year. Most schools need time to find their way forward.

Objection 2: 'Faithfulness to one partner is a naïve suggestion'

Some think it is hopelessly naïve even to mention the option of being faithful to one person, let alone staying with one partner for life. It is interesting that in almost every class I have been into pupils have worked out the options of abstention and monogamy for themselves—and the benefits.

When you ask them what 'safe sex' is, there are usually two reactions. If you ask who has seen the slogan 'condoms mean safe sex' or 'for safe sex use a condom', you will often find every hand shoots into the air. Almost always they have misread official slogans by dropping the 'r' off the end of 'safer' to remember 'safe'. However, when you ask pupils what they think, those with an ounce of common sense tell you that safe sex is certainly not using a condom. They know friends or relatives who became pregnant using them.

I would argue that it is hopelessly naïve to expect that pupils are going to decide after your lesson to use condoms every time they have sex until the day they die, when the alternative of a test in a long-term relationship is so simple. Also, many people are searching for love that lasts.

Objection 3: 'Suggesting celibacy or monogamy as options is moralistic'

Some say that you should not make any suggestions at all about behaviour, nor propose any role models. 'Pupils should be totally free from any proactive or directive approach.' They say it is moralistic to talk about keeping to one partner or to suggest not having a sexual partner at all.

In reply, three points need to be made. First, medical facts are morally neutral. It is a medical and human fact that it is possible for people to refrain from sexual activity or promiscuity, and that this can be a very healthy way to live—for a start it protects you from sex diseases. Secondly, in the UK there are legal requirements to present sex education 'in such a manner as to encourage those pupils to have regard to moral considerations and the value of family life'.[661] Thirdly, even if such an approach was not required by law, the parents and governors of most schools in the country would insist on it anyway.

Having addressed a number of Parent/Teacher associations, it is obvious that some of the most conservative parents are those who were themselves teenagers in the 1960s and are now deeply concerned about their children living the way they did in a pre-AIDS world. Many still want marriage to work.

Objection 4: 'If you don't show people how to use condoms they won't bother or they will make mistakes'

It is true that people should be encouraged to familiarise themselves with a condom before they need to use one. The best place for this to happen is in the privacy of the person's own home, where the packet can be opened, the condom examined, the instructions read and if necessary experimented with. Demonstrating condoms to children under sixteen years of age could be taken to be encouraging under-age sex, and even over that age you could land yourself in trouble. (See earlier comments about demonstrating condoms on page 307.)

Objection 5: 'Visiting speakers are dangerous because they do not fit into the overall work of the school'

We have already discussed the importance of each educator becoming, in effect, an extension of the head teacher's own staff in the school. Nothing is worse than a hit-and-run approach with no continuity, no follow up and little impact.

We have also noticed the huge advantages many schools see in outside carer/educators. They have impact because they are involved in care. They are respected experts. They are seen as non-threatening and not part of the establishment. They are often easier for pupils to talk to. They bring a fresh perspective to the school.

Objection 6: 'Not enough time is given to gay issues'

As we have seen, AIDS prevention is about preventing HIV transmission through risky sexual practices and drug injecting, not about sexual orientation. This important area is a part of overall sex education, as well as personal lifeskills and social education.

Objection 7: 'You fail to point out that you are almost 100% safe unless you inject drugs or have anal sex with a gay man'

Objections 6 and 7 are almost opposites of each other. If we spend time on the relationship between a gay lifestyle and AIDS, we also create the impression that AIDS is just a gay problem, when as we have seen, AIDS is an increasing threat to heterosexuals in European countries and a huge risk in developing countries. If we spend no time on gay lifestyles we create the false impression that all in our society are equally at risk.

It is 'politically correct' to say there is no such thing as an 'at risk group', but only 'at risk behaviour'. While it is important that we teach people not to hide behind labels and prejudice, we may be in danger of splitting hairs. It is certainly true that the risk of a gay man picking up HIV from a sexual encounter in a gay bar in London is hundreds of times greater than the risk of a heterosexual man picking up HIV from a girl he meets at a party in Newcastle. However, in the classroom we have a very short time to put across a simple message that AIDS is real, HIV is spreading and these are the ways to protect yourself and those you love. Although the risks are low, it is a fact that some have become HIV-infected after a single episode of unprotected sex (see Chapter 6).

Objection 8: 'Fear of getting AIDS is a very negative way to motivate change'

People object if you talk about the illness as it really is. We know what we are talking about. AIDS is a very unpleasant illness, with many unpleasant symptoms which are difficult to treat. People do not just live with AIDS, they die too.

I often say to classes in schools that I hope we do not ever have to look after any of them. After all, that is why I am there: to try to save their lives if I can. If they carry on behaving like some of those who left the school over the last few years, then it is likely that doctors or nurses will be caring for some of them too. This is a frightening thought and it greatly disturbs me too.

A few years ago people were reluctant to talk about dying with AIDS because it created a negative image. This is ridiculous. If you create the impression that to have AIDS is to be a hero, that living with AIDS can be fun, that you can live for many years and there is a lot of hope for a cure, then don't be surprised when people decide there is nothing to worry about.

Objection 9: 'You are creating a negative view of sex'

Some say that if we talk a lot about the dangers of unrestrained sexual activity, then a new Victorian age of sexually-repressed people will emerge. I have met some HIV educators who have openly told me that one of their purposes is to help teenage boys and girls feel happy about their bodies and about their sexuality, so they feel free to enjoy themselves.

Half the emphasis of their presentations is therefore on sexual enjoyment—for example, teaching young girls about orgasm—and the other half is on how to have fun more safely. They say this is realistic and fits in with what the pupils are doing anyway. As you can imagine, they very rarely get the chance to give such presentations in UK schools. This approach certainly fits well with our culture. You only have to wander into a video shop to see what I mean.

Western culture has produced conditions for the rapid spread of HIV and AIDS by encouraging a casual view of sex, through mass communications with a global influence. Our culture is out of date and needs to change in a post-AIDS world. There is no such thing as free sex without cost. At the same time, Western influence has had a huge effect on liberalising sexual constraint in many traditional tribal cultures. In many people groups, where premarital sex or adultery was prohibited and rare, promiscuity is now common.

As we have seen, surveys show that the younger someone is when they first have sex, the more likely they are to have multiple partners. There is also a strong relationship between the age at which a girl first has sex and her risk of cervical cancer.[662] This cancer is often caused by a virus which is sexually transmitted. It appears that the immature cervix of a young teenager is particularly vulnerable to infection. Deaths from cervical cancer are increasing, despite intensive screening programmes.[663]

Other sexually-transmitted diseases are emerging for which treatment is difficult or impossible. For example, genital herpes, which produces clusters of highly-infectious and painful blisters from time to time throughout life, and genital warts, which require repeated treatments with caustic substances. In the last twelve months alone, 250 million people worldwide became infected with a sexually-transmitted disease.[664] The highest incidence is in twenty- to twenty-four-year-olds followed by fifteen- to nineteen-year-olds.

In these circumstances, I feel as a doctor that we do our young people a gross disfavour by making out sex is always wonderful. This is totally ignoring the pain and devastation felt by many pupils in almost every class as a result of marriage break up, or the collapse of stable relationships outside of marriage. On many occasions, unfaithfulness is at the root of the problem. It is always the children who suffer, caught up in conflicts with split loyalties, and with possibly two 'mums' or 'dads'.

A national UK survey showed that children of divorced parents often continue to suffer well into adult life, when they are more likely to be unemployed and experience psychological difficulties.[665] There are real costs attached to so-called sexual freedom and these need to be clearly taught and understood.

It is also vitally important to give a very positive message about sex as a wonderful experience; something which gives great pleasure and can be very fulfilling, especially when it is an expression of love, respect, appreciation, care and commitment. Sex is something well worth waiting for. The UK Population Trends survey shows that couples living together before they get married are more likely to be divorced fifteen years after marriage than those who do not.[666]

At this point we start hearing objection number 3 again, with suggestions that the previous sentence contains highly moralistic, right wing, Christian propaganda. No wonder schools are voting with their feet.

Objection 10: 'You should teach people other ways to have sex'

The AIDS industry continues to churn out large numbers of guides to safer sex which give long lists of 'low risk' or 'no

---

Annual total of sexually-transmitted infections

World Health Organisation 1990
250 million new cases

Trichomaniasis	120 million
Genital chlamydia	50 million
Genital papillomavirus	30 million
Gonorrhoea	25 million
Genital herpes	20 million
HIV infection	1 million*
Syphilis	3.5 million
Chancroid	2 million

*1990 figure—possibly greater than 2 million per year today

---

risk' activities. Examples of 'safe sex' given include rubbing each other's thighs, mutual masturbation and 'talking dirty' on the phone to each other while masturbating.

Some seriously suggest we should be discussing some of these options in schools. They have obviously never tried such an approach with pupils. Laughter is the only response you are likely to get from a class if you seriously suggest that rubbing each other's thighs is the same thing as having sex. That certainly is naïve. The suggestion may be valid for gay men who know there is a one-in-three chance that their next partner could be infected, but it does not go down too well with teenagers in low-incidence countries.

Why should they bother with such a feeble substitute for the real thing when they know they can enjoy rubber-free, anxiety-free, penetrative sex for life, with the help of an HIV test if they or their partner has been at risk in the past? As we have seen earlier, deciding whether to have a test is a delicate business and all those wanting a test should be carefully counselled first (see p 120).

Over-promotion can be a problem

Having looked at ten of the commonest criticisms ACET has faced, we need to look at the opposite problem: over-promotion of a church programme by well-meaning Christians who want to help. A lot of damage can be done. For example, if someone known to be a moral campaigner goes to the head teacher and begins a campaign to get you in, it would be better if that person had never started.

Setting up a schools programme

As we have seen above, you need to take very great care indeed before rushing in as an AIDS educator. The reason is that an amateurish and clumsy approach to this sensitive area could jeopardise the work of many other agencies.

If you are already established as a youth or schools worker supported by churches in the area, then you may be able with care to include some aspects of AIDS in what you are doing. However, you will need to make absolutely sure you get your facts and general approach right. The ACET/ABI teacher pack may help in this, together with ACET's training courses. You will have greatest impact, as we have seen, if you have been involved in caring for those with AIDS.

13

Needle and Condom Distribution?

Although schools are an ideal place in most countries of the world to meet the adults of tomorrow, schools programmes are too late for adults taking risks today. We can try to target the whole population with general messages, or we can try to spend most of our effort reaching those most at risk.

National programmes are usually the preserve of the government, while targeted prevention is often most effectively carried out at a local level by community groups, and churches can have a key role to play. Whatever approach is taken to targeted prevention, it will involve us in hard decisions. Which way should we go, and how will this affect church programmes?

While a church organisation can find doors open easily into schools, and the general approach required fits well with Christian values, when we look at other areas of community prevention things can become much more difficult.

It is far easier to bring HIV or AIDS into other aspects of existing work than to set up new programmes. Examples of this might be detached youth work, work in pubs and clubs, among the homeless or among prostitutes.

Walking the streets

Detached work can be very successful in reaching all kinds of marginalised groups. Two or more people go out onto the streets, heading for areas where people are known to hang out, especially in the evenings. It might be outside a takeaway food shop on a big estate, or at the bottom of a particular tower block.

Friendships are formed and in that context other things can happen. For example, people can be invited back to someone's house, or literature given out about HIV on the streets. The aim is to create a situation where individuals or groups become interested, and ask questions about how they can protect their own health.

In Dublin, Ireland, detached workers from ACET have made contact with a drug-using community who are, to a large extent, outside contact with health services. A number are ill or dying, and many are infected with HIV. Others have become friends. While other agencies or care workers are sometimes unwilling to go into certain areas, with great fears for personal safety, we have found this community accepting and protective in attitude.

Giving out clean needles?

In Dundee, Scotland, we find drug users gather round as soon as we drive onto various estates with our (unmarked) van. Often they will talk to us about friends who are unwell and need help. When in their homes, there is also a chance to talk to others about safe injecting and how to save their own lives or the lives of their partners and friends.

This brings us straight into another area of difficulty. Some are injecting with shared equipment because they have no needles of their own. They do not want to give up. Should we issue them with clean needles on an exchange basis—in other words, take a blunt one and give them a fresh one? Are we back onto the argument of just teaching people to 'sin safely'?

Needle exchange programmes have been very successful in the UK and other nations, dramatically lowering the incidence of needle sharing.[667] However, one problem is that needles do not always come back—sometimes only half do—raising fears that while HIV infection rates may fall, the numbers injecting may rise.[668] The whole issue is very controversial in many countries.[669]

Encouraging a habit or saving lives?

Christians find it is easy perhaps to decide what is right or wrong behaviour, but when confronted by different situations, it can be less easy to know what to do. Let us imagine that you are an ACET worker visiting people ill and dying with AIDS on a big housing estate in Scotland.

Over a period of months, you gradually get to know a group of drug injectors who have no contact with any other source of help. Several need care, and several want to break the habit. You organise help for these people. However, despite your conversations about the dangers of injecting with shared equipment, three of them tell you they will do so again tonight because they only have one needle and syringe between them.

There are several options open to you. You could inform the police and get them all arrested following a raid on the flat. If you do that, you will violate the trust of the group, you and your organisation will never be asked to help again, and those dying on the estate will die without any help at all. Drugs are also freely available in most prisons, so you will have done nothing to solve the basic problem.

You could just turn your back on the situation and walk out, leaving them to infect each other with a warning about the danger, knowing that one or two of them may receive a death sentence that very night from HIV infection.

There is another option: you could decide to help them on their own terms. Despite all your efforts, they are going to continue to take big risks. They are addicted to the habit and are happy to remain so. You could explain that rinsing the needle and syringe with a freshly-made solution of bleach in water (one part in ten) before passing the equipment on will reduce the risk of death from AIDS enormously. This is not just a matter of morals; this is quite literally a matter of life and death.

If you decide not to tell them this and walk away, and a few years later you are cradling one of them in your arms as he dies, because he became infected that night you walked away, will you not feel an element of responsibility for his death? Perhaps you can distance yourself from this situation, but what if it was all much closer to home?

What if the drug user was your own teenage son or daughter? Would you not do all you could to encourage your own child to use bleach if he or she was determined to continue injecting with shared needles or syringes? If your own child was about to go to the house next door to borrow a bloody needle from someone you knew had AIDS and you happened to have a clean needle in the house, would you not feel perhaps a need to offer a clean needle? If your son is infected that night, will you not feel you could or should have prevented the tragedy? These are not hypothetical situations. Similar agony or conflict is an ever-present reality for many Christians caring in the community, and unfortunately for some Christian parents.

We need to find the way of Jesus. What would he do? Jesus was always honest, open and hard hitting in what he said, yet compassionate and loving in what he did. I cannot believe that Jesus would sit watching the person injecting death without a warning to stop, and, if disregarded, then giving advice on at least how to clean the needle properly, taking care of hygiene. If he knew there was a box of new needles in the corner, I can imagine him mentioning it. Not to promote the practice, but to save life until a time when the person may be looking for help out of addiction, and for reconciliation with God.

I have met a Christian who told me that he would rather sit and watch his son die than tell him how to inject safely. What kind of a dad is that? Some parents are so severe with their children—no wonder so many teenagers of Christian families reject their parents' faith. Often teenagers are saying: 'If this is Christianity, then you can keep it. It's horrible.' Life in the home is vitally important, because it is there that people see the reality of how we are. What kind of gospel are we living? We need to recognise that even where parents have been wonderful examples, children can rebel, rejecting not only parental authority, but also parental values and faith. We also need to see that doubt is a big issue for many people.

Another churchgoer told me that if her son ever showed any signs of growing up with a same-sex orientation she would throw him out of the home, disinherit him and never see him again—even if he was celibate. What has such harshness got to do with a loving heavenly Father? I shudder to think what would happen if God judged these parents with the ferocity with which they are judging their children.

Jesus said: 'Do not judge, or you too will be judged. For in the same way as you judge others, you will be judged, and with the measure you use, it will be measured to you.'[670] So take care. You had better be near perfect or you may be rightly accused of hypocrisy. Of course, as we have seen in Chapter 8, there are clear standards and we are called to challenge, rebuke and confront where necessary.

We need to understand that Jesus often behaved in a way that people thought might appear to be encouraging others to do wrong. As far as the spiritual leaders of the day were concerned, he showed a profound lack of judgement and gross indiscretion in the relationships he formed. Jesus was heavily criticised for encouraging either financial corruption or sexual immorality by publicly associating, eating, drinking and making friends with 'tax collectors and sinners'.[671]

They felt Jesus was giving out a very dangerous signal that wrong behaviour was acceptable, and that despite what he said about God's standards, he was actually encouraging these lifestyles. It is the same today. There are some in the church with rigid black-and-white views on what is absolutely wrong and what is absolutely right in absolutely every situation. They would have had exactly the same problems accepting Jesus as the Son of God as the passionately committed Pharisees did 2,000 years ago.

After much careful consideration and prayer among the ACET team, we felt that we should issue a limited number of replacement needles on an individual basis to some we knew who were injecting, whose needles were blunt, who were unwilling to stop and who would be using other people's needles unless replacements were found. This was not an easy decision and some will criticise us for it. Perhaps the reasons will become clearer as you read on.

It is interesting that Christian doctors, nurses, social workers and missionaries living in the real world usually understand, with many coming to the same conclusions. It is usually those whose lives are most sheltered from the daily lives of those at the margins of society who have the greatest difficulty. Yet that was exactly where Jesus was always found: with the marginalised, the poor, the outcasts, the oppressed, those who had dropped out or rejected the common view of what was right or wrong.

The issue of needle exchange is an entirely different issue to giving out condoms to children in schools. We would not give out needles in school corridors either. The equivalent of needle exchange regarding condom distribution might be a church running a Christian pregnancy advisory service.

We do need to help people find ways to say no if they are feeling under pressure to have sex, and to help them understand the risks they may be taking. However, most Christian doctors I have spoken to in General Practice do recognise that there can be circumstances under which they feel it might be appropriate to provide people with condoms.[672] The issue of contraceptives for under-sixteen-year-olds is far more controversial, especially if this is done without parental involvement. If refused, the next request could be for abortion.

Incidentally, I would always prefer advice to be given, if

possible, in the context of the family doctor's surgery, but young people are not always willing to go there because they are afraid that Mum or Dad will find out.

Contraceptives for unmarried people?

Ethical dilemmas are faced by Christian doctors and nurses every day. I am not saying it is possible to be certain about all the answers, but it is important that we face the questions. It is too easy to hide behind a sermon or to withdraw into the Christian ghetto of church social life and hope these things will go away. We need to preach practical faith that helps people to live in the real world; not platitudes that just comfort us when we return to our homes at night.

We face conflicting ethical issues when someone who is unmarried asks for contraceptives. In the past, family planning clinics in the UK would only help married women. I am not sure many Christians would want to insist on such a rigid approach today, any more than they would want a law passed making sex outside of marriage illegal, as is the case in some Islamic states. However, it could be argued that giving free contraceptives to people who are living together is directly encouraging immorality.

Exactly the same thoughts can apply to helping those with a drug habit. We need to be consistent. What is the answer? It seems to me that first we need to provide the best possible rehabilitation facilities for any who would like to come off drugs. Secondly, we also need to offer the best health advice for those who want to continue injecting.

If we follow the same line as with unmarried men and women who want protection against pregnancy, then we will be willing to supply not only clean needles, but also bleach for sterilising.

Some say that we are then being inconsistent about condoms in schools. I think there is a huge difference between agreeing to make condoms available to adults wishing to reduce the risk of pregnancy or HIV, and promoting such methods to children or young teenagers.

We agree that adults, by definition, are of an age and maturity to form their own judgements and to make their own choices. In contrast, we accept that young teenagers have a developing maturity which is particularly susceptible to influence and pressure. For good reason, there is widespread concern that giving out free condoms in schools will send a powerful message that pupils are expected to have sex at a young age. There are enough pressures on young people to say yes to sex. Why add to them?

We are all involved in 'grey' areas

Christians are divided on these issues. All I am saying is that we need to be consistent and compassionate. All would agree that needle exchange is not ideal.

The fact is that in many situations, we are faced with limited choices, each one of which will mean thinking through some important principle. The choice to do nothing is no way out because it breaks another principle, which is our duty to respond to human need.

We are being dishonest with ourselves if we think we can avoid these dilemmas, these shades of grey, and live in a world of black and white decisions. Jesus faced dilemmas in his own day—for example, over the issue of whether it was right to heal people on the Sabbath, or whether it was right to condemn a woman who had committed adultery.

All the options may feel wrong

In reality, from time to time we all have to choose options we do not like very much, when something is disturbingly wrong with every option. The reason for this is that we live in a fallen world. Take the example of a child we think may be at slight risk of sexual abuse. We are caught between the desire to protect children and the need of children for parents, knowing how difficult short-term fostering can be and the dangers present in many children's homes.

Another example is the response of the United Nations in the past to Somalia, Bosnia and Iraq. In each case the autonomy of the sovereign state, and the call to live at peace with each other, is balanced against the need to protect lives, to fight aggression, or to prevent mass genocide. In every situation we need to pray for wisdom and humility, recognising that whatever we decide is the best, there will be others who might take a different line.

Prostitution makes us think

We face the same complex issues when talking with prostitutes, or commercial sex workers as many prefer to be called. As we have seen, there is a strong link between prostitution and drug abuse. In Glasgow, for example, a survey of 208 street-working prostitutes showed intravenous drug abuse by 59%.[673] Many sell their bodies for sex because it is the only way they can generate enough money to feed a drug habit. Their pimps may be paying them in kind with drugs, food and accommodation.

We can offer those on the street a way out through drug rehabilitation programmes and helping them find new housing and jobs, but many will choose to remain. If they do, then I believe we have the same obligations to teach them to protect their own health and the health of others as we have to educate any other members of our community.

Missionaries make difficult choices

Once we become deeply involved in the community we find very difficult situations to which there are no right answers: every choice open to us presents further difficulties. Missionaries overseas have always encountered these situations and still do so today.

For example, I was talking to someone recently who had been working as a missionary in Thailand. Young girls cross the border from neighbouring countries to work in the cities as prostitutes. Sending a daughter to the big city to work in the bars and sell her body can be as much a natural way of life in some countries as sending children to university is in the UK. Many young girls are expected to work this way and to support their families back home, returning after a few years to settle down and marry.[674] In addition, in some places large numbers of children as young as eight are being sold as sex slaves to brothel owners in neighbouring countries.

The problem now is that many of these sex workers have become infected with HIV. Those from neighbouring countries cannot return home because they have heard reports that those returning are tested for HIV at the border and those found to be infected are led away to be shot or injected with cyanide.[675] The girls are effectively owned by brothel keepers in the city and cannot run away. If picked up they would be deported anyway, as they are often there illegally.

Life-and-death choices

A number of churches have programmes reaching out to such girls, many of whom are becoming ill. Some of the girls have formed close friendships with people in the church—the only friends they have—and have become believers. However, it is hard for them to stop being prostitutes for fear of violence or death at the hands of their masters.

The church is faced with a choice: do we encourage them to stop because their work is against God's law? If so, the church cannot risk sending them back across the border. Does it then hide a growing number of illegal immigrants? Where do you hide them anyway as they are bound to be discovered by the intricate communication network between brothel dealers in the city? If they are taken deep into the country, it is still likely that they will be found eventually. The church will have broken the law and will be in big trouble.

I have been told that at least one church has come to the conclusion that the girls will have to stay where they are for their own safety. They are effectively slaves owned by the brothels since they cannot escape. Therefore, most if not all of the moral responsibility for what they are doing lies with those who are threatening to kill them or to beat them if they do not obey. These are very difficult areas, but just the sorts of things that face us once we move out of our comfortable Christian ghettoes and get involved in what life is like for the rest of the world. (See also p 273 for African perspectives.)

Befriending or confronting?

So then in summary we need to define goals: are we wanting to befriend and help people to continue more safely or do we want to confront and offer a way out? There can be a middle way, which is to provide both approaches in the same team or person, but the exact way you go about it is critically important. You cannot expect to drive into a residential area week after week to meet drug users with disapproving comments, and expect to build friendships and become a source of advice.

In any case, HIV spread among drug users means we need to have a big rethink about drug rehabilitation. People like Jackie Pullinger in Hong Kong have caught the imagination of millions of Christians with wonderful accounts of how God has delivered drug users from addiction—usually from heroin use.[676] The only treatment used is prayer and friendship. They have found no need for medically-supervised withdrawal and they see a very high success rate.

Similar programmes have grown rapidly all over the world. They all work in part by using those who have been through the programme to reach, help and support others.

Unfortunately, while in the past such miracles of new life could sustain a growing work, now many of those who have been through such programmes are found to be HIV-infected.[677] Indeed, many may be ill or dying before their first contact with members of the church.

Drug rehabilitation goals changed by AIDS

We need to redefine our aims. If a drug user is going to die in the next six months with AIDS, is there the same point in weaning the person off? It is true, however, that if a person continues injecting with shared equipment, then he may be adding further damage to the immune system, and may die more quickly.

Is the aim to enable the person to have a good quality of life and to die well, or is the aim to provide a long-term stable and secure future?

In summary, then, community prevention is a vitally important area for the church to be involved in, but it often raises far greater ethical questions than AIDS education in the classroom does. The basic principle of unconditional love leads us to offer help in a broader way than we might initially feel comfortable with. We need to have a clear moral framework ourselves for our own lives, understanding God's standards and his design for living, but we may need to be prepared to offer a modified approach to prevention when helping those who do not share our values.

We want people to be fully aware of health risks so they can make their own choices. We want to encourage people to avoid HIV risks completely as far as possible, rather than just carry on as before with latex rubber, clean needles or bleach as partial protection. Part of teaching people the truth about AIDS is teaching them how to reduce risks. While Christians can then be accused of simply teaching people to 'sin safely', we also have to recognise the need to save lives. The key is how advice is given, placing risk reduction in the context of relationships, commitment and empowering people to make their own choices about saying no, taking a long-term view and thinking through what is important to them.

14

Special Issues in Poorer Nations

Once we become involved in developing or assisting programmes in poorer nations, we may find there are other equally complex issues and questions to face. It is not just a question of setting up community care programmes or reaching young people in schools.

For example, testing becomes vitally important in towns or villages where large numbers of all adults may carry HIV. When people realise how many of their friends are infected, they may have one of two reactions. They can become fatalistic, reckoning they may already be infected so not bothering to take precautions. Others may become very worried, wanting urgently to get hold of a test for themselves and their partners.

Pre-marriage testing—a social time bomb

Any church leader involved in pre-marriage counselling in such a situation will find couples wanting to be tested. In many countries, access to testing is very difficult with long travel to a testing centre, long delays, lost results and sometimes even doubt as to whether the result you have been given is really yours, or whether the result is accurate.

A church mission could order some of the newer testing kits which produce a result in a few minutes from a sample of blood or saliva without using costly laboratory equipment.

Prices are falling and it is likely that soon instant saliva testing kits will be available costing less than £5 each.[678] Testing should only be carried out after careful counselling, for reasons which will become apparent below. It is also important to know the limits of accuracy of these tests. Positive results may need confirmation to rule out a false positive result (see Chapter 5, p 121).

Married couples want tests too

Once testing becomes available, other problems can emerge. Married couples also want to be tested. A wife may be worried about the safety of having sex with her husband, since she is aware he has been unfaithful to her or that he had many partners before they married.

She may be even more worried when she hears that in one African country at least one in three of the women who are now dying with AIDS were virgins before they got married and have always been faithful, yet were infected by their husbands.[679]

When testing of married couples begins, it will be found that in some cases both are already infected. At least in this situation there is no risk of endangering the other person's life, although children born to the couple may turn out to be infected (see p 98).

For some couples it will be found that both partners are free of infection, but other couples will emerge where only one partner is infected. How are such situations going to be handled? Before you know where you are, a small testing programme involving fifty couples could have completely destroyed the marriages of ten of them, with partners walking out or being rejected or insisting on divorce.

So you can see that many churches and Christian groups in developing countries are sitting on a social time bomb which could be triggered by indiscriminate testing. Yet access to testing is vital to help contain spread.

Counselling before and after testing

Part of the answer is to provide careful counselling to people before offering a test, and afterwards irrespective of the result. Where one partner is infected, the advice will be to use condoms carefully every single time, recognising that there will be a small risk of an accident (see Chapter 6, p 168). Condom quality can vary in different countries and few people realise that latex rubber, as a naturally-occurring substance, tends to weaken with time so the expiry date on the packet is very important. In a country with a hot climate, condoms in storage can deteriorate quite rapidly.

There is some debate about appropriate advice to people where both partners are infected. It has been suggested that since the virus mutates rapidly inside each person, and since each time two people have sex there is a chance of a fresh inoculation, it is possible that those continuing to have unprotected sex may die more quickly. However, there is no real evidence to support this suggestion at present. It is certainly true that if other sex diseases are passed on, then the combined effect of these on someone whose immune system is already weakened could be great.

Engaged couples or those at the start of a relationship may be faced with difficult questions about their future if one tests negative and the other is infected.

Condom promotion in Africa

Africa has been targeted, as has much of the rest of the world, with the condom message, which varies in expression and emphasis from country to country. I have already challenged assumptions about condoms and safe sex in Chapter 6.

However, even if you believe condoms to be 100% reliable, there are some serious problems to be considered in developing countries: cost, distribution and culture. It is a sobering fact to realise that, as we have seen, many African nations only have less than £2 to spend on total health care for each person per year. This has to cover hospital care, clinic treatment, vaccination programmes, provision of glasses and dentistry.

Condoms can wipe out the health service

The entire health budget for a person would be used up in less than three months just in the cost of providing condoms. A couple of years ago, an international exporter faxed ACET offering us 140 million condoms at a few pence each, delivered free to any African port. The trouble was that even if we had had £10 million, the entire consignment would have lasted the continent just one night—possibly two or three—and then what do you do?

The cost of rubberising all sex in Africa would be at least £250 million a year—more than the World Health programme spends on AIDS for the whole world.

Distribution can be difficult

The distribution difficulties are even greater. Let us assume for a moment that the funds are available. We still have a problem. If you give out supplies free, experience has shown with other kinds of programmes that supplies can quickly disappear. They are often bought up quickly by traders. Supplies are hard to get hold of, and as the price rises, a limited supply becomes available again in the markets.

To get over this problem, another approach has been used called social marketing. This has been tried in Zaire. With this approach, condoms are not given away, but are made available to wholesalers and retail outlets at low cost for them to sell at reasonable profit.

Condoms are then always in the shops and markets, but at a low price. However, while this approach can work well in towns and cities, it is harder to make it work as well in rural areas. (See pp 282–284: does education work?)

A further hurdle to overcome is perhaps the most important

of all. Even if condoms are available throughout a country at low cost, people may still choose not to use them. We are assuming that this is despite a comprehensive health campaign operating at every level.

Condoms are a Western 'hi-tech' solution

Many African people live very simply. If you visit homes up country, you may find that the only factory-made item in the hut is a plastic petrol container being used as a water carrier, and a plastic washing-up bowl. There might be in addition one or two pots and pans and a few utensils. There may be a small battery-operated radio, but possibly not.

In comparison, a condom is real hi-tech: here is a very sophisticated item which is made to precision standard, yet is thrown away after each use. It requires great care in how it is put on and how it is removed, and requires overcoming possible cultural embarrassments or religious objections in order to talk about its use, or even to produce it. They need to be supplied regularly to places where nothing else is supplied, and where there may be a twenty-five-mile walk to the nearest clinic.

So then, condoms can provide excellent protection if used carefully every time, but may only be part of the answer to the explosive African AIDS epidemic.

'Condom dumping' by the West can be resented

The perceived obsession of the West with condoms has caused some ill feeling in Africa. When I have travelled or taken part in radio phone-in programmes across Africa organised by the BBC World Service, it is clear that a number are sensitive, first to being blamed for AIDS—people say it came from Africa and it is their fault.

They are also often very sensitive to 'Western imperialistic' suggestions that there are 'far too many people in Africa', and that over-population is the reason for famine.

They are especially sensitive to people who seem to have

population control as a hidden agenda in AIDS-control programmes. Many are deeply suspicious and angry when they find Western nations willing to pump millions into condom distribution, while their own governments are struggling to provide clean water or adequate food.

I am not saying that population-control programmes are necessarily inappropriate or a waste of time. On the contrary, anyone who has seen a graph of the world population will realise that current rates of growth cannot be sustained. Population control is an urgent issue. The World Bank has recently estimated that the 1990 world population of 5.4 billion (12% African) will rise by 2150 to 12.2 billion (24% African). This is even after the effects of AIDS.

It is also true that the more people there are in the world, the more conditions are set for new epidemics and plagues to evolve. As we have seen, each person represents a new chance for a dangerous new mutation to emerge. The next century will undoubtedly see further new epidemics: we can only hope that they will turn out to be as uninfectious as HIV, and less harmful.

Population control and AIDS

It is ironic perhaps that at a time when a killer plague such as AIDS is out of control, the world population should also be spiralling upwards. Perhaps that is why I have heard people dare to say that they think AIDS is a good thing to keep the population down.

When the two effects combine together, as in a country like Uganda, the end result is that population growth is slowed, while the age distribution becomes grossly distorted. The World Bank estimated that the population of Uganda (8 million adults and 8 million under fifteen in 1991) without AIDS would rise to 37 million by the year 2010.

Because of AIDS, the estimate has been revised down to 22 million—note that even this figure shows a remarkable growth of 6 million at a time when one in six of the entire country may be HIV-infected. However, when you look more closely at the forecasts, you find that the middle-age group has been decimated. The twenty- to forty-year-olds on which the future of the whole nation depends will have been severely depleted by then.

People often use Uganda as an example because it is the most open in discussing AIDS. However, other countries are at least as badly affected. Recent reports suggest similar infection rates as far south as Zimbabwe.

There is a strong link between population control politics and AIDS-prevention programmes. You must remember that African nations are largely dependent on massive foreign government handouts for AIDS. In Uganda such funding supports a major part of the economy, together with other development programmes. As you travel you notice that many of the vehicles driving round Kampala are owned and run by relief agencies.

Rich pipers call the tune

Attending a recent meeting of the World Health Organisation in Geneva I had rather a shock. As an international AIDS agency, ACET has official observer status and can take part in debates. Round the massive circle of desks and microphones were represented a large number of countries, each with four or five delegates. The scene was just like one of the United Nations meetings you see on the news. There was one big difference. Almost every delegate was white.

Most developed nations were there, but only two African nations were represented, and two from Asia. To be there and have a vote, your country needed to be a donor to the World Health Organisation AIDS budget, which of course means that the only countries deciding world policy are likely to be industrialised nations. Because Africa and the Far East would not otherwise be represented at all, the WHO agreed that each continent could appoint two representatives for free.

The results were striking. After a long discussion by nations like Germany, the UK and the US, there was a plea for realism by an African delegate. He was listened to respectfully, but the points he made were lost among the many others present. No wonder overseas aid for AIDS is so often seen as imperialistic.

Now many Western donor nations are refusing to give via WHO, preferring to give handouts direct to individual countries. In many cases this means even more nation-to-nation control, which suits the donor well. We have already seen how many countries have been reduced almost to economic servitude by the crippling burden of foreign debt (see pp 278–285: debt and other issues).

Why condom programmes look good

One big advantage of condom programmes is that Western executives thousands of miles away, with no understanding of African tribal life, can then be dazzled by graphs showing millions of condoms distributed or bought each month. They can see data showing how sales are boosted by advertising campaigns and radio broadcasts. This helps keep donor nations happy, knowing that their 'prevention campaigns' have reached millions of people (see p 284).

So condoms are not necessarily the easy answer you might think when it comes to Africa, although their use may be measurable and attractive to fund.

Despite all I have said, we must recognise their important role in HIV prevention directly and also indirectly by reducing other sex diseases which help transmission. Finally, at a time of great unsustainable population growth, condoms also enable families and nations to control fertility.

Testing can form part of the answer too, while encouraging people to be celibate or faithful. The treatment of other sexually-transmitted diseases is also important. Testing and encouraging no-risk lifestyles do not pose any difficulties for church missions, but treating sexually-transmitted diseases can raise a few Christian eyebrows.

We must treat other sex diseases

As we have seen, one reason why heterosexual HIV has spread so fast in some countries may be because facilities for treatment of other sexually-transmitted diseases are poor, increasing the risk of transmission.

In the UK there are around 580,000 new cases of sexually-transmitted diseases treated each year. Contact tracing on a voluntary basis allows previous sexual partners to be counselled, tested and treated. In many countries such programmes are very limited and sex diseases spread rapidly.

One of the most effective ways we could reduce HIV spread in developing nations might be to set up a large number of clinics to treat these other infections. For many churches this is less attractive than, say, suggesting people reduce their number of partners or abstain. Yet this is something we also need to think about.

Mission hospitals have always treated sex diseases as a normal part of overall community health care, but here we are talking about rapidly expanding the number of services as a deliberate anti-HIV strategy. Are supporters in countries like the UK going to be willing to fund such work? Will they see it as simply encouraging promiscuity—yet another example of helping people 'sin safely'?

Sex disease clinics in Christian missions

Setting up a successful service to treat sexually-transmitted disease means providing a walk-in, friendly environment where people feel very comfortable to explain what they have been up to and with whom (see p 188).

If there is the faintest whiff of moralising, then experience shows that people may stay away, defeating the purpose of the clinic which is to encourage people to come forward for treatment. This atmosphere may be difficult for many Christian agencies to provide.

Different messages for different countries?

In all our community prevention we need to take great care to find the right message for each section of our society, each tribe, each ethnic group or each country. Within each country there can be unique problems. For example, in one African nation ACET has been working with a particular tribe which has an elaborate circumcision rite using a communal knife likely to spread HIV. Radio campaigns and leaflets in tribal languages were useless in changing the practice.

The answer was to build a relationship of trust and respect with the village chief. When the delicate discussions were over, the chief called the village together and announced that the ritual would now be modified so that it was safe. The process took some time, but the practice has stopped in that village at least. The person who carried out the negotiations was a national of that country.

In another area there has been concern about a tradition that the brother of a dead man should have sex with or marry his widow. If the man died of AIDS, it is likely that the wife could pass on HIV to the dead man's brother. In each locality the way of life needs to be respected, understood and incorporated into every aspect of prevention.

In some parts of Thailand it is common for teenage boys to be sent into brothels as part of an initiation ceremony into manhood. It is also socially accepted—or even expected—that adult men will have sex regularly with prostitutes. Even with extensive government campaigns and the efforts of many other agencies such as ACET, these deeply-rooted social practices may require a generation to change completely.

In Eastern Europe, AIDS campaigns are swimming against a powerful tide of Western permissive culture, which is being sucked into former Eastern bloc countries at an alarming rate. Ever since the collapse of communism in many countries, there has been an insatiable demand for pornography and sexual freedom. While many Western nations are just beginning to question the benefits of liberated sex in the light of marital breakdown, increasing juvenile delinquency and AIDS, many East European countries are enjoying the first tastes of previously forbidden fruit.

In addition, opened frontiers and mass migrations due to economic chaos and civil unrest have accelerated spread of sex diseases such as HIV. These countries have also become major corridors for illegal drugs passing from East to West. Most early AIDS cases in countries like Romania were caused through infected blood or contaminated medical treatments, but the stage is now set for rapid spread among adults. Changing medical practice as a result of intensive training of health care workers has been far easier than changing the sexual behaviour of a whole country.

Faith—the ultimate weapon against HIV?

Whether we try to prevent HIV with condom distribution, or by encouraging testing, celibacy and monogamy, we are faced with a problem. We know education encouraging these things will have a limited effect. The reason is that most people do not want to change. Therefore the only secular motivation we can possibly provide is fear.

I have often heard AIDS educators say you must not give a negative message based on fear because it will be counter-productive (incidentally, that statement is itself a similar negative). However, the fact is that all successful health promotion works by creating anxiety about what could happen if you ignore the message.

The faith motivation is totally different and ultimately much more powerful, as social psychologists are beginning to recognise. Faith creates hope, new expectations about behaviour and gives people purpose, self-worth and mean-ing. Christians also believe that faith in Jesus Christ releases God's power in our lives, enabling us to change.

I will never forget meeting the Minister of Health of an

African nation ravaged by AIDS, who told us that although he himself was an atheist he particularly welcomed the involvement of the church in fighting AIDS. He told us the reason was that we could give people hope so they could bear to hear a painful message, and we could also give people the power to change.

Before the communist regime fell in Hungary, secret approaches were made by the communist leaders to a friend of mine who was heading up an evangelical organisation based in the UK. His work was to smuggle Bibles and other items for persecuted Christians behind the iron curtain.

The authorities asked to meet him because they needed help in dealing with a rapidly worsening drugs problem. They knew that those finding faith often came off drugs rapidly and permanently. A wonderful, low-cost, 'infectious' weapon against drugs was too good to turn down. Instead of threatening him with arrest as before, they unofficially invited him to bring others in. The gospel was proclaimed and programmes set up. They too had seen the power of faith.[680]

As Christians we can have confidence in who we are and what we stand for. We have an answer which we feel is *the* answer. We can offer sensitive, practical approaches to prevention, based on medical facts. We can also seek to influence behaviour through the rapid spread of faith in the world today. An important part of the answer to AIDS is for the church, as the most powerful organisation in the world, to combine efforts with governments and communities to help save people from themselves.

We now need to turn to an urgent question which faces every health care worker in developing countries, especially where there is a high incidence of HIV. This issue is seen vividly in the letters missionaries send home to their supporters. How can we help prevent AIDS deaths among doctors and nurses?

Missionaries die of AIDS too

I am often asked for advice by those about to be sent overseas by missionary societies. What is the risk of occupational infection?

Why some missionaries are going to die

There has been increasing concern for the health of those going out; not just from such hazards as multi-drug-resistant malaria, but also from HIV. It is true that the AIDS epidemic has serious implications for missionaries overseas, as it does also for members of the countries who are involved in health care.

The main areas of concern are from blood transfusions or contaminated equipment if the person is needing care, or from medical accidents if the person is caring for others.

Making medical treatments safer

The risks from receiving medical help can be greatly reduced with a few simple measures. First, make sure no one gives you blood from an uncertain source. People working in developing countries often make a point of finding out their blood group before they go so that another in the group can donate blood in an emergency, or so they can donate to someone else.

Many embassies operate an informal blood transfusion service in this way. Obviously just because the donor is an expatriate there is no guarantee that the blood will be uninfected unless you can trust the person's history, or a recent test result—and even that is not a 100% guarantee because it will not detect infection that has taken place in the last few weeks (see pp 120–121).

It is common for people travelling or living in high-incidence countries to take with them a small number of items for their own emergency use—needles, syringes and other items. These can be obtained ready packaged from organisations like SAFA or the London School of Hygiene and Tropical Medicine (see back of book for details).

However, if a missionary society sends someone out with needles and other items to a situation which is badly resourced, they may find that by the time the emergency comes the family has used up its precious supplies to help save the lives of others. When you are living and working alongside nationals from the country and one of them needs care, it is hard not to reach in your bag for your own supplies if you think otherwise there could be a high risk that your friend will die.

Missionaries are becoming infected at work

I received a letter recently from a missionary who explained that the senior nurse at his hospital was now dying of AIDS. She had come out from the UK some years ago and served the people faithfully, becoming infected in the process.

So what are the risks and how can we avoid or reduce them? Fortunately, the risk of infection from a single accident such as a needle jab is known to be very small—even if the person is known to be carrying the virus. Numerous studies from different countries following up people who have jabbed themselves with needles, or otherwise injured themselves while giving care, have shown that there is around a 1 in 200 chance of transmission from a single accident.[681] This is much lower than for hepatitis B, which carries up to a one in three chance of transmission.[682]

However, for someone working day in, day out as a surgeon or midwife, for example, in areas of highest incidence, the cumulative risk soon begins to mount (see pp 190–191).

Exposure to HIV is common

Even assuming your hospital has enough pairs of gloves for you to operate with a good quality pair each time, the chances are that you may tear gloves during long operations several times a week. You hope you do not cut your finger at the same time, but it happens.

In many places, doctors testing patients on their wards using reliable testing methods have found that around half of their patients are HIV-infected.[683] The percentage may be lower for surgical than for medical cases. Let us assume that a busy general surgeon tears one or two gloves each week and that once every month he cuts himself, or spray from a cut artery spurts into his eyes, or there is some other blood contamination of a wound. Let us assume that only one in four of his surgical patients are HIV-infected (it could be higher). A quarter of the time, on average, the blood could be from an infected patient.

Surgeons are working under tremendous pressures. Every time they begin an operation they know that one careless move or unexpected problem could mean HIV infection, with terrible consequences; not only for them, but also for the health of their husbands or wives, for the future of their marriages and for their families.

How big is the risk for surgeons?

The surgeon in our example will be exposed potentially to HIV around three times a year. Each time is like a pull on a fruit machine with 200 possible combinations. How long before you hit the fatal result? The average surgeon working in such an environment will be infected in sixty-six years, but it could happen in the first three months.

To put it another way: if a missionary society is supporting fifty surgeons in high-incidence countries, then it is possible that every two or three years perhaps one or two more of the team might become infected. This has colossal implications for those going out, their families, for churches supporting them and for missionary organisations.

We may debate about exact percentages, but the risk must be acknowledged. So much will depend on local infection levels, the quality of gloves, operating lights and other equipment, the skill of the surgeon and the nature of his work. Some operations are far more likely to expose a surgeon to injury than others. Some surgeons in Rwanda did their own calculations based on their own practice. They estimated that one in four of them would become infected after thirty years' operating in their town which had a seroprevalence of more than 20%.[684]

Unless those going out are tested regularly, we could have a situation arising where a significant number have become infected before anyone realises, because of the delay between the time of the accidents and the development of symptoms.

A missionary society may miss an increasing number of future tragedies by just hoping for the best. However, people might argue that once you have taken reasonable precautions, all you can do is trust God for protection and there is therefore little point in regular monitoring of infection. Even if that is so, we need to think now about our responsibility to care for missionaries who may be returning home infected and unable to carry on working as surgeons as a result. These are big issues that all larger missionary societies need to address now.

Reducing the risks to surgeons

There are a number of simple steps that can be taken to reduce risks in surgery. For example, always sewing away from your other hand rather than towards it, using blunt needles for sewing fascia or skin,[685] possibly considering eye goggles in operations where your experience is that you often get sprayed, double checking gloves before reusing them, and just being extra careful about being jabbed by splinters of bone or other sharp objects. Covering minor skin abrasions on the hands or arms with a waterproof plaster may add further protection. By following all the above, a surgeon may be able to reduce exposure by three or four times.

Perhaps if careful measures are taken, our group of fifty surgeons would only see one colleague infected every three to five years on average. These are all guesses and will depend on local factors, including the stage of illness of the patients, the nature of the operations and the skill of the surgeon. As we have seen, infectiousness increases as AIDS develops.

Testing all patients before surgery may not be helpful since the test will miss those infected less than twelve weeks ago (a lot of people in countries where HIV is spreading fast). If funds are scarce, many surgeons may prefer the luxury of a new pair of gloves for each operation.

Midwives are in the frontline too

Nurses are also very much at risk in certain situations, particularly midwifery. Some time ago I visited a hospital in one African country where a number of midwives had died from AIDS. The death toll seemed to be far higher than in nurses from other parts of the hospital, suggesting that many had been infected through delivering babies. We will never be certain, since there were no testing facilities.[686]

The difficulty for midwives is that their exposure to blood can be even greater than in the operating theatre. If labour is difficult, or if a piece of the placenta is left inside the womb, the midwife may need to have not only her hand and wrist inside the mother, but also much of her forearm. No glove covers that much, although waterproof armsleeves and gloves have been described.[687] Midwives can finish a delivery with arms completely soaked in blood. Unfortunately, in many hospitals across Africa there are not enough gloves for midwives, so many deliveries are being assisted without glove protection. Although HIV cannot cross intact skin, there may be slight cuts or abrasions on the hands, or less commonly on the arms, which can be an entry point for the virus.

Therefore if you are supporting or praying for those working as doctors or nurses in high-incidence countries, pray for their protection. There have always been risks to the health of those serving in the neediest situations. Countless missionaries have willingly laid down their lives to bring the gospel to nations where Jesus has never been known. Many have died in service, often of the very diseases they spent most of their lives treating.

Deaths of missionaries have been rarer since the era of antibiotics and other medical advances, so perhaps it is a shock to find their lives so much at risk again today. These are pressures people live with every day, alongside drug-resistant malaria and other things.

Ten ways to reduce risks in medical and nursing practice with limited resources

1. Sterilise cleaned equipment after each treatment. Use autoclaves, boiling, 70% alcohol or a freshly prepared one in ten bleach solution in water.

2. Use undamaged latex gloves for operating or midwifery.

3. Use eye shields if spray is likely in theatre.

4. Use blood transfusions sparingly.

5. Get hold of instant HIV testing kits if you have no laboratory equipment—and use sparingly when needed to help save lives.

6. Cover cuts on hands with waterproof plasters.

7. Sew away from, not towards, your other hand, using blunt needles where practicable.

8. Never resheath needles, and dispose of used needles carefully—or keep in secure safe container until washed and sterilised.

9. Use gloves for any procedure where (extensive) contact of skin with secretions is likely, including handling laboratory specimens. The threshold for using gloves will depend on availability.

10. Ensure good standards of general hygiene, with spillages carefully cleaned up.

. . . and pray.

352 THE TRUTH ABOUT AIDS

Before drawing the different parts of this book together by looking at a global Christian response to what we have seen, we need to ask one thing. What should the government be doing?

15

A Ten-Point Plan for the Government

At the end of many talks I give on AIDS, people often ask what I think governments of various countries should be doing next. Here are some suggestions. Things are moving fast and I hope that by the time you read this some of these decisions will already have been made.

1. Determine the extent of the problem

We need to get it right: governments do not have resources to squander on problems that do not exist or are being exaggerated by those with vested interests in increasing their own budgets. However, we do not have time to adjust plans if the AIDS epidemic becomes worse than estimated or changes its character in any way. For example, has education reduced heterosexual spread but not affected drug addicts? Are new HIV viruses spreading in different ways? After all, as things stand, a person infected tomorrow will probably die. *You have possibly five to fifteen years to plan his or her terminal care, but only today to prevent a death.*

All discarded blood samples from selected hospital laboratories should have identifying markers removed and be sent to public health laboratories for testing. Only the hospital of origin should be stated. Results will give an indication of spread across the country and will enable us to detect local increases. Hospitals giving cause for concern should then be asked to send regular batches of blood samples with age and sex recorded on each bottle, but no other information. The UK government has recently implemented this proposal. Uganda has completed a full survey already.

2. Target people especially at risk with further new campaigns

As we have seen, education is most effective when targeted at those most at risk. A prolonged, aggressive campaign needs to be aimed at the drug-addict populations of major cities where drug abuse is a problem. They are a prime target for HIV spread in the near future. In addition, a further hard-hitting campaign needs to be aimed at all men who have had sex with other men in the past or may do so in the future—not just at the so-called gay community. Much of the momentum for change in the gay community is coming from the coffins of loved ones who have died.

Young people also need to be targeted before they begin taking risks. It is far easier to prevent risk-taking behaviour before it becomes a life habit, than afterwards. Travellers abroad also need targeting. In some countries travellers may be several hundred times more likely to become infected from a casual sexual encounter than in a country like the UK.[688]

In the UK there has been a great debate over where AIDS should fall in the plan of teaching in schools. Should it be part of sex education—decided by parents and governors of each school with options for parents to withdraw children and for schools to teach neither sex nor AIDS? Should it be out of optional sex education and a compulsory part of the science curriculum—or is this just compulsory sex education via a back-door route? (See Chapter 12.)

In practice, while the great and mighty debate these ponderous issues, schools tend to do what they feel comfortable with anyway. The remarkable success of

ACET's schools programme reaching up to 300,000 a year shows schools do not need laws. They need practical help.

Government campaigns will be insufficient without continued high-profile publicity for a prolonged period afterwards. Education is easy. Changing behaviour is extremely difficult. Smoking kills several hundreds of thousands each year, numbers which dwarf the current AIDS problem, yet public health campaigns have taken years to produce change. Sexual drives are stronger than the power of nicotine or the needle. Only 14% of New York drug users have changed sexual behaviour, for example, while 59% are using clean needles.[689]

All educational literature should be clearly marked with date of issue and leaflets should be promptly withdrawn when out of date.

3. Get an army of health educators on the road

The economics of health education are simple in many industrialised nations: hospital costs for caring for one AIDS patient alone are so high that a health educator only has to prevent one person a year from developing AIDS to save the government or health insurance companies his entire salary.[690] If he or she succeeds in preventing one person a month from becoming infected, the government or other agencies make a fortune. (See Chapter 12.)

The argument for teaching prevention is overwhelming. After all, a human life is worth more than a few thousand pounds. From travelling around to schools and colleges myself, I am convinced that an effective communicator can save hundreds of lives a year.

One important factor has been left out of most school information packs and is also missing from youth education: the personal factor. It is almost useless for a teacher to spend an hour just telling the facts or showing a video. Young people are bored rigid with facts. Where is the action? Who is actually dying? Is anyone dying at all? 'It's all an empty scare story. I'm not gay, so I won't get it.' When I go into a school or college everyone is on the edge of their seats. Why? Because I know people personally who have died of AIDS, people who are dying right now, and I often see people who are dying of it. It is real, so prevention and encouraging positive attitudes are easier.[691]

The biggest asset an educator needs to have is the credibility that comes from personal experience. Even if only to be able to say he or she has visited an AIDS ward would be a tremendous help in earning the attention of students. At ACET, all our schools educators have worked in our national home care programme so they have a real impact in the classroom.

A lot is being done,[692] but it is not enough. An army of health educators needs to speak to all school children over the age of eleven or twelve years.[693] It needs to happen soon. This army needs to go into colleges, universities, factories, workshops, bars, clubs, pubs, leisure centres, churches, youth groups, housing projects, community centres—anywhere people congregate. Obviously they should go in with the agreement of those in charge, with a high-impact, short message—'I want to tell you about three friends of mine who have just died of AIDS. I'm telling you because the person you are sitting next to right now may well be positive and all of you here in ten to fifteen years' time may have been to an AIDS funeral—unless something changes drastically'.

4. National training programme for all health care workers

Never has there been a disease that has spread so quickly. Consider cancer care: cancer has been around for centuries, and hospices for decades. Even so, there are acute training problems to keep pace with the new hospices which are opening each year. Existing units are under strain with conflicting demands from patients and from the need to train more carers.

The explosion of AIDS cases in many countries and the rapidly-changing appearance of the disease—with new treatments and research likely to make most knowledge obsolete in a year or two—means that a vast, crash-training programme needs to be established. If every week terrorists blew up four civilian aircraft on domestic flights killing 1,000 US citizens, a national state of emergency would be declared. Why shouldn't governments treat the AIDS epidemic with the same seriousness? After all, possibly the same number are doomed every two or three days in the United States alone through new HIV infections.

In the United States, AIDS day courses for family doctors based on voluntary attendance have had appallingly low attendance.[694] Those who come are usually those most qualified, most recently informed, and least needing the training. Where is the silent majority? Nothing but regulations will ensure that all medical personnel are effectively educated, and encouraged to have a positive attitude to AIDS patients.

An hour or half a day is totally inadequate. A full day's training should be the absolute minimum for doctors and nurses, particularly in high-incidence areas. ACET has shown the value of 'train-the-trainer' programmes with health care professionals in a country like Romania.

5. Provide a network of specialist advisory teams

Governments should fund without delay full-fledged multi-disciplinary teams to advise and support health care workers in the community and various hospitals in high-incidence areas, as well as giving twenty-four-hour advice to families and friends. One aim would be to channel the latest information and techniques on treatment from research centres to those in the field. Each team could comprise one full-time doctor, two specialist nurses, a full-time social worker and an administrator. Such workers can have a remit to cover other illnesses as well, particularly in poorer nations.

6. Establish a network of hostels

Some governments need to slash through miles of red tape to allow the swift establishment of safe housing for AIDS patients who have nowhere to go, nowhere to live. Often these people are trapped in hospitals.[695] It is not unusual for a recently diagnosed person with AIDS to come back home to find his bags outside the door and that his partner has changed the locks. Urgent planning needs to be made for the hundreds of infected drug addicts who are appearing now in many major cities. Failure to provide adequate care may force many onto the streets and increase the spread of infection. Many may die of AIDS in the streets of some nations.

7. Recruit extra community nursing staff

People with AIDS are heavy users of nursing resources.

Health authorities need additional resources for community nursing that are increased in line with their numbers of people with AIDS.

8. Work in partnership with the church

The church is the largest non-government organisation in many nations and perhaps even globally. With its many different branches and groupings, it represents a massive untapped resource. In many countries the church has a long history of care provision, particularly so in developing nations.

Governments should actively seek partnership programmes. The church represents not only an effective resource organisation, but also a powerful influence for behaviour change. The essential government task is to provide overall strategy, leadership and co-ordination. We all need to work together. The problem is too great in many countries for governments or secular agencies to solve on their own.

9. Increase spending on prevention in developing countries

In an age when a traveller from the UK can be in Uganda more quickly than it takes to drive from the North of the UK to the

South, we must recognise the need to invest in international prevention efforts, even as a matter of self-interest. We cannot allow the AIDS epidemic to rage ahead unchecked. At a time when the care of one AIDS patient costs Western governments as much as an African nation spends on total health care for 25,000 people, it is obvious the worst-affected nations have few resources for prevention.

It is a scandal that in 1993 the UK government spent more on AIDS, with a tiny domestic problem (only 6,000 alive with AIDS) than the entire World Health Organisation budget for the Global Programme on AIDS. No wonder the world epidemic is out of control.[696]

10. Research into long-term relationships as well as vaccine/cure

In addition to these points, governments and international agencies need to fund further major research into vaccines, cures and better ways to prevent spread. Incentives need to be provided to encourage drug companies to direct their vast research operations towards vaccines. A comprehensive study of marriage is greatly overdue: what makes a happy marriage, how to choose the right partner and how to prevent breakdown. Results can then be fed into schools' education programmes on AIDS, sex education and marriage counselling.

How can I help turn plans into action?

The future of your own country is in your hands. You can write, phone, or otherwise make your views known to those in local or national government, to health planners and to church leaders. You can make sure copies of this book get to the right people—all royalties go to ACET. You may feel that your contribution is small and not worth much, but thousands of others are doing the same. Together we can help turn the tide and build a better place for those who come after us. We are too late to prevent a disaster, but not too late to prevent an even bigger one.

Petitions are useless in comparison to individual letters, so get others to write too. Write to your Member of Parliament or other appropriate government official. Even if not read, your letter will be counted as yet another part of a big vote on the issue. Write to TV producers who have made AIDS programmes. Commend them for good content and criticise the bad. Remember that in the past, thirty letters after a programme have been enough to influence the producers.

Write to your local legislators asking them what provisions they are making for those with AIDS. If you are dissatisfied with the reply, say so, and send copies of the correspondence to your newspaper.

Having looked at how the government can respond, we now need to return to our overall Christian vision for responding to AIDS. Is there more needed than just prevention and cure? Is there anything more we need do? Is the church in danger of just becoming an expert provider of AIDS programmes almost identical in many ways to government ones? Are we in danger of losing our way?

16

A Global Christian Challenge

In earlier chapters, we have looked in detail at how the church can care for its own members with AIDS, care in the community, save lives of young people and develop community programmes for different cultures and situations. However, we need to look again at the call of Jesus. Is this enough, or is something missing? Is this the sum total of a global response to AIDS, or is there another dimension?

Care and prevention are not enough

Many would say the work is complete. We are expressing love to our neighbour and we are also teaching people the medical facts about AIDS, so what more do you want? Surely that is more than enough?

If Jesus had just lived on the earth as a remarkable man, occasionally healing people or using his carpentry business to help people out, he would never have been crucified. If Jesus had merely mobilised great numbers of people to help the poor, to help feed the hungry, to care for those who were oppressed, he would have lived till a ripe old age.

The problem people had with Jesus was not what he did, but what he said and who he was. They loved him for what he did and hated him for what he said. Jesus said he was the light of the world.[697] John's Gospel tells us that the light shines in the darkness and the darkness has never overcome it.[698] Light is always visible, always directional. Its source is obvious, threatening to darkness. In a dark cave you can strike one match and be blinded. The greater the darkness, the brighter the light.

The darker the city, the brighter the light

Jesus said we should let our light shine so that people could see the good works we are doing and give glory to our Father in heaven.[699] Being light then is about explaining, about proclaiming, about being prophetic, about high profile. Jesus said that no one places a light under a table, but we should hold it up so the light can shine on a wide area.[700] While we are to be filled with humility, we are to take every opportunity to explain and show what God is doing so that people give honour and glory to him.

Letting the light shine

This means being happy to be known as believers, identified very publicly as belonging to Christ, willing to teach what he says. It means we welcome it when in a media-dominated world we find press, radio or TV wanting to report what we are doing, describe what we are, or broadcast what we are saying, recognising that if everyone followed a Christian lifestyle, HIV would disappear as an epidemic in thirty years.

Huge reaction to Christian view of sex

Christian views on sex can provoke a huge reaction. Recently I was approached by a major publisher and invited to submit a one-page idea for a book, challenging the supposed benefits of the 'sexual revolution', based on a survey of scientific data on AIDS, other sex diseases, and on the economic, social and psychological consequences of the breakdown of marriage and family life.

The editorial meeting rapidly became a highly-charged

debate, with passionate heated arguments over personal lifestyles and personal morality.[701] Clearly the idea had touched a raw nerve, a deeply painful area. They realised such a book would cause a massive media storm: 'AIDS expert calls for new moral code'. But they feared big publicity might not result in sales of a book 'no one will want to read'. One participant was unable to recall such a fierce and stormy debate over any other book. Another publisher took it.

Many people are very sensitive to hypocrisy, double standards (for example, church leaders falling into immorality), attempts to put behind closed doors the reality which has only recently come into the open, bigotry, lack of reasonableness, and blind negativism, which they may suspect is based on a fear of sexuality, prudery and a lack of normal, healthy, emotional and sexual development.

Some psychologists might say that the stronger an anti-Christian reaction, the more they might also suspect that deep dark shadows of latent guilt are being disturbed. In my experience, many of those who fight the most seem to be people who feel insecure and threatened by another world-view. Those secure about their own values and lifestyle are generally far more relaxed in open discussion.

Some who have rejected the Christian faith may also be angry for the guilt they still feel, blaming the church for a moral code they are unable to shrug off from their childhood. However, many Christians would argue that God's framework for living is constant and absolute, and that even without the teaching of the church there is a 'natural law' of conscience which is an innate part of every person. A sense of right and wrong is a God-given part of our being.[702]

Where is the body of Christ?

So who is the voice of Jesus today? Who are his hands and feet? No single person has the capacity to represent the heart and mind of God. We are told that together as believers we are his body.[703] That is why Jesus prayed so much that those who believed in him would be one.[704] Together we show his love, together we seek to express his voice, together we seek to present his challenge to the world and together we seek to reconcile the world to God.

That is why I am so encouraged to see God's people joining together across the nations, with barriers breaking down, whether as millions of people praying for our world as in March for Jesus,[705] or whether it is at the sharp end of providing unconditional care to those with AIDS who are dying.

Daring to be different

We are called to fight discrimination, stigma, prejudice, bigotry, intolerance, oppression, injustice and cruelty. We are to encourage love, care, consideration, compassion, understanding, responsibility, commitment, faithfulness, truth and righteousness.

Jesus promised we would be identified, targeted, challenged, mocked, misunderstood and persecuted. The trouble with the church is that so often we have deserved a rapping on the knuckles for strident moralism based only on an empty call to stand as light, without being prepared for the loving sacrifice of being salt. The more fully we represent Jesus, the more we may find that some people love what we *do*, but sometimes hate what we *are*.

Called to be wise and innocent

We need to be sensitive and wise. For example, when ACET started home care in London, it became clear from comments made by members of other groups that a number of people were hoping a volunteer would overstep the mark; that we would be 'caught' as it were, insensitively 'Bible-bashing' someone with Christian faith in the home. We acted with integrity: what we said we did in public was what we actually did in private. But we took great care to ensure this really was so (see pp 237–244, 252–256, 264–266, 386, 391–392 about appropriately meeting spiritual needs).

Criticised for being Christians

At the end of the day quality of care is critical, and so is the quality of training and prevention. If mud starts flying, you want the only accusation that sticks to be that you are followers of Jesus and have perhaps a different worldview and a different motivation.

We need to be clear about our purpose: if it is to challenge the moral climate of our nation, then we had better watch out. If this is more than just an occasional comment, we may find we have caused so many insecurities in the minds of those we care for, that they do not want us to look after them any more. It may be better sometimes to leave such weighty matters to other church leaders.

Once said, comments cannot be unsaid. Off-the-cuff remarks can be a disaster: you need expert advice from those experienced in media matters and used to handling sensitive issues as Christians in the area of AIDS.

An alternative view of AIDS

If our purpose is to present a clear, common-sense, no-nonsense independent view of the epidemic, then that is relatively straightforward. I am often asked for an accurate informed comment on AIDS by press, radio and television. People seem to want a fresh and different perspective from the rest of the AIDS industry—much of which is beginning to look very tired after years of predictable and increasingly irrelevant responses.

Jesus was always something of a puzzle: people could never quite work him out, or predict how he would respond. If we are to be his light, then we will find we are like that too. We have a God-given responsibility to contribute to public debate, just as Jesus did in his day, for example, over the emotive issues of imperial taxation and allegiance to the Roman occupying forces.[706]

In conclusion then, a growing number of believers are waking up to the explosive destruction of AIDS. They have clearly heard God's call to care unconditionally for all those who are ill, regardless of how they came to be so and to do all they can to save lives, challenging societies to think again about what is ultimately important and the future of life on earth.

Time for a confession

In many countries I believe the church needs to acknowledge its own failure to give a clear moral lead in situations where it would have been possible in the past. We need to confess our corporate neglect of the oppressed, the poor and the marginalised, many of whom have turned to dangerous lifestyles in their isolation and need. We need to confess our apathy and slowness to respond to the AIDS crisis, our blindness to the needs of other nations, and our judgemental attitudes to those outside the church, particularly in view of the frequency of divorce and sex outside marriage in many church networks and denominations.

We need to honour the work of those who have a very different worldview to ourselves who got involved years ago, starting AIDS initiatives and setting standards of excellence at a time when the church was wallowing in its own confusion as to how to respond.

Hope and comfort in tragedy

We need to recognise the part we must now play. We can begin to mobilise the vast network of church resources around the world, bringing hope and comfort at a time of terrible tragedy. We can speak of the God of love who never intended the beautiful world he made to end up in such a mess as this.

We can continue to do all we can to fight injustice, fear and prejudice. We can speak of God's purpose in creating us, and of friendship and forgiveness.

A global movement

We need to see the church's response to AIDS in the context of rapid church growth. There has never been a time in history when so many have turned to Christ each year, at a much faster rate than the growth of the population. In almost every continent of the world the church is growing rapidly, as idealism and faith in political systems have died, where in many people's lives there has been a spiritual vacuum. It is no coincidence that both HIV and faith are spreading so fast: in different ways both are temperature gauges of sick societies which have lost their way.

While HIV spread can be an indicator of the loss of traditional values that have held societies together for centuries, spiritual awakening is an indicator of recent rediscovery of purpose, meaning and ultimate destiny.

The pendulum of history is moving

The lesson of history is that fashion and behaviour both change constantly. What one generation counts odd or foolish is often seen as sensible orthodoxy to the next. The great pendulum is never still for more than a moment. It swings from side to side with unfailing regularity, surprising and shocking each generation which is ignorant of all that has gone before. It turns as it swings—tomorrow is unique.

Therefore it seems inevitable to me that we will see in many parts of the world the emergence of a new sexual culture early in the next century. Unless a widely available vaccine or cure is found fast, the effects of AIDS will be long lasting on the psyche of many of the worst affected nations, with a ricochet effect in many other countries.

Even if a cure is found in ten years, it will not be in time to prevent a scarred generation which has learned through painful experience that having multiple sex partners is an efficient way to kill yourself and those you love (see p 54).

Children born in the 1990s are inheriting a new kind of world with scarce resources, a tendency to epidemics, and with the increasing threat of organised crime, terrorism, civil wars and ecological disaster. They may see worrying pressures grow in some places for a new national, regional or world order almost totalitarian in strength, to give security in a world increasingly torn apart by market and military forces beyond the control of democratically elected governments.

In all this we are called to pray that 'God's kingdom will come and his will be done'. I believe the church needs to take hold of God's answer to AIDS with confidence; to tell people about the God who invented the wonderful gift of sex and who loves it when we love and are faithful to each other. It is time to proclaim a clear message based on facts and God's purpose for us all. It is time for us to reach out and care for those who until now we hardly realised were there.

Writing words is easy, and reading them is even easier. How are you going to respond? What is your church going to do about AIDS? Are you going to put this book away now on the shelf, or are you going to respond to what you believe God is calling you to do? For perhaps tens of thousands around the world, this is a call to move out of the secure comfort of our churches and into the problems and pain of the city, a world stricken and dying with AIDS.

You are either part of the problem, or you can be a part of the answer.

Action list

Ten things you can do in and through your church:

1. Become a link person for your church for ACET. You will be sent a special information pack, literature, prayer

requests and news about AIDS and the Christian response from around the world, and details of how your church can make a practical difference.

2. Invite someone from ACET, or a similar Christian organisation involved in AIDS care or prevention, to speak during a Sunday service.

3. Form a prayer group or add AIDS to the things your prayer group is praying about. Pray for the work of ACET and other church groups.

4. Support Christian AIDS initiatives financially yourself on a regular basis and encourage the church to do so. Remember Christian AIDS organisations in your will—have you made a will? It will probably be the biggest gift you will ever be able to make and reduces the tax liability on your estate.

5. Help promote AIDS prevention in schools and make them aware of resources available. Use the ACET schools materials, available in bulk free of charge at the time of writing.

6. Encourage your leaders to include teaching about sex and AIDS as part of the programme for adults and youth in the church.

7. Consider helping those dying with AIDS in your area, perhaps by becoming a volunteer in a Christian organisation.

8. Write to missionaries you know in high-incidence countries with words of appreciation and encouragement. Do all you can to ensure missionary societies you support are resourcing their work properly in the light of AIDS, and make sure your church is supporting its overseas workers properly.

9. Hold a fund-raising event—it will educate people and help the cause.

10. Lend your copy of this book to a friend or a church leader—or buy one to give away. All royalties go to ACET.

APPENDICES

APPENDIX A
How Many People Need Help in Your Area?

So how do people get the facts they need to decide if there is justification for a home care team? Here is an approach I have found helpful.

1. National annual infection figures. These will show the current situation and how quickly things are changing. The figures will only reveal the numbers known to have tested positive. An adjustment needs to be made for those who have not been picked up through testing, who may have no idea they are carrying HIV. In many developed countries it is probably reasonable to multiply the figure for known HIV infection by two or three to obtain an estimate of the total infected.

In developing nations a World Health Organisation or government estimate is often available.

2. National annual figures for AIDS cases, particularly the number of new cases of AIDS reported each year and the number of deaths. Figures for the last eighteen months are usually incomplete due to some reporting delays or missed deaths—up to 80% of AIDS deaths are missed in some developing countries. These omissions may be offset to some extent by those diagnosed incorrectly as having AIDS who are ill or dying for other reasons.

One can tell roughly how many are alive with AIDS at any given time by subtracting total AIDS deaths from total AIDS cases.

3. For each person alive with AIDS there will be at least one other unwell with early HIV illness.

4. In many countries around 25% of those unwell with AIDS are likely to be at home at the moment, experiencing sufficient problems to need intermittent or regular support in order to enjoy a good quality of life at home.

5. Around 12% of those unwell are likely to need care at home this week.

6. Around 2% of those unwell are likely to need daysitting or nightsitting or other intensive help at home.

These are rough estimates which help give me some kind of feel for a particular area—even if the numbers need adjusting due to local factors. The calculations are based on a developed country and need reworking for particular situations in other nations with the assistance of local experts.

Example (using approx figures from March 1994). Adults:

1. Number known to be infected in UK:	21,718
Estimated total infected:	30,000

2. Total UK AIDS cases to date less deaths
    = numbers alive
    New diagnoses average 150 per month
    Deaths average 100 per month
    Increase in numbers alive 50 per month
	3,000

3. Total (est) with HIV illness 3,000 3 2 5	6,000
4. Total (est) ill at home needing practical support—even if only from time to time	1,500
5. Total needing help this week	750
6. Total needing daysitting/nightsitting etc this week	125

Local example:

One can make a rough calculation of the numbers needing care locally by going through the same process as above but with local figures, or by just working out more simply that there are, say, 2% of all AIDS deaths in a given area each year, so take 2% of all figures above, eg:

Total needing practical support:	30
Total needing help this week:	15
Total needing intensive help:	2–3

Offering care to those who need help

If there are no other services available (in the UK we would need to include community nurses, social workers, care assistants or those from other voluntary or statutory agencies who are providing help) then you can see that a small group of, say, thirty volunteers with a part-time co-ordinator, could provide a useful service in such a situation.

However, that assumes of course that every person in need knows of the service and how to contact it, and also that every person wants it involved.

In some countries many of those needing help have their needs met already from existing services. Some of the remainder may also prefer for the moment to struggle on without help, or they may be hidden as 'missed cases'. For all these reasons it is essential to know who else is in the field.

Estimates may be altered if a new AIDS programme is begun, or if government or development agency spending on AIDS changes. This can be particularly difficult to predict.

To estimate hospice needs it is perhaps reasonable to calculate that for each person needing intensive care at home there may be a need for another to be cared for in a hospice, or in a hospital with an emphasis more on symptom control and emotional support than on diagnosis and active treatment.

Also remember children: by 1 February 1994 in the UK, for example, there were 354 reports of confirmed or possible HIV infection in those fourteen years or under who were still alive, with 110 AIDS cases.

APPENDIX B
Setting up Community Care

This brief outline is a summary of some of the lessons learned by ACET home care teams in various places, but particularly drawing on the experience of the UK. Many of the principles are important in different situations, but all need adapting to one degree or another to each situation, particularly in developing countries. This cannot in any sense be regarded as a blueprint for success. Clearly the best resource of all is likely to be ongoing personal contact with those who have experience of setting up and running similar projects locally.

In whatever country ACET has operated there have been a number of general principles found to be helpful. Some of these apply not only to community care, but also to prevention or training:

1. Church backing

In most countries we have found the first move has come from national believers. This is certainly the case in the UK, where in many towns and cities people came to us with a desire to respond practically to AIDS.

In Uganda the first visit took place as a result of an invitation by a particular church to help them in the fight against AIDS. Through that contact, meeting many other leaders and returning a second time with the international agency TEAR Fund, a series of local initiatives was begun, working alongside local churches in an equipping and facilitating role.

Each country is different however. In Romania, when the communist regime fell and borders opened, the churches were overwhelmed by the immediate needs and the problem of adjusting to freedom after severe persecution. There was little creative energy left to consider starting AIDS projects, yet HIV education was necessary in churches as in the rest of the country.

ACET was approached by the Romanian government and UNICEF to

376

help as an international agency. While ACET staff in Romania were members of the Romanian churches, and while the Romanian Evangelical Alliance endorsed the work, it was left to ACET to get on with it. Now the emphasis is beginning to change, with hopefully an increasing sense of ownership by local Christians.

We have found that in general the greater the church backing, the stronger the programme is likely to be. However, the backing ideally needs to be across a number of different church groupings, or the work may be hindered by sectarian interests.

We might ask if local leaders share and own a common vision. When starting a new home care service in a town or city in the UK we have been particularly concerned about local support for staff and volunteers. Becoming deeply involved in the lives of those who are dying with AIDS can be very costly and painful.

It is always more traumatic to look after young people who are dying, and with AIDS most are young. While there is often a richness and a personal growing in those who are caring, there is always grief as the person dies. We have found that support is essential, practically and pastorally. It can be more difficult sometimes in a big city like London, than perhaps in a place like Brighton where the team is smaller and there is a greater sense of support from one or more larger churches.

2. Communication with others

Sometimes we have had to learn the hard way that people like to hear in advance of new ideas or projects rather than afterwards, or just the week before. Consultation and communication are very important.

3. Clarity about motives

We have needed to be clear about our motivation—to honour Jesus by working together, laying down the temptation to build an empire or to be sectarian. The alternative is isolation.

Because our motives are broader than our own personal work, we will want to work together if at all possible. Our prayer is for God's kingdom to come and for his will to be done across the whole town, the entire city, the region, the nation, the continent, the world, so we need to work together.

4. Working together

Sometimes we have found our ability to work together has been hampered by incidentals. For example, in the London office there are many staff from differing church backgrounds. An act of corporate worship has sometimes created tensions because there are represented different styles and personalities of churches which together form the rich tapestry of church tradition and life.

When a project draws together churches locally there can also be other issues, such as church structure or recognition of leadership, which can make unity difficult. For example, in one country there is very limited recognition of the role of women in positions of responsibility. This has sometimes made the role of female trainers more difficult.

The two pillars of a Christian response, unconditional care and effective prevention, respecting and upholding the historic teachings of the church, are ones that the vast majority of those from different denominations can unite over. This has been one of the most exciting things about ACET's work since we started. Christians who could never work together in any other context are working happily side by side, discovering a new vitality and dynamism in the process.

5. Partnership and parallel programmes are both valid

We have found that sometimes it is right to work separately—but in parallel, not in competition. There are good reasons for this when the nature of the work is distinct.

The Salvation Army and TEAR Fund

The Salvation Army is a magnificent organisation second to none in pioneering compassionate care throughout the world, together with the proclamation of the gospel. The Army has a great number of AIDS initiatives and ACET enjoys a good working relationship with them. We may be in partnership over some joint projects in the future, yet the organisations will always be separate.

TEAR Fund is the fifth largest overseas development agency in the UK, with programme assistance in over 100 nations, working through churches. ACET is working in partnership with TEAR Fund in several different countries, joining expertise and resources to further God's work. Partnership allows us to help get the job done more quickly and more efficiently, and speaks of unity and co-operation.

Sometimes we have found that one area of activity can affect another adversely, so it has seemed wise to separate or to keep separate. An example could be a group of people within a care agency whose vision is primarily to lobby parliament on various issues. Campaigning can confuse and damage care. Better to encourage those who campaign to join a campaigning group.

6. A need to ask whose needs we were meeting

Another question we have had to ask is: Whose needs are we meeting? We needed to be brutally honest: our needs, those in the church, service planners', or those with AIDS and their carers? It is so easy to start a project feeling we have something to offer, rather than because there is proof of a real need.

From time to time people in the UK have written to us offering redundant church property which they hope will be useful for those with AIDS. Unfortunately so far the places have been in the wrong parts of the country or unsuitable for various reasons. Yet when it was suggested that the property be sold and the proceeds used to purchase a suitable property in the right area, the answer was always no.

Whose needs are we meeting? What are we creating? Are we just growing our own empires or are we primarily concerned to meet the needs of others? Often buildings have limits on use and disposal created by ancient trust deeds. This is an area the church needs to look at urgently.

In the UK we have a large surplus of underused or disused church buildings costing millions to maintain, while we have desperate needs for other kinds of buildings in other places—or even in the same areas. This is particularly true with church-planting initiatives such as Dawn 2000, which is hoping to establish 20,000 new churches by the year 2000 in the UK alone.[707]

7. We needed to be sure a specialist team was justified

We have had to get an accurate picture of what local needs are before progressing with service plans. So often I have heard people say that there must be a local problem so they are setting up a small programme to help— or they think ACET should do so. The trouble is that the size of the problem may be too small to justify a specialist AIDS team. For example our own research suggests there are few areas in the UK where new teams are needed at the moment.

8. We needed to be clear why we were expecting people to come to us for help

We have needed to ask a further question: Why should people come to us for help? People with AIDS are often extremely cautious about offers of assistance—one breach of confidentiality could result in loss of job and home within days. It could also result in intimidation, death threats, or even attempts at blackmail.

People who work in sex disease clinics, on hospital wards or in social services may feel they are taking a big risk with their own reputations in referring people to a Christian agency. How are we going to prove our credentials? People with AIDS often know each other well and are part of social networks, so good news and bad can travel very fast. People vote with their feet. We have found that if we have cared well for one or two, it is very likely that others will begin knocking at the door.

Overcoming doubts when first starting up can be hard and can take time. It has been helpful to form a larger network with a track record, although a service working well in one town, city or country has not always guaranteed acceptance in another.

9. Grants and equipment loans have been important

In the early days of ACET Home Care, we found the best way to win trust fast in a new area was to make available small hardship grants to help with things like heating bills, bedding and telephone installation. These things do not cost a lot, yet can be real lifesavers. They are also low-risk requests for the referrer. When a service is getting off the ground and is unproven we have found it is often easier for people to ask for grants than to ask for volunteers.

Grants and equipment loans speak louder than any words or literature about a commitment to people with HIV, and have been helpful in building relationships. Referrers or recipients have often come back and asked for additional help.

Telephones are lifelines

We have found that telephones are very helpful when caring for people at home. If someone who is dying at home has no phone there are three problems. First, the person cannot call for help. Secondly, if there is a volunteer in the home and the situation deteriorates, the volunteer has to leave the home and go looking for a vacant phone box in working order, which is often difficult in a crisis. Thirdly, it is impossible for people to phone in, either as a routine check to see how the person is, or to communicate a change in plan.

In some countries such telephone access may be impossible or too costly, resulting in a need to visit more frequently. It is then even more important to try to place your office where the telephone exchange is reasonably reliable. This means that if someone has gone to enormous time and trouble to try and phone you then they are likely to get through.

Practical help louder than words

Grants need to be set up carefully so that sufficient information is obtained without being intrusive, to ensure the person qualifies, ie they have serious HIV illness and practical needs which they cannot meet from their own finances.

We have found it essential to verify diagnosis, as it has not been unknown for people to pretend they have HIV or AIDS in order to claim benefits, or for other reasons including a desire for attention. Verification is difficult without risking breach of confidentiality. We developed a special two-part form with the diagnosis confirmed only on one section with a unique number on it. If the form is opened or lost in the post, confidentiality is still preserved.

10. We need to listen to those who are ill

We need to take every opportunity to listen to those who are ill with AIDS. People with HIV who are well also have important perspectives, but those who are most ill will have had the greatest insight into practical problems.

As we have seen, caring for the carers is a vital part of helping someone ill at home. If carers become exhausted and cannot manage any longer, then there may be a crisis. We have needed also to listen to what their needs are, since they also need our support.

Long before ACET starts in any new area, we begin by researching needs and talking to others already involved. This informal survey is vitally important. We have a flexible approach so that as the service evolves we continue to learn more about what we need to provide. The day we stop listening is the day the service will begin to die.

I cannot emphasise the listening aspect too much. As medical director I took particular time in the early days to ask the people we were caring for what they thought about the service. Did what we were offering match what we were actually providing? What should we be offering in addition?

Twice recently ACET has carried out a formal postal survey which was made anonymous so that answers could not be traced to individuals. The results have been essential for our own planning and service development, but also for communicating to those who fund us—what better way to convince people of the value of our service?

User groups can give misleading views of those dying

User groups with committee meetings and other forums can tend to provide a distorted view of the needs of those who are dying. This is because they are likely to be dominated by the voices of those who are least exhausted and ill. Yet it is precisely those who are least able to get out of bed and attend meetings whose views we most need to hear.

Of course if we had been providing a different kind of service, for example a drop-in counselling and advice centre, then a regular meeting of users would have been invaluable.

11. We have needed to be ready for opposition

Whenever we have begun to talk about a new service we have found there are reactions. Some have welcomed us if they also recognised the need and saw the beginnings of an excellent team. Others have been opposed if they thought we might be in competition with what they were already doing, or with their future plans.

Our surveys of unmet need have sometimes been incorrectly perceived as a criticism of what others have been doing. Surveys can cause big problems if they show that there is no effective service provision despite all the funds received to provide care.

In many towns and cities in industrialised nations we have to face the fact that when members of the gay community were ready and willing to get involved in supporting those with AIDS, the church was nowhere to be found. There has therefore been a natural suspicion at times of this new-found enthusiasm. Will it last? What is behind it? Do we want them? Will they get on with us? Do they understand us? Will they compete for funding? Will they wreck all we have set out to do?

Coping with different agendas

While Christians are often accused of prejudice, it is also true that those who say they are opposed to prejudice are often very prejudiced themselves against Christians. In other words they may have a fixed view of what our service will be like, and that view may be very negative.

Some groups already in existence may have a hidden agenda. For example, an AIDS group that began as part of a local gay phoneline may well see part of its mission to fight anti-gay prejudice and to encourage acceptance of gay lifestyles as normal, including in schools.

These secondary aims may be seen to be vulnerable if a Christian group like ACET seems to be muscling in, especially if they find most of the support is drawn from churches that would be very traditional in their views on sexuality. They may suspect, rightly or wrongly, that just as they have a hidden agenda to promote gay rights and lifestyles, we may be wanting to promote Christian morals or to evangelise.

There is no easy way to overcome these things. The key is always relationships and discovering a common concern for those ill with AIDS. We hope and pray that when we meet representatives of other groups there is mutual liking and respect. Although there are areas where we would take a different approach, we can still be united in a common goal, which is to help provide the best possible support for those ill with HIV and AIDS.

12. Defining service limits

Limiting what is offered at first

In the mid-1980s a great flurry of secular AIDS projects were set up in the UK, many poorly researched and badly run. By 1988 there were over 300 separate initiatives, many of which have since collapsed. In contrast, ACET started in 1988 as a co-ordinated network of local initiatives, each well researched and well managed. As we have seen, ACET has grown rapidly in response to almost overwhelming demand.

One of the reasons for success (apart from the sovereign grace of God) is that after much prayer and careful research we felt it right to restrict severely what we were going to offer and where we were going to provide help. The alternative is to be drawn into many different areas with few resources or without specialist know-how.

It is so much better to say we will only be able to meet certain needs because of limited resources, and to state clearly what they are. We can always offer extra help if other needs arise. Much better to do it that way round than to promise more than we can reliably deliver, creating an image we cannot live up to and blowing away our reputation. Our service definitions describe the kind of support available, what area we are covering, and how ill someone has to be.

13. Making it easy to get in contact

It has been important to make it as easy as possible for people to contact ACET services. Nothing is more frustrating than wanting to get in touch urgently and getting an answerphone or no answer at all. Message machines are a wonderful help to those receiving calls, but are no help for those phoning in who may be out themselves later, or may be using someone else's phone. Sick people can't wait. If we cannot receive the call quickly we could find the person we have been helping for months to stay at home is suddenly in hospital, because someone was worried, could not get through and took the person to hospital.

An ideal service provides a telephone number as an out-of-hours contact point, possibly using a radio paging system if available. Most people become ill and need help outside of the forty hours of a normal working week for the simple reason that a full week is 168 hours long, so a service that only answers the phone during office hours only provides 25% cover. A service where the phone is only answered for two out of five days a week is only covering one hour in ten.

In practice, however, twenty-four-hour access is very costly in time and effort, unless provided for a large number of people at home over a large area. A radio pager means the person on call does not need to sit by the phone. It also means that person can be contacted when out visiting someone else.

We have found it is perfectly in order to provide an out-of-hours telephone advisory service, backed by volunteers who can be asked to provide extra help if needed. Even in London, where we are covering up to 240 people with our on-call service twenty-four hours a day, it has been very unusual for the person on call to need to visit.

14. Training people to turn up on time

When someone ill with AIDS has only a week or two to live, he or she does not want to waste half a morning waiting for someone to turn up. As people become weaker, their world becomes smaller. The room or home becomes the world. Time takes on a new significance and things that would previously have appeared trivial can become overwhelmingly important.

If it takes you an hour to wash and dress and you want to be dressed for a visitor, you may begin to think about getting ready two hours before the person is due to arrive. As the hour approaches you may be sitting thinking about the visit—hopefully looking forward to it. If the person is ten minutes late you can easily become convinced that he has got lost or has forgotten. After an hour you may be feeling exhausted, having now been up for three hours. You may want to get back into bed again. The trouble is that getting back into bed, after making a drink and going to the toilet is probably going to take you another half an hour. And then the person arrives.

We emphasise in training that people should never be late by carelessness or thoughtlessness. If someone is made late by incident or accident, and the person with AIDS has a telephone, we try to phone immediately. It is better to be ten or fifteen minutes later still, but to arrive and find someone settled at the other end who has been able to use the time to do something else.

15. Teaching people about servanthood

When we go into a home we do so to provide an extra pair of hands or feet to the person who is ill. We go in on the person's own terms. When someone is very ill or vulnerable, it is easy to want to take over, to make decisions, move the furniture about, call the doctor or clean the kitchen. In all these things we need to be sensitive. For example, the person may genuinely prefer that we do not do the washing up because he or she is unable to face the thought that we need to do it.

Sometimes there is a time and a place for confronting a situation gently, if failure to do so is going to have grave consequences in the future. We were involved in caring for a mother recently with three young children. What was happening was so painful to her that she found it almost impossible to think about the future. We had to ask her to think about it and to make some decisions while she had the strength to do so. As a result, she was then more settled, and the children were later cared for as she wished.

It is our privilege to help. We need to be flexible. Someone's condition can change for the better or worse quite rapidly. The priorities of the person and his or her feelings about things can also change.

16. Taking care about image

The public perception of any service is important. We have needed to think about image. Promoting a new service has meant having a first-class piece of literature to hand out and to give to people after we have met them.

We have found it helpful to have something short and easy to read for people who are ill and those who care for them, and some kind of a brochure explaining in more depth who we are for those who want to know. In the church it is common to spend many hours praying and planning, and a lot of money on buildings or people, but very little of either when it comes to literature.

Credibility and relationships are important, so it has been helpful to list names of key supporters whose association has provided security for users and funders alike. Sometimes this has been difficult because the name of a particular person on the list has been attractive to church supporters while being controversial to other agencies, or the other way round. The answer has been a large list which is broadly based. The list has been quite separate from the management committee, trustees or board, all of whom share the same faith and values enabling us to maintain distinctives with unity.

17. Investing in volunteers

An organisation run or supported by volunteers should be just as professional and well-organised as a well-run government agency. Co-ordinating offers of help without chaos has required great skill, dedication and hard work. We have not always managed it.

Selection

Careful selection of volunteer workers has been essential. In the UK we have found a detailed questionnaire, given to all enquirers, to be helpful. What motivates them? Seeking to work out problems of their own? Guilt? Confused sexuality? Homophobia? Recent unresolved grief? Do they think they might be infected themselves? If so, are they going to be able to cope when seeing people with AIDS die? What are they hoping to achieve? What will they find most rewarding? What will they find most difficult? Do they have adequate support at home or will partners and friends be antagonistic? Is there any church support? Does the volunteer have a church commitment?

Someone once said to me that all she wanted to do was to 'get onto an AIDS ward and tell them all about Jesus'. The trouble is, if she had found her way onto a volunteer programme (as she might have if selection procedures were sloppy), in five minutes she could have destroyed five years of goodwill, making it almost impossible for any Christian organisation to continue working in that area. In many countries people are sensitive, and rightly so, to someone coming in and 'Bible-bashing'. It only takes one insensitive, over-zealous person to damage a whole organisation. There is a right time and a right place.

The important thing is to be a servant. If someone asks us why we are doing what we are doing, there may well be the opportunity to share the hope that we have. However, we would be crazy if we thought a medical agency was going to refer people with AIDS to us for help if we abuse that position of trust by preaching or moralising. We would destroy the credibility of the service. The behaviour of volunteers should be just as professional as hospital staff.

References from employers, ministers or church leaders are important. All these form the basis of a preliminary interview. We always delay a final decision on accepting a volunteer until after they have completed training. Our hope is that those who emerge as unsuitable during training will gradually recognise this without us having to reject them. Some people are unsuited to visiting those who are very ill. It is helpful for them to have the chance to come to this conclusion themselves. Even if they are not able to help as home care volunteers, they will often be well placed to help in other ways as a result of being trained.

It can be hurtful and distressing to someone to find they have not been accepted. It is vitally important that we are clear with people from the start about how selection and training is carried out so that there are no misunderstandings later. Sometimes people ask why they have been turned down. Our policy has always been not to disclose the reasons, as this may in fact give more offence—nor do we usually give reasons why job applications have been unsuccessful. We have had to have a standard policy for all.

Volunteers are as important as paid staff

Somehow there is the notion that because someone is offering free time without asking for a salary, it is rude and offensive to turn the offer down. However, we have always taken the view that a volunteer in the home has a role at least as important as a paid member of staff. Therefore we do not just want to increase numbers of volunteers; we are also looking for the very best and most suitable people we can find.

Whether or not to accept someone can be a hard decision. Clearly things may have emerged during small group training which may raise a question-mark. For example, if the person has recently been bereaved, there is a danger that he or she will find it hard to cope when confronted so soon by others who are dying.

A volunteer who is ill may also find it hard to cope. I am not saying that people who are ill with cancer, AIDS or other conditions should be turned down. I am suggesting that it may be unhelpful to send in a volunteer who in fact may need support later on from the very person they are meant to be helping. We always need to remember whose needs we are supposed to be meeting.

We also have to think about the psychological effect on someone who is visiting day after day a person who is now dying of the same illness they themselves have. In a cancer hospice we would, I think, take great care before appointing a new ward sister or doctor with terminal cancer. I expect we would suggest he or she found a job in a specialty that did not face them with their own disease every day. Clearly each person needs to be considered individually, but we do need to think these things through.

Sensitive questions

Many AIDS organisations in different countries have faced near collapse as a result of selectively recruiting staff and volunteers with HIV or AIDS. We need to take care if we want to have an organisation which is still going to be able to care effectively in the future. Some ask if it is our policy to ask about HIV infection or sexual orientation at interview. We ask about neither of these. HIV is a personal and confidential matter. Sexual orientation is irrelevant in giving care, or in living the Christian life. Lifestyle, however, *can* be an issue, depending on the situation.

There may be doubts over a potential volunteer's ability to cope in the home when faced by death, about their reliability, their emotional stability or the degree of support at home or from their church—perhaps they do not even belong to one. If someone at home is deeply hostile to those with AIDS we may suggest the person waits a little before going ahead as a volunteer. Support from those at home is very important.

Another question we need to ask is whether the volunteer is the sort of person we want to represent our service in the community. What is the person like under pressure? How is the person likely to respond to sensitive situations? For most people who are ill, or for their carers, their impression of ACET's service will be made by their impression of the volunteer.

When the pressure is on it is tempting to accept all kinds of offers, but ultimately it may damage the service. The ideal volunteer is the sort of person we would be keen to employ if the person was available and we had the funds.

Training and sending

Most people with AIDS in the UK are well informed about their condition—they have to be with so much misinformation and ignorance around. Training needs to cover a broad range of medical facts about AIDS.

It is rude, insensitive and unfair to send in a volunteer who is ignorant about the disease. Training therefore includes not only clear factual presentations, but also opportunity for people to work through hidden reactions to homosexuality, fear of dying and fear of disease.

Facts can be communicated formally or informally in large groups or small. However, we have found small groups are the best forum in which to cover such things as death and dying, grief and loss, and sex and sexuality. Reactions, responses and prejudices also need to be explored. People need to be familiarised with the drugs culture where relevant, and the need to understand how to prevent cross-infection. Videos can be an excellent way to open up issues and to stimulate discussion. ACET has used videos in small group training since the earliest days. One-to-one counselling is sometimes necessary following a group session, together with church-based pastoral support and prayer.

Support

A useful part of ACET's training programme is developing friendships between volunteers and existing team members. The work is stressful. It can be harrowing to visit someone a few hours before death and spend time with them as they pour out their anger in the face of doctors' false promises, dead hopes and dashed aspirations. It can be hard to stay with someone who keeps asking, 'Why me?'

It can also be very difficult to support someone with a major psychological disturbance due to HIV damage to the brain (encephalopathy). The person may be withdrawn and deeply depressed, or wildly elated, overactive, with torrents of continuous speech, unpredictable and uncontrollable to the point of putting himself at risk. The person may be confused, forgetful and disorientated.

It can be distressing to be with a dying person for several hours and have to leave, knowing that they may then die alone. It can be particularly difficult when someone dies who has become quite a close friend through several months or even years. Grief is a reality and is part of the cost of what we do.

Support is essential: a network of caring relationships between like-minded people who have experienced similar things and can understand. It is good to encourage local church support, and volunteers to pray for each other.

Communication

We have found it is important that volunteers report back after visits, unless they are routine—for communication and for support. It is also important that arrangements for future visits are made with the office, not with individual volunteers, for two reasons. First, so the office knows what is going on, and secondly to prevent undue pressures on one person.

It is hard to say no when you are in a home and someone needs more things to be done, or another visit. Volunteers are by their very nature people who like to say yes, and they need to be protected. If an individual is becoming quite ill, we have found it is helpful to ensure the person is known to several volunteers so that the load can be shared among a number of familiar faces.

Co-ordinators can usually spot a volunteer who is getting out of his or her depth or is becoming over-involved to the detriment of personal well-being.

Volunteers cost money

Volunteers are not free: they are expensive to train, and take time to book in and out, and time to support. In some countries where many live at a subsistence level, the whole concept of volunteers needs adapting. If people are helping us instead of growing food then we need to help them in return.

Even in industrialised countries volunteers are usually only able to commit themselves for a limited time. Each year we have to train some to replace those who have moved on in addition to those needed because the service is growing.

Continuity of care can also be more difficult to provide using volunteers if round-the-clock help is needed. Over a weekend, for instance, it would be unfair to ask the same volunteer to stay in the home for more than one night, or for more than half a day. Therefore we could end up having to use up to twelve different people in three days alone.

Employing care assistants can be a way of reducing that number considerably. ACET has always been fortunate in having a number of medical students, nurses in training, people training for the ministry and others from overseas who are keen to learn by spending up to three months with us. They also make an enormous contribution in return for some formal teaching and training. In addition, they go back as a new resource to their communities and countries; some to set up their own services.

Volunteers need careful organising, and finding suitable volunteers available at short notice can be difficult—especially for daytime requests. ACET tries to match volunteers to tasks and people. Volunteers vary a lot in what they are able to do and in whom they are good at relating to.

ACET has had to keep quiet about the location of different offices because they are not geared up for drop-in callers—and it is important to avoid the possibility of being broken into, with the threat of harassment or blackmail of those whose names and addresses are taken. In the UK we have used PO boxes extensively for these reasons.

The sorts of things volunteers do

This depends on experience, personality and availability. Each volunteer has special potential which needs to be harnessed creatively. A nurse provides a different type of help from a builder.

Shopping, laundry, gardening, cleaning, cooking, walking the dog, mending things around the house, driving a person to and from clinics, and being a good friend are important ways to serve any sick person. A good attitude is that of a servant, basically saying, 'I am here. I am available now and at these times in the future. What can I do that would be helpful?' Suggest some things that you would be willing and able to do.

Sometimes it has been helpful just to have a volunteer sit in the home to allow a friend, partner or relative to go out. The carer may feel trapped, unable to leave the room or the house with a sick person needing constant attention. After a while exhaustion sets in. Sometimes the main carer may have taken so much time off work already that a job may be in jeopardy. Nightsitting is also important when the person is weak or afraid.

Some guidelines given to ACET volunteers

1. Communicate with others frequently.
2. Always be utterly reliable and punctual.
3. Respect the privacy of the person you are visiting. It is his/her life and home.
4. Remember that touch is important and that a hug can mean more than a thousand words.
5. Be sensitive to the needs of the patient.
6. Be careful not to overstay your welcome.
7. Be a servant, caring unconditionally in a non-judgemental way.

---

17. Careful about counselling

People I talk to often think first about setting up counselling services. This is probably because in each country infection precedes illness so the first needs are often to support those who have recently discovered they are infected.

However, I will never forget one of our first patients who said he felt he was being counselled into his coffin, and described how a counsellor had arrived for a weekly chat. After he had gone the ACET volunteer arrived. The person with AIDS lifted up the sheets and smiled. Underneath he had been lying in his own faeces for several hours, unable to tell the counsellor because of his embarrassment.

The volunteer cleaned him up and helped him have a bath, changed the bedding and took it to the laundry. Sometimes actions speak more than words. Words and a listening ear can cost less than getting your hands dirty—although it is also true that sometimes we can hide from harrowing conversations by making ourselves busy.

There are many forms of counselling: pre- and post-HIV test, bereavement, anticipatory grief and so on. Counselling is very important but there are often many other agencies willing and able to provide such help. Counselling is also a sensitive area, since Christians may wish to provide directive counselling, helping people find faith in God or to follow Christian lifestyles, while those wanting help may be looking for a non-directive approach.

Because of all these sensitivities, ACET has tended to steer clear of a formal counselling role, particularly in the UK. Emotional support, however, is an integral part of caring for those ill or dying, whether making a cup of tea, holding someone's hand or just being there to listen. The companionship of a sensitive person can make all the difference to those coping with grief and loss.

APPENDIX C
Professionally-Based Home Care

You may be intending to set up a home care team following the Christian care principles outlined elsewhere, or you may be involved in a team already. Here are some brief thoughts on the structure and function of successful, rapidly-growing, professionally-based teams, based mainly on my experience of the ACET home care team in London, of working at St Joseph's Hospice and as part of the Community Support Team at University College Hospital. As with the notes on setting up community care, these perspectives will need careful and sensitive adaptation to your own situation.

My definition of professionally-based care is care with a component provided by health care professionals, such as nurses, doctors or social workers. Since the key here is to cover medical problems, the role of nurses or of a doctor is critically important. This kind of care is very expensive in comparison to just using volunteers or paid care assistants, but is in my view essential in a team of any size.

Our primary aim is to provide whatever people need in order to have a good quality of life at home and to live and die well. A strong team will be able to fill from its own resources most of the major needs people have. The exact role of the team may vary according to the person and what else is available, but we are there as a back up, an insurance policy, a safety net to help fill gaps as far as we can. A large team without any professional involvement is going to be unable to help if someone is deteriorating at home with medical problems, such as uncontrolled symptoms or infections.

In London our role has been to support and enhance what other health care workers are doing, not to take over. Therefore although there is a small element of doctor cover for the team we do not prescribe medication, just as we do not provide community nursing. Occasionally those guidelines are broken for a particular reason at a particular time—usually because of an unexpected crisis—but it is the exception.

Our aim is redundancy. In theory the need for specialist teams should grow less with time if the teams are doing a good job—even if the problem is growing. As we help other care workers gain experience in HIV we hope that problems like the relief of pain can be dealt with increasingly by them. We want to normalise HIV so that those with AIDS are integrated into all the normal channels of health care. There will always be a role for specialist advisors in the community in helping sort out the more difficult problems, available on a twenty-four-hour basis.

In some countries this approach may be impossible due to cultural factors or lack of other resources. The principle still applies that wherever possible I believe our long-term aim should be seeking to integrate HIV care into whatever other services exist. This will give the greatest benefit to those with AIDS by reducing marginalisation and offering the widest choice.

Communication and planning

The two greatest keys to successful care are communication and planning. Therefore the most important event of the week is the team meeting when staff members discuss each person they are caring for. The central record must always be the patient's notes (or client if you and they prefer this term).

It is vitally important that in addition to a full account of past history, medication, treatment, social situation, insight into diagnosis, list of main problems and list of others involved, there should be a log of every contact. This is best maintained in the form of a diary. The log is to enhance care but will also be a great help in recording workload for funders.

Each time someone is telephoned or visited, or there is some other communication, it should be logged in the notes by the person concerned. Notes should be written up at the time or immediately following a visit. It is much better to have the notes open with pen in hand ready to write when sitting down to make important telephone calls. When things get busy, people are tired, and emotions run high with many dying, it is easy for things to slip and for important facts or requests to be forgotten.

The test of good records

The test of good notes is that somebody should be able to be on call over a weekend having just come back from holiday—with the minimum of handover time. If someone calls, the person covering should be instantly in the picture just by opening the notes. They should know exactly what is happening and be able to give exactly the right input.

Effective team meetings

During the meeting each care worker brings the team up to date with any changes and plans for future action. New referrals are also presented and discussed. A well-run team meeting will create discussion so that problems and concerns can be shared and solutions found. It is essential for the health of the team that all members feel they have a special contribution to make. It is therefore an opportunity to affirm and encourage people in their different roles.

It is easy for a two-tier team membership to develop, where the professionally trained members are responsible for care and the care assistants are being used as nothing more than full-time volunteers. This is always likely to damage team spirit and care, because nurses will tend to be overburdened while others are likely to feel undervalued.

In my experience, those who have professional training can oscillate at times from thinking their training is hardly being used and their qualifications are being wasted, to thinking that you have to have letters after your name to do anything other than menial tasks. The truth lies somewhere between the two, and an effective team meeting can enable safe delegation with effective oversight.

Sorting out a growing caseload

People cared for can be grouped in three ways: those who are quite ill and need regular nursing advice and support in addition to practical help, those whose condition is stable and whose needs are mainly practical, and those who are reasonably well at the moment and who do not need help this week or next.

The sickest patients need nurse supervision of care, preferably with each nurse having his or her own group of people to look after. Those needing only practical help can be delegated to a care assistant to look after. The care assistant ideally will work very closely with the nurse who did the first assessment, reporting back anything new which might indicate a further professional visit is necessary.

A simple checklist can be drawn up for a care assistant to use when visiting. It might cover some standard enquiries about new or existing symptoms, changes in medication and changes in mobility. Change is the key. Is the pain the same one you have always had, or is it new? The cough which started last week and which was assessed by the doctor at the hospital, do you think it has got better or worse?

Short-term placements

People joining the team on short-term training attachments are also an invaluable resource. Training requires investment on our part, so we want to make the most of their contribution; not just using them for driving or cleaning. Medical students on electives may be close to qualifying and may be very helpful in some reassessments, or in liaising with other health care workers or agencies.

Nurses and doctors on short-term placements can also play an important role, recognising that their lack of specialist knowledge may limit their symptom-control advice, as well as their ability to network with other agencies to build a package of care. In that context we also need to make sure we are using the professional expertise of some of our volunteers. Sometimes our own professional pride can prevent us from fully using the resources God has given us in our staff, our volunteers, or from other sources.

Why fill gaps that others can fill?

One rule when making assessments is that we ourselves never provide what can be found elsewhere. Often we find that a massive list of needs compiled during the first visit can be almost entirely met from other sources. Our main role may be as co-ordinator or organiser of care, backed by a twenty-four-hour call out facility.

However, a word of warning is needed. Never assume that what is promised by others is actually being delivered. Recently the London Home Care team carried out a survey of symptoms in patients whose clinical monitoring was supposed to be fully covered by others. We all had something of a shock to find how many we were caring for had uncontrolled symptoms such as pain, diarrhoea, nausea, vomiting or itching. In some cases all treatment options had already been offered and refused, or had been tried with limited success. However, in a number of other situations we found there were urgent steps which needed to be taken.

Be clear about active or palliative plans

One of the problems of coping with advanced HIV at home is that many symptoms can only be alleviated by diagnosing and treating an underlying infection—a process which may require hospital admission. However, if we are not careful we can move to a situation where whenever a new problem emerges the person goes back to hospital, eventually to die there.

We have seen earlier how pressures are growing for legalised euthanasia, driven in part by the AIDS lobby. Those pressures are magnified if the response to every new problem is active treatment. Gradually the person with AIDS accumulates more and more chronic conditions, each of which produces a number of unpleasant symptoms which may or may not be controllable. There must come a time for each person when further active treatment is questioned, with the alternative being partial treatment at home (say with antibiotic tablets but not with intravenous therapy), or symptomatic treatment only.

Ideally then everyone in the team meeting will have some notes in front of them of people they feel responsible for and will be presenting to the others. Each week some notes will be passed across to others as the person's needs are reclassified. Only those requiring active input soon need to be discussed each time (in London this might be half of those on the books). The remainder who are 'low dependency' do need monitoring, perhaps with a monthly phone call.

If you just wait for people to contact you again you may find people have died with all kinds of problems that you knew nothing about. This is particularly true for people referred too early when they do not really need care. Although we say they can ring us any time they feel the situation has changed, in practice many may feel a slight hesitation. They may have had high expectations before our first visit, and a feeling of disappointment, or even of being let down, when we told them they were not really suitable yet for our involvement.

Recording team decisions

When discussing each person's care in the meeting it is important to record decisions made. Three important things need to be noted on a regular basis: main problems, agreed action to be taken, and likely problems in the future. The latter is very important. How is the person going to die? Where is it likely to happen? Is that what the person wants? What is likely to be the next problem we face along the way? How are we planning to meet this? AIDS is an uncertain illness and it is easy to be lulled into a false sense of security by someone who looks reasonably well today. A recent survey showed that half of all those referred to London Home Care were dead in fewer than twelve weeks.

It is important to record team decisions in the notes, possibly in a different colour so they can be clearly found among the log of other entries.

All team members including care assistants should be writing in the notes, including short-term secondments. This ensures the record is complete, and also sends out a further message that their contribution is an essential part of the care.

Allocating discussion time

A well-run team meeting will allocate time wisely with a gentle but firm leader, ensuring that those discussed at the end of the meeting are not skipped over, and that longer is spent on those with complex problems. Time also needs to be given to support for team members when care has been traumatic, to discussion of new referrals and to a review of recent deaths. It is important to look back. We cannot go on caring for large numbers of the dying, forgetting about them the moment the funeral is over.

Care 'post-mortems' can be a deeply meaningful part of a team meeting. They can be a time when hopefully we can pat each other on the back and tell ourselves we did well. They can also be a time when we comfort each other because we feel, for reasons possibly out of our control, that things turned out badly.

This might be true for someone who died unexpectedly quickly, or where support in the home collapsed towards the end and the person ended up in hospital when they wanted to be at home. Sometimes there are lessons to be learned. Did we communicate well enough with others? Could we have anticipated the need for extra symptom control over the weekend? Sometimes symptoms can be severe and very difficult to control. The problems can be far more complex to manage than in the cancer patient.

Adjusting structures

With a growing caseload, the structure of the team may need adjustment. This should be done in a way which maintains a sense of family, continuity of care and a feeling of stability. If the caseload is too big to handle in one group, a large number of people may have to sit through a never-ending list of reports. Tiredness results, and discussion can become almost impossible due to time constraints. We have faced this recently in London.

A growing team may need dividing into two sub-groups which are reasonably self-contained, but providing on-call cover for each other, and care for each other. Inter-team communication can be maintained by continuing to base all members in the same offices, and by having the two care meetings overlapping by an hour so that all are aware of those who are most ill or who are likely to call.

Providing care for the carers

In Chapter 10 we looked at how important it is to care for the carers: others in the home on whom the person who is ill depends. However, adequate team support is also essential. This needs to happen on three levels. First, by friendship between team members, caring for each other and praying together. Secondly, by those responsible for the oversight of the team, preferably people not involved in the day-to-day running, who meet with the whole team and with individuals as needed. Thirdly, by the churches that team members belong to. Sometimes it is hard to unravel personal needs from home, and needs arising from the strains of the work.

One thing is clear: terminal care of any kind is draining and traumatic. There is a cumulative load with time. Emotional survival in the longer term may require a degree of emotional detachment and breaks from close involvement with certain individuals.

Recognising the roots of anger

Anger can be a real problem in any team caring for the dying. Anger, as we have seen, is often close to sadness and tears. It is often a defence mechanism. Therefore we can expect to find a lot of angry feelings emerging in those visiting people at home. The trouble is that anger can destroy a team if the reasons for it are poorly understood.

Sometimes anger among a group can be directed at some unwitting outsider, whether senior management, a person from another agency or a representative of local government. While this may act as a relatively safe outlet as far as the group is concerned (because it is better than attacking other group members), it can still be very damaging. It can also create tension between people who are trying to support the team from outside and team members themselves. Distancing can then create further resentment and difficulty.

Preventing burnout

The answers to preventing unbearable stress and burnout may include giving people extra time off—especially after an 'important' death or a busy weekend on call—redeploying them for a while into other areas of work, taking steps to reduce caseloads by recruiting more staff or by reducing service levels, providing a listening ear, encouraging local church support by contacting leaders, and finally sometimes by helping someone see the need to have a complete break by getting a different kind of job for a while.

As with anger from those we care for, the issues raised must always be taken very seriously, and be responded to quickly. Nothing is more infuriating than to be told the reason you are so upset is because three of your favourite patients died last week. Those who are doing the caring are at the sharp end and deserve every ounce of support and encouragement we can give them. Just as with carers in the home, it may be more helpful to roll up your own sleeves and get involved than just sit and listen (see p 401).

Everyone can help

There have been times of particularly great pressure when almost every member of the ACET staff in London has given time to help in the home, including our accountant, educators, secretaries and members of the executive team. The boost to morale is out of all proportion to the level of the contribution. We are in this together. Caring for people in desperate need at home is what we are all about. It sharpens all we are doing in prevention. As a byproduct, extra staff involvement ensures that we are all in touch with the heart of our work.

And finally . . .

Just to show you how complex home care can be, here are just a few of the issues raised during a single team meeting recently:

Clients' forgetfulness (leaving taps or gas on or cigarettes burning—one person we cared for in Scotland died in a terrible fire); incontinence; verbal abuse of volunteers and staff by emotionally disturbed clients; difficult symptoms (pain, itching, diarrhoea, loss of sight); volunteer helper upset by very explicit pornography on walls (change person going in?); chaotic client not keeping appointments—visits cancelled at last minute, sudden discharge from hospital, rapid deterioration at home; massive skin infections (herpes); multiple drug-resistant TB; home intravenous infusions, eg glanciclovir; total parenteral nutrition (feeding via a vein); children about to be orphaned; fostering; client terrified of death; homelink telephones (pendant around neck to press in case of fall or emergency); six people died at home or in hospital this week; eight more referrals to see . . .

APPENDIX D

Burnout among AIDS Care Workers —How to Spot it, How to Avoid it

'Burnout' is a loose term used to describe what happens to some people in the caring profession when they have given out too much for too long, have become too drained and have been lacking support, quality time off and opportunity for understanding.[708]

It starts when a warm caring person begins to distance himself or herself from people, in order to gain protection from further suffering. The person may become profoundly depressed, bursting into tears for little apparent reason, taking time off work, sleeping badly, not coping at all. Over-involvement is another danger sign. When a volunteer is asked to go in from 10.30 to 12.30 to help with housework, but regularly stays at the home until 11.00 pm, I would say that volunteer is a good candidate for burnout.

Now there are times when we all switch off. But if I burst into tears at the scene of a major car accident I would not be much use as a doctor. As a medical student I used to faint at the sight of blood and sometimes I still do, but I have to harden myself in order to get a job done. Nor are we emotionally capable of identifying fully with every person's suffering. Jesus was able to—and is able to now—but we are more limited. Dame Cicely Saunders, founder of St Christopher's Hospice, once said that the most important thing you can ever give your patient is your tears and the knowledge that you will miss him when he is gone. That is true. Tears are a part of my life as a member of a home care team and a part of my life as a leader of a church. If we cannot laugh and don't know how to cry, then what are we made of? The shortest verse in the Bible is this: 'Jesus wept.'[709] He was grief-stricken.

However, there are times when I need someone to point out danger areas. I remember when working at St Joseph's Hospice in Hackney, I was looking after a young woman who had shown great courage over many months with

401

pain that was sometimes very hard to relieve. After much suffering she developed a pneumonia. I prescribed antibiotics and was confronted by the ward sister whom I respected enormously. She felt strongly that I had made the wrong decision. I backed down only after the intervention of a senior medical colleague. Eventually I realised that I was too emotionally involved with this patient to be capable of any rational decisions regarding her treatment.

The patient was a very strong character who had often been hard for us to care for, but over time I grew fond of her. Having wished sometimes that her suffering would end, I now found myself unable to let go and let her die.[710]

In actual fact, as in so many of these things, I do not think antibiotics would have made any difference—she was very near death and deteriorating rapidly. I found the whole thing very distressing. Now if that sort of thing was happening two or three times a week, you can see that in a month or two I would become emotional jelly. Should I have not cared about her? Not at all. But let us care for each other, care for the caregivers, listen to each other, protect each other and share the load.

Support teams crack up and pack up with monotonous regularity due to lack of care and personality clashes. Together we can avoid these things.

APPENDIX E
HIV Prevention Objectives (US and UK)

The US Public Health Service HIV infection prevention objectives for the year 2000:[711]

- the confining of annual incidence of diagnosed AIDS to no more than 98,000 cases (from an estimated 44,000–50,000 in 1989) and prevalence of HIV infection to no more than $800/10^5$ (from an estimated $400/10^5$ in 1989);
- a reduction in the number of adolescents who engage in sexual intercourse and to increase the number who use condoms (for example for young women aged 15–19, by their partners, from an estimated 26% in 1988 to 60% in 2000);
- increasing the number of iv drug users in treatment or who use clean equipment;
- increasing the provision of counselling on HIV and STD prevention, the proportion of services that screen, diagnose, treat, counsel and provide partner notification services, the provision of education in schools and colleges, and the number of cities providing outreach programmes.

Similar goals for prevention of HIV are included in the UK 'Health for the Nation' document.[712]

HIV/AIDS and sexual health (UK)[713]

- To reduce the incidence of gonorrhoea among men and women aged 15–64 by at least 20% by 1995 (from 61 new cases per 100,000 population in 1990 to no more than 49 new cases per 100,000).
- To reduce the percentage of injecting drug misusers who report sharing injecting equipment in the previous four weeks by at least 50% by 1997, and by at least a further 50% by the year 2000 (from 20% in 1990 to no more than 10% by 1997 and no more than 5% by the year 2000).
- To reduce the rate of conceptions among the under 16s by at least 50% by the year 2000 (from 9.5 per 1,000 girls aged 13–15 in 1989 to no more than 4.8).

APPENDIX F
Checklist of Countries[714]

Some people still think you can only get infected with HIV if you are in the United States, Europe or Africa. However, almost every country in the world is affected. The update of these figures since the first edition in August 1987 and again in 1989, 1990 and 1993 has been an alarming and depressing task. African countries are reporting huge increases as are those in Western Europe. Figures in Western Europe have increased more slowly than predicted in 1987.

Please note that the following figures show only those cases of AIDS reported up to January 1994. Figures are in reality often much higher due to unwillingness of governments to admit the extent of the problem, and failure of each government's information agencies to hear about many who have died. Numbers in themselves do not reflect the size of the problem in any country, and need to be seen in the context of the size of the country. The Bahamas, for example, have only reported a few cases. However, its total population is tiny, giving a high rate. Remember to multiply any estimate by between two and five to give total numbers of people who are actually ill (early disease). See also graphs and tables in Chapter 1.

The current global situation of the HIV/AIDS pandemic[715]

As of January 1994 851,628 cumulative AIDS cases in adults and children have been reported to WHO.

WHO estimates that over 3 million cumulative AIDS cases have occurred to date. This estimate is based on the available data on the distribution, spread and penetration of HIV throughout the world, and is consistent with the effect of under-diagnosis, under-reporting and delays in reporting of AIDS cases. Again as a consequence of such reporting biases, whereas 50% of *reported* AIDS cases are from developed countries, about 75% of all *estimated* AIDS cases are from the developing world.

405

In the developing world, two-thirds of all estimated AIDS cases to date are thought to have occurred in sub-Saharan Africa. However, HIV infection trends have been rapid in South and South-East Asia, with over 2 million cumulative HIV infections estimated to have occurred to date. The January 1994 worldwide total exceeded 14 million adults HIV-infected since the pandemic's start, with an additional 1 million or more HIV-infected children. The distribution of adult HIV infections in other regions of the world is as follows: Australasia over 25,000; East Asia and the Pacific over 25,000; Eastern Europe and Central Asia about 50,000; Latin America and the Caribbean about 1.5 million; North Africa and the Middle East over 75,000; North America over 1 million; Western Europe about 500,000. The unstable political, social and economic environment in Eastern Europe and Central Asia suggests that the evolution of HIV/AIDS in that part of the world may potentially be rapid; current estimates are based on relatively limited data. AIDS rates per 100,000 below are 1992 (highest only).

Country/Area	Rate per 100,000	Number of cases	Date of report
Africa			
Algeria		138	31.03.93
Angola		608	26.05.93
Benin		566	10.12.93
Botswana	28.9	439	22.12.92
Burkino Faso	11.2	2,886	31.12.92
Burundi	27.4	7,225	10.12.93
Cameroon	11.3	2,870	10.12.93
Cape Verde		143	10.12.93
Central African Republic	13.5	3,730	30.11.92
Chad		899	31.12.92
Comoros		3	31.05.93
Congo		5,267	31.12.92
Côte d'Ivoire	28.3	14,655	19.02.93
Djibouti	33.3	355	09.06.93
Egypt		64	09.06.93
Equatorial Guinea		31	31.05.93
Eritrea		372	31.12.92
Ethiopia	6.6	8,376	30.09.93
Gabon	14.1	472	10.12.93
Gambia		240	10.06.93
Ghana	16.3	11,044	30.04.93
Guinea		397	31.12.91

Country/Area	Rate per 100,000	Number of cases	Date of report
Guinea Bissau	11.2	288	20.12.92
Kenya	36.6	38,220	09.07.93
Lesotho		219	31.03.93
Liberia		28	30.09.92
Libyan Arab Jamahinya		10	09.06.93
Madagascar		4	31.05.93
Malawi	51.6	29,194	28.08.93
Mali		1,479	31.03.93
Mauritania		40	31.12.92
Mauritius		16	01.02.93
Morocco		145	09.06.93
Mozambique		737	30.04.93
Namibia		311	31.03.90
Niger		795	31.12.92
Nigeria		552	31.12.92
Reunion		65	20.03.92
Rwanda	37.5	10,138	10.12.93
Sao Torno and Principe		12	31.03.93
Senegal		911	31.05.93
Seychelles		1	30.04.93
Sierra Leone		95	31.05.93
Somalia		13	09.06.93
South Africa	1.7	1,803	01.02.93
Sudan		727	09.06.93
Swaziland	18.4	248	19.01.93
Togo	18.3	1,953	02.03.93
Tunisia		136	09.06.93
Uganda	22.3	34,611	01.11.92
United Republic of Tanzania	15.5	38,719	07.01.93
Zaire	3.0	21,008	10.06.93
Zambia	14.0	29,734	20.10.93
Zimbabwe	79.0	25,332	30.09.93

Americas

Country/Area	Rate per 100,000	Number of cases	Date of report
Anguilla		5	31.03.93
Antigua and Barbuda		6	31.12.90
Argentina		2,767	30.06.93
Bahamas	103.7	1,329	30.09.93

Country/Area	Rate per 100,000	Number of cases	Date of report
Barbados	29.4	397	30.09.93
Belize		53	30.09.92
Bermuda	29.8	215	31.03.93
Bolivia		60	31.03.93
Brazil	6.5	43,455	02.10.93
British Virgin Islands		6	31.03.93
Canada	4.6	8,640	30.09.93
Cayman Islands	23.5	15	31.12.92
Chile		723	31.03.93
Colombia		2,957	30.09.92
Costa Rica		470	31.03.93
Cuba		168	31.12.92
Dominica		12	30.06.90
Dominican Republic		2,179	30.09.93
Ecuador		253	31.03.93
El Salvador		470	31.03.93
French Guiana		232	30.09.90
Grenada		35	31.12.92
Guadeloupe	14.0	353	31.03.93
Guatemala		434	31.03.93
Guyana		359	31.03.93
Haiti		3,086	31.12.90
Honduras	13.4	2,865	30.06.93
Jamaica		576	30.09.93
Martinique	12.6	237	31.03.93
Mexico	3.5	16,091	30.09.93
Montserrat		1	31.03.93
Netherlands Antilles and Aruba		110	30.06.92
Nicaragua		39	31.03.93
Panama		460	31.03.93
Paraguay		56	31.03.93
Peru		614	31.03.92
Saint Kitts and Nevis		38	31.03.93
Saint Lucia		49	31.12.92
Saint Vincent and the Grenadines		49	31.03.93
Suriname		128	31.12.92
Trinidad and Tobago	21.2	1,404	30.09.93
Turks and Caicos Islands	40.0	25	31.12.92
United States of America	24.8	339,250	30.09.93

Country/Area	Rate per 100,000	Number of cases	Date of report
Uruguay		359	31.03.93
Venezuela		2,342	31.12.92
Asia			
Afghanistan		–	09.06.93
Armenia		2	31.12.92
Azerbaijan		–	31.12.92
Bahrain		11	09.06.93
Bangladesh		1	04.06.93
Bhutan		–	04.06.93
Brunei Darussalam		2	19.12.91
Cambodia		–	01.04.93
China		11	26.10.92
Cyprus		24	09.06.93
Democratic People's Republic of Korea		–	04.06.93
Georgio		3	31.12.92
Hong Kong		63	26.09.92
India		495	30.11.93
Indonesia		31	04.06.93
Iran (Islamic Republic of)		60	09.06.93
Iraq		13	09.06.93
Israel		234	31.03.93
Japan		543	17.02.93
Jordan		27	09.06.93
Kazakhstan		–	31.03.93
Kuwait		8	09.06.93
Kyrgyzstan		–	31.12.92
Lao People's Democratic Republic	1	31.03.93	
Lebanon		44	09.06.93
Macao		4	26.09.92
Malaysia		83	31.03.93
Maldives		–	04.06.93
Mongolia		–	04.06.93
Myanmar		133	30.11.93
Nepal		18	04.06.93
Oman		29	09.06.93
Pakistan		26	09.06.93

Country/Area	Rate per 100,000	Number of cases	Date of report
Philippines		92	05.05.93
Qatar		34	09.06.93
Republic of Korea		13	30.04.93
Saudi Arabia		50	09.06.93
Singapore		58	23.04.93
Sri Lanka		24	04.06.93
Syrian Arab Republic		21	09.06.93
Tajikistan		–	31.12.92
Thailand	1.2	3,001	30.11.93
Turkey		99	31.03.93
Turkmenistan		1	31.12.92
United Arab Emirates		–	09.06.93
Uzbekistan		1	31.12.92
Vietnam		–	07.04.93
Yemen		2	09.06.93
Europe			
Albania		–	31.03.93
Austria		943	30.04.93
Belarus		8	31.03.93
Belgium		1,364	31.03.93
Bulgaria		18	31.03.93
Croatia		49	31.03.93
Czech Republic		36	31.03.93
Denmark		1,182	31.03.93
Estonia		2	31.03.93
Finland		128	31.03.93
France	7.3	26,970	30.09.93
Germany	2.1	10,447	30.09.93
Greece		757	31.03.93
Hungary		120	30.04.93
Iceland		26	31.03.93
Ireland		334	31.03.93
Italy	6.6	18,832	30.09.93
Latvia		4	31.03.93
Lithuania		3	31.03.93
Luxembourg		62	31.03.93
Malta		27	31.03.93
Monaco	25.9	24	30.09.93

Country/Area	Rate per 100,000	Number of cases	Date of report
Netherlands	3.1	2,783	30.09.93
Norway		319	30.04.93
Poland		137	30.04.93
Portugal	2.5	1,575	30.11.93
Republic of Moldova		2	31.03.93
Romania	1.7	2,545	30.11.93
Russian Federation		127	31.03.93
San Marino		1	30.09.92
Slovak Republic		6	31.03.93
Slovenia		25	31.03.93
Spain	8.7	21,205	30.09.93
Sweden		817	31.03.93
Switzerland	6.8	3,415	30.09.93
Ukraine		14	31.03.93
United Kingdom	2.2	9,025	31.03.94
Yugoslavia		268	31.03.93
Oceania			
American Samoa		–	18.11.92
Australia	4.0	4,258	09.11.93
Cook Islands		–	31.03.93
Federated States of Micronesia		2	01.09.92
Fiji		5	05.04.93
French Polynesia		30	12.03.93
Guam		14	23.03.93
Kiribati		–	11.03.92
Mariano Islands		4	20.05.93
Marshall Islands		2	26.05.93
Nauru		–	17.12.91
New Caledonia and Dependencies		22	26.08.92
New Zealand	1.6	413	30.09.93
Niue		–	14.05.93
Palau		–	15.10.92
Papua New Guinea		47	31.03.93
Samoa		1	18.02.92
Solomon Islands		–	15.04.93
Tokelau		–	18.02.92
Tonga		4	15.03.93

Country/Area	Number of cases	Date of report
Tuvalu	–	22.11.90
Vanuatu	–	01.05.93
Wallis and Futuno Islands	–	24.05.93

Distribution of estimated cumulative HIV infections in adults (Africa, 1992)[716]

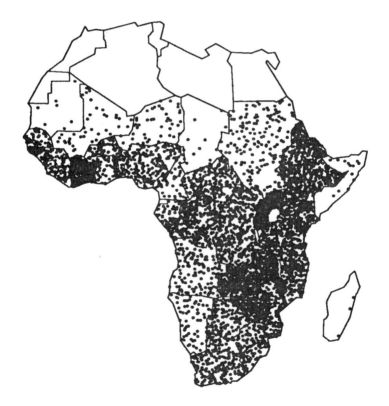

Estimated global distribution of cumulative HIV infections in adults, by continent or region (mid May 1994)[717]

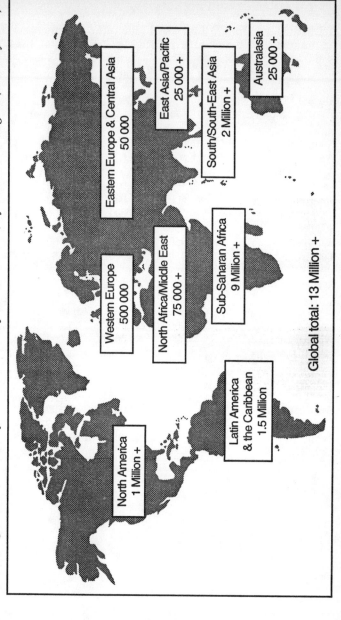

Eastern Europe & Central Asia
50 000

East Asia/Pacific
25 000 +

South/South-East Asia
2 Million +

Australasia
25 000 +

Western Europe
500 000

North Africa/Middle East
75 000 +

Sub-Saharan Africa
9 Million +

North America
1 Million +

Latin America
& the Caribbean
1.5 Million

Global total: 13 Million +

Global estimates and projections

Compiled by the Global AIDS Policy Coalition (Dr Jonathan Mann of the International AIDS Centre at Harvard School of Public Health). The figures give estimates and projections for HIV infections and AIDS for 1992 and 1995.[718] Estimates are higher than WHO figures.

Region	HIV infections			
	1992		1995	
	Children	Adults	Children	Adults
North America	16,000	1,167,000	29,000	1,495,000
Western Europe	8,000	718,000	19,500	1,186,000
Australia/Oceania	500	28,000	1,000	40,000
Latin America	40,500	995,000	84,000	1,407,000
Sub-Saharan Africa	969,500	7,803,000	2,030,500	11,449,000
Caribbean	16,000	310,000	37,500	474,000
Southeast Asia	24,000	675,000	72,500	1,220,000
Elsewhere	1,950	103,000	5,500	183,000
Total	**1,076,450**	**11,799,000**	**2,179,500**	**17,454,000**

Region	AIDS			
	1992		1995	
	Children	Adults	Children	Adults
North America	9,000	257,500	21,000	534,000
Western Europe	4,000	99,000	12,000	279,500
Australia/Oceania	200	4,500	500	11,500
Latin America	21,500	173,00	56,000	417,500
Sub-Saharan Africa	520,000	1,367,000	1,338,500	3,227,500
Caribbean	8,000	121,000	23,500	121,000
Southeast Asia	9,500	65,000	40,500	240,500
Elsewhere	800	9,500	2,900	36,500
Total	**573,500**	**2,018,500**	**1,494,900**	**4,918,000**

APPENDIX G
Organisations

This is a very incomplete list; a fuller list in any country can be obtained by contacting some of the organisations below. Inclusion in this list is not necessarily a recommendation. There are a very large number of Christian AIDS programmes across the world, many of which are small, linked to existing church initiatives or missionary agencies. Some organisations listed here are secular, with a different worldview.

ACET (AIDS Care Education & Training)
  PO Box 3693, London SW15 2BQ. Tel: 081–780 0400. Fax: 081–780 0450. ACET is a Christian national and international AIDS charity with the following objectives: (1) To develop appropriate local responses to the global problem of HIV/AIDS. (2) To provide professionally-based practical home care to men, women and children at home with HIV/AIDS-related illnesses, irrespective of race, religion, lifestyle or any other factor. (3) To reduce the number of new infections through professional training, education and awareness initiatives.

African Medical Research Foundation (AMREF)
  PO Box 30125, Nairobi, Kenya.

AHRTAG (Appropriate Health Resources and Technology Action Group)
  1 London Bridge Street, London SE1 9SG. Tel: 071–378 1403.
  Useful publications, information consultancy and annual directory of training courses in community health.

AIDS Intercessors
  c/o Joy Thomas, Midcroft, Chorleywood Road, Chorleywood, Herts WD3 4EU. International network of praying groups.

Association of British Insurers
  Education Liaison Officer, 51 Gresham Street, London EC2U 7HQ.
  ABI/ACET schools booklets and teacher packs available free at time of writing.

415

British Medical Association
  Tavistock Square, London W1. Tel: 071–387 4499.
Body Positive
  51b Philbeach Gardens, Earls Court, London SW5 9EB. Tel: 071–835
  1045. Many services including drop-in centre, counselling, support groups.
Bureau of Hygiene and Tropical Diseases
  c/o CAB International, 56 Queen's Gate, London SW7 5JR. Tel: 071–225
  0069. Fax: 071–589 3861.
  Caroline Akehurst will advise on a wide variety of very useful AIDS
  bulletins.
CARE (Christian Action, Research and Education)
  53 Romney Street, London SW1P 3RF. Tel: 071–233–0455.
  Christian campaigning and care group.
CASA (Christian AIDS Service Alliance)
  PO Box 232, 77 Washington DC 20026. Tel: 410–268–3442.
  International Christian Association of AIDS initiatives. Literature,
  networking.
Crusaid
  1 Walcott Street, London SW1P 2NG. Tel: 071–834 7566.
  To raise and distribute funds for the support and care of people with
  AIDS/HIV.
CHESS (Community Health Support Services)
  Department of International Community Medicine, Liverpool School of
  Tropical Medicine, Pembroke Place, Liverpool L3 5QA.
  Advice on setting up programmes, writing proposals and evaluating
  projects.
Christian General Store
  2130 Fourth Street, San Rafael, California 94901, USA. Tel: 0101–415–
  457–9489.
  Excellent list of Christian books and videos on AIDS, mainly for US
  market.
Christian Medical Fellowship
  157 Waterloo Road, London SE1 8XN. Tel: 071–928 4694.
  Has a growing range of AIDS booklets.
Christians in Education
  16 Maids Causeway, Cambridge CB5 8DA. Tel: 0223 66225.
ECHO
  The Joint Mission Hospital Equipment Board Ltd, Ullswater Crescent,
  Coulsdon, Surrey CR3 2HR. Tel: 081–660 2220.
  Supplies for missions.
Evangelical Missionary Alliance
  Whitfield House, 186 Kennington Park Road, London SE11 4BT. Tel:
  071–735 0421. Association of many UK mission societies.

Grandma's
  PO Box 1392, London SW6 4EJ. Tel: 071–731–0911.
  Christian agency providing support for families affected by HIV/AIDS.
Health Education Authority
  Hamilton House, Mabledon Place, London WC1H 9TX. Tel: 071–383 3833.
International Planned Parenthood Federation (IPPF)
  PO Box 759, Inner Circle, Regent's Park, London NW1 4LQ.
Links International
  Oasis House, Essex Road, Chadwell Heath, Romford, Essex RM6 4JA.
  Christian relief and development agency.
London Lighthouse
  111–117 Lancaster Road, London W11 1QT. Tel: 071–792 1200.
  A residential and support centre for people affected by AIDS which provides an integrated range of services.
London School of Hygiene and Tropical Medicine
  Keppell Street, London WC1. Tel: 071–636–8636.
Medical Assistance Programme (MAP International)
  Box 50, Brunswick, Georgia 31520, USA.
  Christian development agency.
Mildmay Mission Hospital
  Hackney Road, London E2 7NA. Tel: 071–739 2331.
  A Christian charity providing residential/palliative care and day care.
National AIDS Helpline
  Tel: 0800 567 123.
  AIDS helpline for UK.
National AIDS Trust
  6th Floor, Eileen House, 80 Newington Causeway, London SE1 6AS. Tel: 071–972 2845.
  Promotes voluntary activity across a number of AIDS programmes.
Pan-American Health Organization
  525, 23rd Street, NW, Washington DC 20037, USA.
  A health resource centre for the Americas.
Panos Institute
  9 White Lion Street, London N1 9PD. Tel: 071–278 111.
  An AIDS and development information unit for developing countries.
Salvation Army
  101 Queen Victoria Street, London EC4P 4EP. Tel: 071–236 1403.
  Large network of AIDS programmes in churches.
Save the Children Fund (SCF)
  17 Grove Lane, London SE5 8RD.
SCODA (Standing Conference on Drug Abuse)
  Waterbridge House, 32–36 Loman Street, London SE1 OEE. Tel: 071–928 9500.

Co-ordinating body for non-statutory services; giving advice on referrals, training, funding, producing leaflets and conferences.

TALC (Teaching AIDS at Low Cost)

PO Box 49, St Albans, Herts AL1 4AX. Tel: 0727–53869.

TEAR Fund

100 Church Road, Teddington, Middlesex TW11 8QE. Tel: 081–977 9144.

International Christian relief and development agency.

Terrence Higgins Trust

52–54 Grays Inn Road, London WC1X 8JU. Tel: 071–831 0330.

Offers counselling, support groups, helpline, legal advice, health education and volunteer projects.

Tropical Child Health Unit

Institute of Child Health, Guilford Street, London WC1.

Resource centre on all aspects of community health.

UNICEF (United Nations Children's Fund)

UN Plaza 4/1234C, New York 10017, USA.

Large range of resource materials, journals and books. Regional offices provide advice on all aspects of child health care.

Voluntary Health Association of India

40 Institutional Area, South of 11T, New Delhi, 110016, India.

World Health Organisation (Global Programme on AIDS–GPA)

Avenue Appia 1211, Geneva 27, Switzerland. Tel: 010 41 22791 21 11.

Co-ordinates global HIV/AIDS prevention and control programmes.

World Health Organisation (Distribution & Sales)

1211 Geneva 27, Switzerland.

WHO publishes books, journals and reports.

Regional offices:

Africa: PO Box no. 6, Brazzaville, Congo. Tel: 83 3860 65.

Americas: Pan-American Sanitary Bureau, 525, 23rd Street, NW, Washington DC 20037, USA. Tel: 861 3200.

Eastern Mediterranean: PO Box 1517, Alexandria, 21511, Egypt. Tel: 48 202 230.

Europe: 8 Scherfigsvej, DK–2100, Copenhagen O, Denmark. Tel: 29 01 11.

South East Asia: Work Health House, Indraprastha Estate, Mahatma Gandhi Road, New Delhi, 110002, India. Tel: 331 7804.

Western Pacific: PO Box 2932, Manila 2801, Philippines. Tel: 521 84 21.

Yeldall Christian Centres

Yeldall Manor, Hare Hatch, Reading, Berks RG10 9XR. Tel: 0734 404411.

Christian agency providing drug rehabilitation.

APPENDIX H
Further Reading and Resources

Inclusion in this list does not indicate suitability for any particular situation. Resources for education, training or prevention should be carefully assessed first.

Popular journals

The best information by far is produced by the Bureau of Hygiene and Tropical Diseases (CAB International) (Tel: 0491 832111). Two publications:

(1) *AIDS Newsletter*, seventeen issues per year. Four regular sections: News and media—UK; News from abroad; Social and occupational; Science and medicine. Other features include publications, meetings and full indexing. It aims to provide health care professionals with an authoritative, accurate and up-to-date synopsis, in straightforward terms, of the latest developments in AIDS as reported by the lay, scientific and medical press.

(2) *Current AIDS Literature* Monthly annotated and classified bibliography of recent books and reports on AIDS, related retrovirus infections and the agents that cause them. Each issue contains an overview—a look at last month's publications—and editorial commentaries of the main sections—epidemiology, clinical, medical microbiology and social. For health care professionals, public health workers and researchers.

AIDS Action. Free on AIDS prevention and control (international)— AHRTAG. Quarterly: English, French, Spanish, Portuguese.

'AIDS Letter', Royal Society of Medicine: Twenty-five issues a year of practical up-to-date information for people who have AIDS. (1 Wimpole Street, London W1M 8AE.) Strictly confidential mailing list.

EPI Newsletter. Pan American Health Organization. Free. Six issues per year (English).

Future. UNICEF, 55 Lodi Estate, New Delhi 100001, India. Four issues per year (English). An edition for Pakistan is available from UNICEF, PO Box 1063, Islamabad, Pakistan. Quarterly (English, Urdu).

Medicine Digest. York House, 37 Queen Square, London WC1N 3BH. Abstracts and updates on all aspects of medical care with emphasis on tropical medicine. Monthly (English).

Morbidity and Mortality Weekly Report, vol. 35, no. 53 (1986): 119–120. A summary of United States sources of information.

National AIDS Information Clearinghouse, PO Box 6003, Rockville, MD 20850, USA, is a centralised source of information on AIDS.

World Health Forum (available from WHO). Comprehensive coverage on a variety of community health related topics. Each issue is about 100 pages. Quarterly (English). WHO also publishes other journals (address in Appendix G).

Books

Adler, Michael, *ABC of AIDS* (British Medical Journal, 1993).

Amos, William, *When AIDS Comes to Church* (US Westminster Press, 1993).

Arterburn, Jerry and Steve, *How Will I Tell My Mother?* (Thomas Nelson, 1988).

Baker & Ward, *AIDS, Sex and Family Planning* (African Christian Press, 1989).

Barber, Cyril, *Your Marriage Can Last a Lifetime* (Thomas Nelson, 1989).

Barclay, William, *Ethics in a Permissive Society* (Fontana).

Barter, Barron and Gazzard, *HIV and AIDS—Your Questions Answered* (Churchill Livingstone, 1993).

Children and HIV: guidance for local authorities (Dept of Health, 1991).

Coates, Gerald, *An Intelligent Fire* (Kingsway, 1992).

Coates, Gerald, *Kingdom Now* (Kingsway, 1993).

Cohrs, Jo-Anne, *Stigma: an AIDS Widow's Story* (Harvestime, 1989).

Crumb, Duane, *Guide to Positive AIDS Education* (American Institute for AIDS Prevention, 1993).

Derita, et al, *AIDS Aetiology, Diagnosis and Treatment* (Lippincott Company, 3rd edition, 1993).

Doyle, D., *Domiciliary Terminal Care* (Churchill Livingstone, 1987).

Facts about AIDS for Drug Users (Terrence Higgins Trust on AIDS: London WC1N 3XX).

Foster, Richard, *Celebration of Discipline* (Hodder & Stoughton, 1978).

Guidelines for developing a sex education policy (CARE Trust).

Hinton, J., *Dying* (Penguin, 1986).

Houghton, John, *A Touch of Love—A Personal Guide to Sexual Happiness* (Kingsway Publications, 1986).

Kubler-Ross, Elizabeth, *On Death and Dying* (Macmillan, 1969).

La Haye, Tim & Beverley, *The Act of Marriage—The Beauty of Sexual Love* (Zondervan Publishing, 1976).

Laukester, T., *Setting up Community Health Programmes—a practical guide for use in developing countries* (Macmillan, 1992).

Lewis, C.S., *A Grief Observed* (Faber & Faber, 1961).

Libman and Witzburg, *HIV Infection—a Clinical Manual* (Little, Brown, 1993).

Murray-Parkes, Colin, *Bereavement* (Penguin).

Olowo-Freers, *In Pursuit of Fulfillment Studies of Cultural Diversity and Sexual Behaviour in Uganda* (UNICEF Kampala, 1994).

Oxford Textbook of Palliative Medicine (Oxford University Press, 1993).

Payne, Leanne, *The Broken Image* (Kingsway, 1993).

Pratt, R., *AIDS—A Strategy for Nursing Care* (Edward Arnold, 1991).

Sims & Moss, *Terminal Care for People with AIDS* (Edward Arnold, 1991).

Watson, David, *Fear No Evil* (Hodder & Stoughton). A description of author's own dying.

Wellings, Johnson et al, *Sexual Behaviour in Britain* (Penguin, 1994).

Wheat, Dr Ed, *Intended for Pleasure—Sex Technique and Sexual Fulfillment in Christian Marriage* (Scripture Union, 1977).

Wheat, Dr Ed, *Love Life*.

Wimber, John, *Power Healing* (Hodder & Stoughton).

Wood, G, *The AIDS Epidemic, Balancing Compassion and Justice* (Multnomah Press, USA, 1993).

Yelding, David, *Caring for Someone with AIDS* (Hodder, 1990).

Yoger & Connor, *A Management of HIV infection in Infants and Children* (Mosby-Year Book Inc, 1992).

Youle et al, *AIDS Therapeutics in HIV Disease* (Churchill Livingstone, 1988).

Videos

Lessons in Love (Steve Chalke, CARE)—recommended for church youth groups.

Compassion Has the Heart (ACET/TEAR Fund video on Uganda).

Make Love Last (CARE)—aimed at schools, includes teacher pack.

In Sickness and in Health: Story of Love in the Shadow of AIDS (CBN Publishing, USA).

Other resources

Strategies for Hope—a series of booklets and videos: 1. From Hope to Fear; 2. Living Positively with AIDS; 3. AIDS Management; 4. Meeting AIDS with Compassion; 5. AIDS Orphans; 6. The Caring Community; 7. All Against AIDS.
Available from TALC (see addresses). Booklets 1–6 also available in French. All are suitable for developing nations.

HIV—Facts for Life (ACET/Association of British Insurers). Booklets and teacher pack available from ACET and ABI (see addresses). 600,000 already distributed free to UK schools, colleges, clinics, hospitals, prisons and church organisations.

Towards a New Sexual Revolution: Guidance for Schools on Sex Education (Christians in Education, 1988).

My Body. Classroom card pack, Health Education Authority (Heineman Educational, 1991).

Let's Talk About AIDS (9–13 yrs), Sanders and Farquar (Aladdin, 1989).

Children and HIV. Guidance for local authorities (HMSO, 1993).

The Sexual Revolution and AIDS in Britain (HMSO, 1993).

Sexual Attitudes and Lifestyles. UK national survey (Blackwell, 1994).

Glossary of Terms

(Abbreviations are listed first: other terms follow)

AIDS:	Acquired Immune Deficiency Syndrome.
ARC:	AIDS Related Conditions (pre-AIDS syndrome), or AIDS Related Complex.
ARV:	AIDS associated retrovirus (old name for HIV).
AZT:	Antiviral drug currently being evaluated. Otherwise known as Zidovudine. Most effective drug discovered so far.
CD4:	New experimental therapy injecting fragments similar to CD4 white cell wall in order to mop up free virus in the blood. Disappointing.
CMV:	See also Cytomegalovirus. Common cause of diarrhoea in AIDS.
CSF:	See Cerebrospinal fluid.
DNA:	Deoxyribonucleic acid: complex making up genetic code (genes) contained in cell nucleus (brain).
ELISA:	Enzyme Linked Immunosorbent Assay—a test used on blood or plasma before transfusion to detect infection with HIV.
GP:	General Practitioner.
HCW:	Health Care Workers.
HIV:	Human Immunodeficiency Virus—name for the virus causing AIDS agreed to by an international scientific committee.
HTLV-III:	Human T-Lymphotropic Virus type III (old name for HIV).
ICU:	Intensive Care Unit.
Ig:	Immunoglobulin or antibody.

423

ICU:	Intensive Care Unit.
IV:	Intravenous—drugs directly injected into a vein. Same as 'mainlining' or 'shooting' for drug abuse.
KS:	Kaposi's sarcoma.
LAV:	Lymphadenopathy Associated Virus (old name for HIV).
LSD:	Drug causing hallucinations. Used to be popular in the sixties. People take it for an exaggerated perception of situations, sound, colour and memories. It causes death due to the person being unaware of risks and having unreal ideas, e.g., that they can fly so they jump out of a window. It may cause repeat 'trips' which can occur at any time without any warning some months after the initial experience. The drug has disappeared long ago from the body but it has damaged the brain in some bizarre way. A cousin of mine was given the drug by a doctor as part of a treatment for depression in the sixties. It has long been rejected for this and any other medical purpose. My cousin had a 'bad trip' which was extremely frightening. He had flashbacks at intervals for years.
NIR:	No Identified Risk, i.e., not drug addict, homosexual, bisexual, no blood transfusions, etc. Often misapplied term—it is just that the person is too embarrassed to admit the truth.
NY:	New York.
OD:	Slang for overdose by drug users.
PCP:	Pneumocystis carinii. Pneumonia.
PGL:	Persistent Generalised Lymphadenopathy—large lymph nodes for several months. Early sign of infection.
RNA:	Ribonucleic acid: carbon copy of DNA which is used to carry instructions from DNA throughout the cell. Retroviruses contain RNA.
STD:	Sexually Transmitted Disease—same as VD.
TMP-SMX:	Antibiotic used to treat pneumocystis chest infections. May affect bone marrow.
VD:	Venereal Disease—same as STD.

Acyclovir:	Antiviral drug currently being evaluated.
Alpha-interferon:	Substance usually produced by CD4 white cells. Disappointing as an anti-AIDS drug.
Amphetamines:	Drugs which stimulate and appear to speed up thinking. Often abused by people wishing to stay awake.
Anal intercourse/ sex:	Insertion of a man's penis into the anus of a man, woman or child. Even in adults can cause slight bleeding.
Antibodies:	Substance produced by white cells to destroy germs.
Asymptomatic:	Person feels well.
Autologous blood transfusion:	Giving and storing your own blood, which is given back to you after an operation.
Azidothymidine:	Anti-viral drug being evaluated (see also AZT).
Bestiality:	Intercourse between an animal and a man or woman. More common these days than many realise.
Biopsy:	Taking a tiny piece of tissue for examination under the microscope.
Bisexual:	Someone attracted sexually to both men and women.
Body-positive:	Someone who has sero-converted HIV (see also HIV).
Bone marrow:	Hollow red spongy core of human bones. It makes blood cells. Can be affected by many anti-AIDS or anti-cancer drugs and by radiotherapy.
Bronchoalveolar lavage:	Collecting fluids from inside the lung. Used to try and identify cause of pneumonias in people with AIDS.
Bronchoscopy:	Insertion of a tube, with a special tiny camera on the end, down the windpipe into the lungs to look and take samples. Patient sedated first.
Buddies:	System of friendships and caregivers for those with AIDS who may be feeling extremely vulnerable, lonely, isolated, rejected and depressed. It has been very successful in providing support and care.
Buggery:	Placing of a man's penis in a boy or man's rectum.
Cannabis:	Leaves of plant smoked like tobacco for mood-altering and relaxing effects.
CAT scan:	Special computerised X-ray machine that can produce excellent pictures of brain, lung, or abodmen for particular purposes. Huge and expensive. Not available everywhere.
Cerebrospinal fluid:	Fluid removed during lumbar puncture. Normally

bathes brain and spinal cord. Can be infected in meningitis. See also Lumbar puncture.

Co-factor: An additional feature that may influence infection—usually making it more likely or rapid.

Cold turkey: Addict may experience severe symptoms with shaking and aches all over as he withdraws suddenly from the drug.

Coming out: For a homosexual this means being open and honest about his or her sexual preferences and lifestyle. Being unashamed.

Condom: Sheath made of latex rubber or animal membrane designed to fit over the erect penis during intercourse to collect seminal fluid and reduce the risk of pregnancy. Also reduces risk of HIV infection greatly (by 85%) but not completely.

Co-trimoxazole (Septrin): Antibiotic used to treat pneumocystis carinii chest infections, or to help prevent same.

Crack: Cocaine. May depress immunity still further.

Cryptosporidium: Common infection in AIDS.

Cum: Slang for seminal fluid.

Cytomegalovirus: (CMV) Common infection in AIDS.

Dope: Loose term used to cover a wide variety of drugs taken for mood-altering properties as part of addiction or abuse.

Doubling time: Length of time for the number of cases of AIDS to double.

Downers: Barbiturates and other sedatives taken to slow someone down after taking amphetamines. See also Amphetamines.

Encephalitis: Inflammation of the brain due to infection.

Factor VIII: Substance required by haemophiliacs (blood extract).

Fibre optic: Name given to cameras used in endoscopy and bronchoscopy which are in fact made of thousands of tiny glass fibres. See also Bronchoscopy.

Fix: Dose of drug given into vein.

Flashback: Reliving of a previous LSD trip. See also LSD.

Foscarnet: Anti-viral drug being evaluated.

Gallium lung scans: Test used to confirm pneumocystis chest infection.

Gay: Alternative name for homosexual (recent use), usually of someone who has 'come out'. See also Coming out.

Hashish: Cannabis. See also Cannabis.

Hepatitis B: Bloodborne disease caused by virus. Can be caught in similar ways to HIV, but much more infectious. Causes liver damage which can be fatal. More than two thousand cases in UK each year.

Herpes Simplex type 1: Causes sores around mouth: cold sores.

Herpes Simplex type 2: Causes painful sores in the genital/anal areas. May increase risk of cervical cancer. Highly infectious when activated.

Heterosexual: Someone whose sexual preference is for someone of the opposite sex.

High: Mental state of an addict after taking drugs.

Homosexual: Someone whose sexual preference is for someone of the same sex.

Immunoglobulin: Antibody. See also Antibodies.

Immuno-suppression: Body's natural defences against disease reduced: white cells and antibodies are less effective or fewer in quantity.

Inosine pranobex: See Isoprinosine.

Interferon: Substance made by infected cells. Protects against further viruses entering cell. Can be manufactured. Has been used in chemotherapy.

Interleukin 2: Substance usually produced by CD4 white cells. Being evaluated as an anti-AIDS drug.

Isoprinosine: Drug tried with little success.

Johnny: See Condom.

Joint: Marijuana cigarette containing cannabis. See also Cannabis.

Lesser AIDS: See ARC.

Lumbar puncture: Insertion of a needle in the lower back under local anaesthetic to remove a sample of fluid from the fluid covering the brain and spinal cord. Usually to try and find cause of a new infection.

Lymph node: Small gland usually too small to feel. Swollen in infections. Filters out germs preventing them from reaching the blood. Full of white cells.

Lymphocyte: White cell—part of body's defence against infection. Two types: B cells produce antibodies. T cells sometimes kill germs directly, others help B cells prepare the right antibody. The CD4 T-lymphocytes are the ones infected by HIV.

Lymphoma: Unusual kind of cancer involving white cells of the body.

Mainlining: Injection of drugs directly into a vein by an addict. This is carried in one big amount through the lungs and into the brain via arteries. The travel time from arm to brain is about one minute. After ten minutes the drug is then diluted throughout the entire body, but the addict has experienced a huge 'kick' or 'buzz' from only a relatively small dose.

The body has virtually no defences against germs entering the blood directly so dirty needles make addicts very ill. If shared, the needles transfer blood and HIV from one addict to another.

Many addicts die from an overdose. They buy heroin 'cut' with anything ranging from salt and sugar to chalk. They measure out the mixture which may have very little heroin in it. One day they meet a dealer who sells them the pure drug. They measure out the same volume and it kills them. The drug overdose stops their breathing about one to three minutes after the injection. Brain damage may start three minutes after that.

Meningitis: Inflammation of the surface of the brain due to infection.

Methisoprinol: See Isoprinosine.

Neonatal: Pertaining to a newborn baby.

Nitrites: Drugs taken to increase sexual arousal. Some claim an association between use of nitrites and developing Kaposi's sarcoma. Nitrites certainly damage immunity which can be lethal in someone infected with HIV.

Oesophagus: Tube connecting mouth to stomach.

Oral sex: Genital contact with the mouth of a sexual partner. Dangerous if one partner infected.

Pentamidine: Antibiotic used to treat pneumocystis pneumonia.

Pleural effusion: Water between the lung and the chest wall, caused by infection or cancer. Can reduce the amount of air in the lung and cause shortness of breath.

Pneumocystis carinii: Unusual organism, causing chronic severe lung infections in people with AIDS. Usually treated with Septrin/co-trimoxazole or pentamidine.

Pneumothorax: Collapse of a lung. Can cause chest pain and sudden shortness of breath. Usually gets better quickly by itself, but may require treatment. Sometimes follows pneumocystis infection or a bronchoscopy.

Poppers: Slang for nitrites (see also).

Pre-AIDS: See ARC.

Prodromal AIDS: See ARC.

Q Substance: Trichosanthrin—experimental drug.

Retrovirus: A virus which makes new DNA code from its own RNA using the enzyme reverse transcriptase. HIV is an example.

Reverse transcriptase: Enzyme used to make DNA in a cell nucleus as a carbon copy of RNA from virus. Many AIDS drugs try to prevent this enzyme from working.

Ribavirin: Anti-viral drug being evaluated.

Seminal fluid: Fluid produced by a man when sexually aroused. Contains sperm.

Septicaemia: Situation where a (bacterial) infection has spread from a localised part of the body into the bloodstream. The result is someone who feels very unwell, may have a high temperature, and may be shaking uncontrollably.

Septrin: See Co-trimoxazole.

Sero-conversion: Time when person begins to carry antibodies in his or her blood indicating HIV infection.

Sero-positive: Antibodies to HIV present in the blood.

Sex-change operation: Mutilating operation to cut off a man's penis and testicles. A section of bowel is cut out and turned into a blind pouch. This is sewn into the skin at a point roughly where a woman's vagina would be expected to be. The result is an opening which can function as a crude vagina. Several such operations are carried out in London each week. It is a major procedure because it involves cutting intestines with risks of infection. It also requires a long anaesthetic. By psychiatrists people are referred to surgeons. Medically the person is regarded as mentally ill. He has a delusion that he is a woman born by accident into a male body. Because psychiatrists sometimes cannot alter this belief, one or two suggest altering appearance. Stage one is giving female hormones to a man so his breasts grow to a woman's size. Stage two is amputation of his penis and the rest. Sex is determined by genetic code as a 'fact of life'. The sex change is a crude cosmetic attempt to enable a man to pass himself off as a woman—especially in bed.

Many doctors, of whatever faith or no faith, consider the procedure to be unethical and wrong. Since when has it been right to reinforce someone's lost grip on reality by agreeing to mutilate the person, especially when the procedure could kill? This is not a minor procedure. If someone went to a psychiatrist convinced that cockroaches were living in his left leg, causing him terrible pains as they ate up his body, do you think it would be good medical care to cut his leg off on the basis that it would probably make him more content?

A friend of mine was worried recently because as a junior doctor one of his patients told him he had changed his mind yet again about 'having it done'. The man already had breasts, had posed successfully as a woman for some months (a condition of the operation), but said he now had had second thoughts. My friend decided not to sign him up for the operation and got into trouble with a senior colleague. The operation was done and the man had a big reaction afterwards. He could not remember if he had agreed to it or not. As many as thirty out of a hundred people are dissatisfied, asking for reversal (impossible) or committing suicide.

A family doctor I know broke partnership with a colleague in her practice after an attractive eighteen-year-old girl had walked into her surgery: 'Don't you remember me?' she exclaimed. 'I'm Roger, you remember?' This had been the adolescent sixteen-year-old boy who was confused about his sexuality. The doctor violently objected to her colleague. Surely to send a teenager for an opinion about a sex change operation was a terrible thing. It cannot be reversed. You cannot replace a man's genitalia any more than a woman's womb.

Medicine cannot alter the code of all your cells, only mutilate your appearance in order to allow deception. A friend of mine (male) was shocked one day to discover that he had been dating another man who was taking female hormones. He felt deceived, cheated and angry with the person and his doctor. He had been thinking of marriage. He was a devout Christian.

Shingles: Painful skin condition caused by chickenpox virus.

Shooting gallery: Place where addicts meet together to inject drugs. Part of the culture which makes the habit even harder to break is the whole ritual of drug abuse: meeting together, mixing the drug, drawing up the syringe, and injecting, often everyone using the same needle. People often feel safer with others—in case someone overdoses or has a bad trip (on LSD).

Snorting: Sniffing cocaine or heroin up the nose.

Speed: See Amphetamines.

Sperm: Tadpole-shaped organisms consisting of a single human cell containing half of a complete genetic code. The other half is contained in a human egg.

Spermicide: Chemicals which prevent tails of sperm moving, and therefore prevent fertilisation of an egg. Spermicides can be irritant and may increase the risk of transmission.

Spunk: Slang for seminal fluid.

Suramin: Anti-viral drug with slight effect on HIV but having serious side-effects.

Surrogate mother: A woman bearing another woman's child. Usually result of a test-tube baby conceived using someone else's egg and donated sperm, implanted in her womb. The developing baby uses her body as a 'hotel' during development. Hiring a womb like this raises enormous emotional and ethical issues.

Systemic infection: Affecting the whole body.

Test-tube baby: Baby conceived by placing a drop of a man's seminal fluids onto a glass slide containing a human egg. When fertilisation occurs, the egg starts to divide, and this is checked under the microscope. At a certain critical stage the rapidly developing embryo is placed in the womb of the woman.

Obtaining eggs is far more difficult than obtaining semen. Because success rates are low, women are given drugs to make the ovary produce several eggs at once—normally it produces one a month. The woman then has an operation to collect the eggs. As many as twelve eggs are exposed to sperm and usually three or four are put in the womb. Because embryos often die without settling in the womb the result can be no baby, one baby, or twins. Occasionally triplets or quadruplets are born.

What do we do with the other developing embryos? At the moment they are used for experiments. The first experiment tries to see if they can be kept alive for longer in the laboratory. The second kind of experiment exposes them to all sorts of chemicals to see what happens. These experiments happen every day in the United Kingdom despite several attempts by medical personnel to stop them.

The way to stop it is to fertilise only the number of eggs that could safely be placed inside a woman. Abortion has so cheapened the life of a baby in the womb that many cannot see the issue of experimenting on these 'things' at all. We distance ourselves by using scientific terms like morula, foetus or embryo when medically there is no distinction between them. What is the difference between life after an hour, a week, a month, or ten years? Logically, there is none.

Thrush:	Fungal infection of mouth, throat, gut, or skin caused by *candida albicans*.
Toxoplasmosis:	Common infection in AIDS.
Transmission:	Passing of infection from one person to another.
Trip:	Experience of an addict after drug taking.
Venereal disease:	Sexually-transmitted disease.
Virus:	Bag of protein containing genetic code, capable of infecting a cell and instructing it to make new viruses.
Withdrawal (of drug addict):	Stopping drug supply to someone who is dependent. Can produce symptoms such as severe shakes and cramps (see also Cold turkey).
Works:	Needle and syringe used by an addict. The habit of flushing remaining drug out of the syringe by drawing back your own blood leaves gross contamination of the syringe as well as the needle, and increases the risk of getting HIV infection enormously as the works are passed around.

Endnotes

1. *Morbidity and Mortality Weekly Report* (United States), 30 (1981): 305–308.
2. One or two are ill with pre-AIDS/AIDS-related complex (ARC) for each person with full-blown AIDS. However, figures quoted are always for AIDS. *Medical Clinics of North America*, 70 (1986): 693–705.
3. *International Herald Tribune* (31st March 1994) p 8. Range 600–800,000. 1989 estimate was 1 million.
4. Dr Robert Gallo co-discoverer of HIV. *Scientific American*, 265 (1987): 39–48. His discovery disputed though—see p. 72.
5. Major damage to the immune system can be detected in two out of ten people infected after only two years. After only five years, half those infected have abnormal immune systems. *AIDSFILE* (June 1987). But this is a slow virus. Other slow viruses do not cause disease until ten, twenty, or even forty years after infection. *Nature*, 326 (1987): 636.
6. UPI (9 April 1993) quoting *Morbidity and Mortality Weekly Report* in US.
7. *Sunday Tribune* (9 April 1993) quoting US Secretary of State for Health.
8. 'Epidemiology of AIDS in the United States' (excellent review), *Scientific American* (October 1988): 52–59.
9. Source: CDSC figures (US).
10. Source: Estimated HIV seroprevalence figures from *The Economic Effect of AIDS in Southern Africa*, Alan Whiteside, University of Natal, Indicator SA, October 1992; South Africa figure from *AIDS Analysis*, Southern Africa, Vol. 3 No. 6. All figures are based on surveys and estimated doubling times to 1992. (Panos Institute 1993.)
11. Isolated case reports from 1962 to date; but only recognised as such in 1980s. *Scandinavian Journal of Infectious Diseases*, 5 (1987): 511–517; also *Canadian Medical Association Journal*, 137:7 (1987): 637.

12. Personal communications. Information from Africa is politically sensitive. Workers have to keep their mouths shut or face imprisonment or deportation. Often the source or even the country cannot be identified, to protect doctors and scientists. Uganda led the way with openness, admitting one in eight of all adults were infected (1 million) in 1990 and possibly one in six (1.4 million) by 1993.

13. Up to 68% of barmaids tested positive in Southwest Uganda. *AIDS*, 1;4 (1987): 223–227.

14. Personal communications. (See endnote no. 12).

15. Predictions of which agricultural systems will be worst affected by AIDS labour loss. *New Scientist*, 117 (14 January 1988): 34–35.

16. *Observer* (19 April 1992): 57.

17. Personal communications. (See endnote no. 12).

18. *Annales de la Société Belge de Médicine Tropicale*, 66: 3 (1986): 345–350. See Chapter 4, p. 99.

19. It is hard to understand how low development agencies place AIDS.

20. *World Health Forum*, 4:3 (1988): 384. *Uganda Report*, 3:2 (1989): 79–85. See p 284.

21. WHO figures (1993).

22. 1994 estimate based on WHO figures.

23. WHO GPA *AIDS Surveillance in Europe* (1993) no. 36. Recent survey of 2,362 children in Romania found 7.3% infected, 97% probably through contaminated needles.

24. *European* (7 February 1993): 2 and *Observer* (21 February 1993): 21. See also *Lancet*, 338 (14 September 1993): 645–49.

25. *Revue Roumaine de Virologie*, 42 (1992): 59–66. Undernourished children were given a small injection of fresh blood as a tonic.

26. Source: Panos. Calculations based on estimated numbers of HIV+ provided by WHO Regional Office for South-East Asia, February 1993. Percentages calculated using population figures from UNDP and World Bank assuming sexually-active population to be equivalent to the population aged fifteen to sixty-five.

27. In terms of infection. Because of the long incubation period, African AIDS cases will dominate the picture beyond 2000.

28. *AIDS Newsletter* BHTD Vol. 7, issue 8 (1992): 2, quoting an estimate of sexually-active adults in India 2.5 times the number of total adults alive in sub-Saharan Africa.

29. *Guardian* (8 August 1992): 7, quoting Dr Iswar Gilada.

30. Dr Michael Merson, Director of WHO GPA, quoted in *Toronto Star* (1 February 1993): 2.

31. *Lancet*, 2 (1981): 1339.

32. *Lancet*, 1 (1985): 1261–1262. (Clinic for sexually-transmitted diseases.)

33. *International Journal of STD and AIDS*, 3 (1992): 4, 267–72, 261–6.

34. *British Medical Journal*, 306 (13 February 1993): 416–428.

35. *British Medical Journal*, 305 (25 July 1992): 219–221.

36. Each prostitute may have sex with several thousand people a year. (See Chapter 7, page 202; Chapter 4, pages 329–331.) 1% heterosexuals reported. *British Medical Journal*, 298 (18 February 1989): 419–422. Figure rose to one in sixty men by 1992. *Daily Telegraph* (27 August 1992). Government figures also show 1 in 500 women in inner London are HIV-infected.

37. Day Report CDR (15 April 1994) 4, 15.

38. 60,000 quoted in *Independent* (9 January 1987). Rees estimated possibly 110,000 in the United Kingdom were infected as early as 1985. *Nature*, 326 (1987): 343–345. Most people thought these were too high.

39. Numbers hard to estimate. *British Medical Journal*, 294 (1987): 389–390.

40. *Independent* (21 May 1993) quoting Day Report.

41. *Sunday Times* (18 April 1993): p. 2, for example.

42. ACET Home Care figures (1991–1993).

43. Part of the Day Report 1993 (Communicable Disease Report). Dr Gordon Stewart, Emeritus Professor of Public Health, Glasgow, has been a vigorous proponent of the view that heterosexual AIDS is never going to be a serious problem. He also has unconventional views on HIV and AIDS in Africa, dealt with in Chapter 5. *Lancet*, 341 (3 April 1993): 898, 863–4.

44. *Sexually Transmitted Diseases*, 18 (1991): 3, 188–191.

45. *Journal of the American Medical Association*, 262 (1989): 1201–1205.

46. Barcelona Symposium on Heterosexual Hepatitis B (May 1990).

47. *Independent* (27 August 1992).

48. *AIDS Bulletin*, 3 (1988): 62.

49. *Independent on Sunday* (9 May 1993).

50. Many are married. *Sexual Behaviour and AIDS in Britain* (HMSO, 1993).

51. *Observer* (10 May 1987).

52. *Lancet*, 2 (1986): 814 (nurse). *Lancet*, 1 (1983): 925 (surgeon). *New York Times* (6 June 1987), (dentist). Total of sixty-four health care workers reported infected (worldwide) through their work. Possibly 118 others. (UK Communicable Diseases report 3, Oct 1993). Numbers increasing slowly. Risk from needlestick injury probably less than 1:200. See pp 189–192 and pp 347–351.

53. See Chapter 4, page 100 for discussions of risks.

54. *Annals of Internal Medicine*, 106: 2 (1987): 244–245 (kidney transplant). *Lancet*, 1 (1987): 983 (skin donor).

55. *Lancet*, 339 (25 January 1992): 246. Happened at a wedding.
56. House of Commons debate (6 March 1990).
57. *Today* (29 April 1987).
58. *Atlantic Monthly* (February 1987): 48.
59. *The Times* (6 January 1987).
60. Boston area of US. *Boston Globe* (18 May 1993): 21.
61. *The Times* (13 July 1987). Clifford Longley: 'Since 1981 the church has continued to recruit to the ministry men who are homosexual and they have continued to engage, if discreetly, in homosexual activities.'
62. Front page of *Sun* newspaper (9 July 1987). Source: the Rev. Tony Higton, Rector of Hawkwell, Essex.
63. Andrew Walker, *Restoring the Kingdom* (Hodder & Stoughton, 1986). Contains extensive review of these new churches. See also *An Intelligent Fire*, Gerald Coates (Kingsway 1992).
64. For both sides of the argument: *New England Journal of Medicine*, 326 (1992): 2, 128–133 and 327 (1992): 7,501–502.
65. Personal communications.
66. Widely commented on in press reports and often remarked on by media delegates at conferences I have attended.
67. Freedom of Information Campaign, Harrow, Middlesex, UK, also linked to the Strecker Group, California. For further discussion of the origins of HIV see Chapter 5.
68. *Daily Telegraph* (7 April 1993): 8. See Chapter 2 for ways to evaluate new treatments.
69. For list of common STDs see page 319.
70. CDSC figures.
71. *New York Times* (1 April 1993) and *International Herald Tribune* (8 April 1993).
72. World Health Organisation figures 1990.
73. CDSC figs.
74. PID is involved with 20% of all gynaecological problems.
75. *Reviews of Infectious Diseases*, 9:6 (1987): 1102–1108.
76. Clumeck's famous letter to *Lancet* in 1983. Many still dispute that HIV first infected people in Africa. What is the evidence? Old blood samples dated from the 1960s from people in Central Africa have been found positive when tested for HIV infection. *New Scientist* (22 January 1987). One sample, dated 1959, was also positive. However, an early AIDS case was recently confirmed in a sailor from Manchester dated 1959. It seems his wife also died of AIDS. *The Independent* (6 July 1990). Some of the African results have been questioned: traces of malaria infection, and other things, sometimes confused earlier testing. The local monkey population is well-known for being infected with viruses which are very

similar to those producing AIDS. Nearly one-third of some species are infected in some areas. 'Field study among African Primates', *Microbiology and Immunology*, 30:4 (1986): 315–321; also 'AIDS in African Context', *Nature* (1986): 324. Spread from monkeys to man could have been from bites, bestiality (common in all countries of the world including the United Kingdom), or the practice of certain African tribes inoculating people with monkey blood as part of a fertility rite. *Lancet*, 1 (1987): 1498–1499; also *New Scientist* (16 July 1987). One report has suggested monkey–human spread was the result of eating green monkeys! AIDS seems common in areas where consumption is high. *Guardian* (19 February 1987). There is also evidence of AIDS in the United States as early as 1968 and possibly as early as 1958 (1988 reports from Washington University and the Medical University of South Carolina). Wherever it first came from, it does not explain why it has apparently spread so much faster in Africa than elsewhere. There is no genetic susceptibility. *AIDS*, 1: 4 (1987): 258–259; also *Lancet*, 1 (23 April 1988): 936—a previous paper's figures were wrongly added. Spread is more likely where other sex diseases result in untreated genital ulcerations. This is common in Africa due to inadequate facilities. Excellent summary of origins discussion: *Scientific American* (October 1988): 44–51. See also Chapter 5, p 138.

77. This sounds terrible, but New York City had over 20,000 cases of AIDS and 500,000 infected (estimate), according to the *AIDS Weekly Surveillance Report* (1987). Gay behaviour changed dramatically in San Francisco between 1983 and 1986, although heterosexual teenagers continued to take big risks. *New Scientist* (7 January 1988): 36–37; also *American Journal of Public Health*, 78: 4 (1988): 460–461.

78. Personal communication.

79. 'AIDS Has Created a New Form of Bereavement', *Canadian Medical Association Journal*, 136: 2 (1987): 194.

80. Five cases of mental illness resulting from fears of catching AIDS have been reported. 'AIDS-Phobia', *British Journal of Psychology*, 150 (1987): 412–413; also *British Journal of Psychology*, 152 (March 1988): 424–475. However, doctors must take care not to miss true disease: a Boston doctor has been sued for $750,000 damages by a woman whom he misdiagnosed as an asthmatic with imaginary symptoms when she had an AIDS-related pneumonia. *The Times* (21 February 1988). See also Chapter 5 on seronegative AIDS.

81. *AIDSFILE*, 1: 3 (1986): 1. Figures vary. See p 86.

82. United Kingdom. Financial consequences are far more catastrophic if you are ill in the United States.

83. *Daily Telegraph* (11 February 1987; also 2 February 1987); also *Sunday Telegraph* (15 February 1987).

84. *AIDS Newsletter*, 5. Bureau of Hygiene and Tropical Diseases (February 1987).

85. *Star* newspaper. Complaint to Press Council dismissed as 'in public interest'. *The Times* (20 July 1987). From 1985 Dan-Air only took female cabin staff for this reason. This was outlawed by the Equal Opportunities Commission in 1987. *The Times* (3 February 1987).

86. *Daily Telegraph* (11 February 1987; also 14 February 1987); also *Sunday Telegraph* (15 February 1987).

87. Personal communication from the person who was thinking of introducing it to prevent collapse of the service.

88. *American Journal of Public Health*, 76 (1986): 1325–30; also 'AIDS Stress Health Care in San Francisco', *Science*, 235 (1987): 964.

89. Middlesex, St Stephen's and St Mary's Hospitals report to the Social Services Committee, *Independent* (5 March 1987).

90. *International Herald Tribune* (13 May 1992): 6.

91. *Los Angeles Times* (16 May 1993): A5, 1.

92. Personal communication.

93. Editorial, *Nature*, 334 (11 August 1988): 457.

94. Several died without ever developing so-called AIDS in San Francisco (personal communication). Also in Scotland, UK.

95. 204% increase in reported cases in first quarter of 1993 compared to same period in previous year. 20% was genuine growth of problem. *Morbidity and Mortality Weekly Report* (1993): 42, 16, 308. See p 97.

96. See Chapter 3 p 86.

97. Source: Panos. Calculations based on estimated numbers of HIV+ provided by the European Centre for Epidemiological Monitoring of AIDS, December 1991. Percentages calculated using population figures from UNDP and World Bank assuming sexually active population to be equivalent to the population aged 15–65.

98. Personal communication.

99. Example: 'The virus . . . is extremely fragile and can only live momentarily outside body fluids.' *London Lighthouse* (AIDS hospice) *Newsletter*, 2 (April 1987).

100. *Journal of the American Medical Association (JAMA)*, 255: 14 (1986): 1887–1891.

101. LAV/HTVL-III. Causative agent of AIDS and related conditions. Revised guidelines (June 1986).

102. Personal communication.

103. *Journal of Medical Virology*, 35 (1991): 4, 223–227.

104. *AIDS Newsletter* 12 (1992): 7, 13, quoting VIIIth International AIDS Conference poster POA 2401 from Central Public Health Lab. in London. It also showed how poor 70% alcohol or bleach were at

disinfecting spilled blood because their effectiveness were diminished by blood proteins. Semen is a hostile environment: 90% loss of HIV infectiousness in twenty-four hours and 99% loss in forty-eight hours. The most effective way to disinfect equipment is to wash it thoroughly first so that agents used are more effective.

105. *Lancet*, 2 (1987): 166. See Chapter 5.

106. It has also been pointed out that figures for known HIV positive people may be underestimates because many are being tested at private clinics which do not send out statistics. Also HIV over-the-counter home-testing kits using saliva could make matters worse. *Doctor* (18 August 1988). See also Chapter 5.

107. Bloomsbury and Islington reporting—*Genitourinary Medicine* (1992), 68 (6): 390–393.

108. Several cases in older people missed in the United Kingdom. *Independent* (16 September 1988); also *British Medical Journal*.

109. Dr Anna McCormick of United Kingdom Office of Population Censuses and Surveys detected 887 more deaths than expected in single men fifteen to fifty-four years old from 1984–1987. On inspection of records only half were diagnosed as AIDS cases although most of the rest died of conditions often causing AIDS deaths. She concluded that recorded United Kingdom AIDS deaths may have told only half the story. *British Medical Journal*, 296 (1988): 1289–1292.

110. *Journal of the American Medical Association*, 257 (1987): 1727.

111. This is a cheap, reliable way to confirm AIDS diagnosis in someone who has all the appearances of it. Because almost everyone in Africa has had some slight exposure to TB, nearly everyone reacts positively to the special skin test. A sign of AIDS is that the person's body fails to produce the skin bump usually seen. The test is cheap and widely available in Africa, unlike AIDS testing kits. Personal communication.

112. President Kaunda's son (Zambia)—*The Times* (5 October 1987).

113. Dissenting voice: 'Point of view,' *Lancet* (1987): 2906–207. Article questions if situation is as bad as feared—based on a personal tour.

114. Unofficial reports of 6 in 100 newborn babies in Soweto testing positive. Personal communication.

115. *AIDS Newsletter*, 2 (1987): 11. Bureau of Hygiene and Tropical Diseases.

116. 'Youth Lifestyles 1993': survey of 869 fifteen to twenty-four-year-olds in the UK. Attitudes no longer wild and unpredictable, but loyal, trustworthy, sensible and responsible—attributed to the recession and AIDS.

117. *Independent* (16 February 1987).

118. A scientist called Duesberg has suggested that AIDS is not caused by HIV but by some other agent. He is regarded as an eccentric and his original paper has been heavily criticised as being full of inaccuracies. *Cancer Research*, 47 (1987): 1199–1220. To read both sides of a confusing debate see *New Scientist*, 118 (28 April 1988): 34–35; also (5 May 1988): 32–33. Also *Science*, 243 (1989): 733. See Chapter 5 for further discussion.

119. Excellent review articles: *Scientific American*, 255 (1966): 78–88; also 256 (1987): 38–48.

120. The Human Fertilisation and Embryology Act 1990 outlaws experimentation on human embryos after a certain period. None has succeeded in becoming law so far, due to lack of government support. See 'Test-tube babies' in the glossary of terms.

121. P. Dixon, *The Genetic Revolution* (Kingsway Publications, 1993).

122. *Ibid.*

123. Examples simplified enormously.

124. *Journal of the American Medical Association*, 259: 20 (1988): 3037–3038.

125. *New Scientist*, 113 (26 March 1987): 36–37.

126. Excellent article: 'AIDS in 1988', *Scientific American*, 259 (4 October 1988): 25–32.

127. *Scientific American*, 259 (October 1988): 34–42.

128. *New Scientist*, 113 (26 March 1987): 46–51.

129. For discussion of vaccine problems: *Nature*, 362 (1 April 1993): 382; *Nature*, 361 (18 March 1993): 212.

130. *New Scientist*, 113 (26 March 1987): 46–51.

131. Thirty-nine minor variations of HIV found in two patients. *Nature*, 334 (4 August 1988): 440–444.

132. 'HIV-2 infection', *Lancet*, 1 (1987): 223; also 'An Unexpected New Virus' (HBLV), *Lancet*, 2 (1986): 1430–1431.

133. These are viruses with differences in shape and character. There are five major variants of HIV-1 and there is also HIV-2. Testing only for HIV-1 can miss HIV-2. New strain reported March 1994.

134. Report of the American Association for the Advancement of Science in Boston. *Observer* (14 February 1993): 1. Also *Lancet*, 341 (8 May 1993): 1171–1172.

135. *Lancet*, 340 (10 October 1992): 863–867.

136. *Nature*, 325 (1987): 765. Chimpanzees, which are commonly used in AIDS research, could easily become extinct because of over-use in laboratories testing AIDS drugs and vaccines. ATLA (*Alternatives to Laboratory Animals*), 15: 3 (1988): 176–179.

137. *Ibid.*

138. This has been done. *Nature*, 331 (1988): 76–78, 15, 79.

139. Further reading: 'Is a Vaccine Against AIDS Possible?', *Vaccine*, 6: 1 (1988): 3–5.

140. *Nature*, 330 (24/31 December 1987): 702–703.

141. Proceedings of National Academy of Sciences of USA, 85: 23 (1988): 9234–9257.

142. Zidovudine (AZT) resistance described in Wellcome press release (March 1989). Also *New England Journal of Medicine*, 320: 9 (1989): 594–595, and other reports.

143. *Ibid.* See also endnote 136.

144. House of Lords question by Baroness Seear to government spokesman (*Hansard*, 29 June 1987).

145. *Lancet*, 341 (3 April 1993): 889–890. Results of Concorde trial from October 1988–October 1991. Three-year survival similar in both placebo and AZT groups. Also *The Lancet* (9 April 1994) 871–875.

146. *Science* (1992): 258, 388. Mother/Baby? *The Guardian* (22 February 1994).

147. Testing can often be difficult due to issues surrounding certain ethical objections and problems related to finding willing volunteers. See *New Scientist* (12 November 1988): 26–27.

148. 'Will an AIDS Vaccine Bankrupt the Company That Makes It?', *Science*, 233 (1986): 1035.

149. Scrip 2–4.9.92 p. 17.

150. 'Settlement on AIDS Finally Reached Between USA and Pasteur', *Nature*, 326 (1987): 533, row continued however, *Nature*, 345 (1990): 104.

151. *British Medical Journal*, 304 (16 May 1992): 1319. Dr Robert Gallo (US), versus Prof. Luc Montagnier (France).

152. Sales were worth $65 million up to 27 February 1988 with profits of $6 million after development costs. Political and social pressures—'AZT should be free'—in the United States led to a 20% drop. Wellcome's total profits were up by 35% in 1988 because of AZT and another drug used in AIDS treatment (Zovirax). *The Times* (11 November 1988). The Queen's Award for technological achievement was granted to Wellcome for AZT. *The Times* (21 April 1990). By 1991 the $65 million AZT sales of 1988 had soared to $255 million. *Financial Times* (18 June 1992): 17. Controversy continues over pricing.

153. 'Testing an AIDS vaccine may be harder than inventing one', *Scientific American*, 258: 2 (1988): 18–19. Some think it likely that vaccines will be tried out in Africa without permission from governments or individuals. *International Herald Tribune* (22 September 1988): 7.

154. Personal communication (May 1990).
155. Countries chosen by the steering committee of the World Health Organisation Global Programme on AIDS. *New Scientist* (26 October 1991): 17 and (2 November 1991): 21.
156. *British Medical Journal*, 303 (16 November 1991): 1218.
157. WHO press release (9 August 1993).
158. *Ibid.*
159. *Ibid.*
160. *Canadian Medical Association Journal*, 137: 10 (1987): 932–933.
161. 'AIDS Prevention Trade Booming', *Journal of Commerce* (international edition) (9 May 1988): 1.
162. See page 138, and endnote 76.
163. *Ibid.*
164. See Chapter 6.
165. *Daily Telegraph* (7 April 1993): 8.
166. *Proceedings of National Academy of Sciences of the USA*, 90 (1993): 1, 25–29.
167. Dr Robert Gallo, US, presenting findings at the IXth International AIDS Conference (Berlin, June 1993).
168. *Journal of the American Medical Association*, 257: 10 (1987): 1327. It seems people are much less infectious when they are well.
169. *Nature*, 362 (25 March 1993): 287.
170. Reports at the IXth International AIDS Conference (June 1993).
171. PO–CO4–2627 paper at IXth International AIDS Conference (1993).
172. See Chapter 5.
173. *New Scientist* (1 August 1992): 8.
174. 'AIDS and the Dentist', *British Dental Journal*, 162: 10 (1987): 375, also *New Scientist* (19 February 1987): 19.
175. In people without AIDS, antibiotics start the job and the body does the rest. If the immune system is damaged, it is sometimes extremely difficult to get rid of the germ completely. An example is syphilis where it seems that prolonged high dose antibiotics are required to prevent relapse. *New England Journal of Medicine*, vol. 316 (1987): 1569–1572; 1587–1589; 1600–1601.
176. *Respiratory Disease in Practice* (October/November 1988).
177. *Sozial-und Proventivmedizin*, 37 (1992): 5, 199–206.
178. 'AIDS Not Gentle on the Mind'—excellent review article, *New Scientist*, 113 (26 March 1987): 38–39.
179. *AIDSFILE*, 1: 3 (1986): 1.
180. Chief Neurosurgeon in San Francisco gave a verbal report on a series of post-mortems of people who died of AIDS. Each showed damage to the brain.

181. *Science*, 233 (1986): 1089–1093.
182. *Cell*, 47:3 (1986): 1.
183. *AIDSFILE* (1986): 1, 3, 1.
184. *Medicine*, 70 (1991): 5, 326–43.
185. *Pediatrics*, 78: 4 (1986): 678–687. The mean lifetime cost (in patient) per child with AIDS in New York in 1988 was $90,347. *Journal of the American Medical Association*, 260: 13 (1988): 1901–1905.
186. Eg spinal cord. *British Medical Journal*, 294 (1987): 143–144.
187. WHO CDSC. 7,000 US births in HIV women each year—not all infected.
188. European Collaborative Study *The Lancet*, 337 (2 February 1991): 253–259.
189. European Collaborative Study update presented at the IXth International AIDS Conference in Berlin (June 1993).
190. *Science* (28 February 1992): 1134.
191. *Pediatric Infectious Disease Journal*, 7: 5 (1988): 561–571.
192. Further reading and colour illustrations: *British Medical Journal*, 294 (1987): 29–32.
193. *Ibid.*
194. *Lancet*, 1 (1987): 280–281.
195. *New England Journal of Medicine*, 328 (1993): 3, 210–211.
196. *Journal of Infectious Diseases*, 157: 5 (1988): 1044–1047. Other data on survival times: *Lancet* (6 April 1988): 880.
197. *Epidemiology*, 3 (1992): 3, 203–209.
198. *Quarterly Journal of Medicine*, 67: 254 (1988): 473–486.
199. *Ibid.*
200. *Journal of the American Medical Association*, 257 (1987): 3066.
201. *American Journal of Diseases of Children*, 140: 12 (1986): 1241–1244.
202. *British Medical Journal*, 302 (26 January 1991): 203, 203–303.
203. *Ibid.*
204. *AIDS*, 6 (1992): 10, 1159–1164.
205. *British Medical Journal*, 303 (9 November 1991): 1185–1186.
206. *Ibid.*
207. *Ibid.* Accepted by WHO in 1992.
208. WHO figures (May 1993).
209. *AIDS Weekly* (2 November 1992).
210. *Lancet*, 339 (23 May 1992): 1298.
211. See p 41. By 1988 AIDS was number nine in the list of causes of death in United States for children from one to four years of age. (Report of United States Health and Human Services—December 1988.)
212. 15%–20% Europe, 25%–30% Africa. AIDS Letter 41 (1994), 1–3. AZT may help prevent (*The Guardian* 22 February 1994).

213. *Lancet,* 340 (5 September 1992): 585–588.
214. AIDS Letter 41 (1994), 1–3.
215. WHO press release: WHO/301 (4 May 1992).
216. *Weekly Epidemiological Record,* 67 (1992): 24, 177–179.
217. *Daily Telegraph* (19 March 1987).
218. *Journal of the American Medical Association,* 256: 22 (1986): 3094.
219. *Trinidad Express* (1992).
220. *The Times* (30 April 1987); possibly two more *The Times* (1 August 1987).
221. *Pediatric Infectious Disease Journal,* 11 (1992): 8, 681–682.
222. *Journal of Pediatrics,* 112: 6 (1988): 1005–1007.
223. *Pediatrics,* 80: 4 (1987): 561–564.
224. *Reuters* (31 May 1993). See also Chapters 12–14.
225. *Newsweek* (31 May 1993): 32–33 and *China Post* (26 April 1993).
226. *AIDS,* 1: 1 (1987): 39–44.
227. *Journal of Infectious Diseases,* 155: 4 (1987): 828.
228. Five million IV drug users in the world (UN estimate, 31 March 1990).
229. *Guardian* (6 July 1987).
230. *British Medical Journal,* 294 (1987): 389–390.
231. One in every 250 people in Merseyside uses heroin or similar drugs. This explosion of drug abuse began in the early 1980s. However, most of the addicts in Merseyside sniff heroin and do not inject. *British Journal of Addiction,* vol. 82 (1987): 147–57.
232. *Journal of the American Medical Association,* 259: 15 (1988): 859.
233. *Guardian* (6 July 1987).
234. *British Medical Journal,* 294 (1987): 571–572; also 297 (1988): 859.
235. Scottish police inspector at conference in Peebles (April 1987).
236. *International Journal of STD and AIDS* (1992): 3(4), 288–290 (Glasgow addicts).
237. Chalk is often mixed with heroin by dealers to cheat drug users.
238. *Lancet,* 1 (1982): 1083–1087.
239. *International Herald Tribune.* High priced prostitutes—only one in seventy-eight infected compared to 9–21% of those on the street. *Communicable Diseases Unit* (14 November 1988).
240. *AIDS,* 6 (1992): 623–628.
241. *New Scientist* (20 February 1993): 12–13.
242. Scottish prison—personal communication.
243. *The Times* (28 May 1993).
244. Addicts may be using clean needles more than condoms.
245. *Journal of the American Medical Association,* 257: 3 (1987): 321–325.
246. *Journal of the American Medical Association,* 258: 4 (1987): 474.
247. *New Scientist* (26 March 1987): 55. Rectal trauma, pre-sex enemas,

scarring, fistulas, or fissures and receptive anal intercourse are high risk factors for HIV. *American Journal of Epidemiology*, 138: 4 (1987): 508–577. Tearing of the anal wall during anal sex is especially likely following fisting, where the hand and sometimes the forearm are inserted into the rectum. Other objects can also be used. Drugs (nitrites or 'poppers') are often used to relax the anal sphincter. 63% of one survey of gay men in London reported anal insertion of objects or hand/arm of a partner in the previous month (*Lancet*, 339 [1992]: 28, 632–635), 34% in the previous year in a US sample (*Annals of Internal Medicine*, 99 [1983]: 145–151). Oral/anal contact (rimming, licking and/or inserting the tongue) is also unhygienic, carrying a risk of infections of various kinds including hepatitis A, practised by 89% of the same UK sample, 63% of the US group. Another US study found 70% of gay men were rimming, with the annual incidence of hepatitis A at 22%, far higher than in heterosexuals (*New England Journal of Medicine*, 302 [1980]: 6, 435–438). Another US survey suggested that 23% of gay men interviewed had had sex as adults with boys sixteen years old or younger, 76% had had sex in public places such as toilets or in a group, eg gay baths. Sadomasochism was also common—37% of sample. 'Water sports' or 'golden showers'—splashing a partner with urine—were reported by 23%. (Large survey of gay men in Jay and Young, *The Gay Report NY* [Summit, 1979]. See also *Psychology Reports*, 64 [1989]: 7, 1167–1179.) Those training AIDS helpline operators sometimes seem to enjoy trying to shock trainees with some of the descriptions of current sexual practices (I went through training, as have some of my colleagues and friends). However, it is true that counsellors do need to be completely familiar with culture, terminology, lifestyle and practices, and they do need to be unshockable!

248. *Ibid.*
249. *Ibid.*
250. See page 25 onwards.
251. *American Journal of Public Health*, 177 (1987): 578–581.
252. *Science* (1987): 382.
253. *Nature*, 360 (3 December 1992): 410–412—preliminary results of the National Survey of Sexual Attitudes and Lifestyles, paid for by the Wellcome Trust. The full results were published in 1994 (Blackwell Publications). Also *Sexual Behaviour and AIDS in Britain*—HMSO, 1993). French study: *Nature*, 360 (3 December 1992): 407–409.
254. Pink Paper (3 January 1993): 11.
255. *American Journal of Public Health*, 82 (1992): 2, 220–224.
256. *Sexual Behaviour and AIDS in Britain* (HMSO, 1993).

257. The other prison risk is widespread drug abuse. *The Times* headlines (27 July 1987); *British Medical Journal*, 297 (8 October 1988): 873–874.

258. 'Could a Prisoner Sue the Authorities for Inadequate Protection?', *AIDS-Forschung*, 2: 2 (1987): 52, 55.

259. All infected prisoners were isolated in Brixton prison in a new unit for protection of and from other prisoners. *The Times* (22 April 1987).

260. Charing Cross Hospital lecture on sexually-transmitted diseases.

261. *New Scientist* (26 March 1987): 56.

262. *Journal of Infectious Diseases*, 164 (1991): 5, 962–964.

263. *Sunday Times* (6 September 1992) reported cases in UK between 1985 and 1991.

264. 'Male Rape: Breaking the Silence on a Taboo Subject', 278 rapes of men by men in South-east England in 1986. *The Listener* (23 July 1987).

265. *New Scientist* (26 March 1987): 56–57.

266. Personal communication.

267. *New Scientist* (26 March 1987): 56–57.

268. *Shanti* is a Sanskrit word meaning peace.

269. Christopher Spence, director of London Lighthouse (AIDS hospice), 'AIDS and the Wind of Change', *Leading Lights* newsletter (April 1987): 3–4.

270. Prof J. Mann (then at the World Health Organisation) at conference in Washington, DC (June 1987).

271. *Independent* (4 February 1987).

272. *Financial Times* (11 April 1987).

273. *Guardian* (16 February 1988): 2.

274. Chief Executive magazine survey reported in *Daily Telegraph* (9 March 1987).

275. *Business Insurance*, 27 (1993): 20, 33.

276. For example, Jeffrey Archer, member of Parliament, and the prostitute libel case. He won but they won: a destroyed political career. All because they suggested he had spent a night with a prostitute.

277. Three risk factors for transmission from an infected man to a woman: STD in the last five years, partner with AIDS, and anal intercourse. Transmission occurred in 27% of 155 heterosexual couples overall and 67% in those with more than two risk factors. *British Medical Journal*, 298 (1989): 411–415. See Chapters 5 and 6 also.

278. The diocesan AIDS office in San Francisco is contacted every week by wives of Anglican clergy who have just discovered their husbands

have HIV infection and have been having sex with men. Personal communication.

279. Heterosexual risks and uncertainties. *British Medical Journal*, 296 (1988): 1017–1020.

280. *Morbidity and Mortality Weekly Report*, 35 (1986): 76–79. Breast-feeding with cracked/bleeding nipples.

281. *AIDS*, 6 (1992): 10, 1181–1185.

282. *British Medical Journal*, 305 (8 August 1992): 364.

283. For example, see *Health Education Journal*, 50 (1991): 4, 166–169.

284. See Chapter 5 for non-sexual risks.

285. *Lancet*, 2 (1987): 40–41. *Annals of Internal Medicine*, 105: 6 (1986): 969. Clinical Infectious Diseases 17 (1993) 6, 1003–1005.

286. *British Medical Journal*, 296 (1988): 1017–1020.

287. *Morbidity and Mortality Weekly Report*, 37: 3 (1988): 35–38.

288. *Christianity Today* (8 April 1988): 39.

289. 'Female-to-Female Transmission of HIV', *Lancet*, 2· (1987): 40–41. Also POC 4196, POC 4560, VIIIth International AIDS Conference (July 1992). Indirect evidence for spread through oral sex from men to female prostitutes.

290. Sevenfold risk of infection where genitalia are ulcerated—*AIDS Newsletter* (1992), 7 (12): 18.

291. *American Journal of Medicine*, 82 (1987): 188–189.

292. Further reading: 'AIDS—How You Catch It and How You Can't', *New Scientist*, 113 (26 March 1987): 38–39.

293. *New Scientist*, 113 (26 March 1987): 37.

294. Testing can be very helpful—other counselling first.

295. *American Journal of Public Health*, 78: 4 (1988): 462–467.

296. *The Times* (25 July 1992): 27. See also Chapter 7.

297. ELISA stands for Enzyme Linked Immunoabsorbent Assay.

298. *New England Journal of Medicine*, 314 (1986): 647–8.

299. *Lancet*, 341 (13 February 1993): 441–442.

300. *Journal of the American Medical Association*, 268 (1992): 8, 1015–1017. Around 1% false positive for HIV when tested an average of twenty-six days following influenza vaccination.

301. *Journal of the American Medical Association*, 226 (1991): 2861. ELISA requires sophisticated laboratory facilities, running water and electricity. Western Blot requires skill in interpreting the colour bands. New 'instant' ELISA kits require little or no equipment and less time, but can be slightly less accurate.

302. *Morbidity and Mortality Weekly Report*, 39 (1990): 282.

303. *Ibid.*

304. *Global AIDS News* (WHO) 1992, no. 1. Number of tests used varies with situation.

Diagnosis of asymptomatic in high-incidence country: 2
Diagnosis of asymptomatic in low-incidence country: 3
Diagnosis of person with symptoms: 2
HIV seroprevalence surveys—high-incidence areas: 1
HIV seroprevalence surveys—low-incidence areas: 2
Blood screening for transfusion: 1
High incidence = more than 10% infected.
1 = single ELISA
2 = ELISA + Western Blot or other
3 = two ELISA tests plus one other—all slightly different tests.

305. Recent survey of 103 labs found 98.2% of positives correctly identified and 1.3% false positives. The rest were indeterminate. *Bulletin of WHO*, 70 (1992): 5, 605–613.

306. *New England Journal of Medicine*, 327 (1992): 1192–1197.

307. *AIDS*, 6 (1992): 9, 953–957.

308. *AIDS*, 6 (1992): 7, 723–733.

309. Friends Provident press release (1 October 1992).

310. Saliva Diagnostic Systems, Oregon, US, has been working for some time on a complete saliva testing kit in one tube, producing a result in less than three minutes, and costing less than $8. They see a big market in developing countries to confirm a diagnosis. See also endnote 678.

311. Individuals with the HLA-Bw4 antigens programmed by their genes seem to have a slower rate of decline of CD4 cells and a slower rate of progression to AIDS. Another HLA gene has also been associated with more rapid progression, although there were signs of progression in all those studied. Research presented by the US National Cancer Institute at the IXth International AIDS Conference in Berlin (June 1993).

312. Research presented by Dr J. Levy, Professor of Medicine, California, at the IXth International AIDS conference in Berlin (June 1993).

313. *Scandinavian Journal of Immunology*, 36 (1992): suppl. 11, 81–83. A survey of seronegative female partners of infected men, half of whom were positive for polyclonal B cell activation test (P-BAT).

314. Findings presented at the 1992 International AIDS Conference in Amsterdam by Dr Gene Shearer, National Cancer Institute, Bethesda, Maryland, US. Also confirmed by him in writing to me on 3 August 1992.

315. *New Scientist* (19 February 1987): 58–59.

316. 'AIDS and the Condom—A Guide to Safer Sex', London Rubber Company leaflet.

317. Channel 4 documentary (UK) *Dispatches* (24 March 1993), produced and directed by Joan Shenton. The same team made a *Dispatches* programme promoting the non-HIV view of AIDS. The *Sunday*

Times also promoted the view of AIDS in Africa as a 'tragic myth' headline of article written by Neville Hodgkinson as part of a long series challenging AIDS orthodoxy (21 March 1993). Also, see reports of the 'alternative Amsterdam AIDS Conference' *Independent* (14 May 1992): 25, *Sunday Times* (3 May 1992): 7 and (17 May 1992): 5.

318. 'Has Duesberg a right of reply?' *Nature*, 363 (13 May 1993): 109; also 363 (11 March 1993): 103–104 for drug issues.

319. John Lauritsen, *Poison by Prescription: the AZT story* (Asklepios, 1993).

320. See *Sunday Times* (26 April 1992, 3 May 1992, 7 June 1992, 31 June 1992) and many other articles since.

321. *Lancet*, 341 (1993): 658–659 and *Nature*, 362 (1993): 103–104.

322. *British Medical Journal*, 293 (27 September 1986): 782–785. *The Guardian* (22 April 1994)—"60 times"—*Lancet* study of 9,389 in southwest Uganda.

323. *New Scientist* (22 May 1993): 17. Some said the number of white cells infected appeared to be too low to fit the HIV theory of AIDS.

324. *Morbidity and Mortality Weekly Report*, 41 (1992): 30, 541–545.

325. Idiopathic CD4 Lymphopenia (ICL). *Nature*, 358 (20 August 1992): 619.

326. *Lancet*, 340 (1992): 1312–1316.

327. It is possible that further research will find that other infections, such as mycoplasma, have a key role in helping HIV infection along—especially in early stages.

328. *Independent* (19 December 1986).

329. *Journal of the American Medical Association (JAMA)*, 255: 14 (1986): 1887–1891. One possible case of spread between footballers, *Lancet*, 335 (1990): 1105.

330. Sports council for Wales lifted the ban in January 1987. *Guardian* (17 January 1987).

331. *British Medical Journal*, 305 (3 October 1992): 835.

332. 'Stability and Inactivation of HTLV-III/LAV under Clinical Laboratory Environments', *Journal of the American Medical Association (JAMA)*, 255: 14 (1986): 1887–1891.

333. *AIDS Weekly* (26 October 1992).

334. *Lancet* (1985): 188–189. Note: This paper suggests the virus is destroyed after twenty minutes' heating at 56°C, but they used an insensitive enzyme test (reverse transcriptase).

335. See endnote 332.

336. *Ibid.*

337. *Ibid.*

338. *Journal of the American Medical Association*, 294 (1987): 1595–1597.
339. *Lancet*, 1 (1975): 188–189.
340. *British Medical Journal*, 294 (1987): 1595–1597. See p 190.
341. *New York Times* (6 June 1987).
342. Safety guidelines: *British Dental Journal*, 162 (1987): 371–373, 375.
343. *Morbidity and Mortality Weekly Report*, 40 (1991): 23, 377–381.
344. Royal College of Surgeons: *Impact of HIV on Surgical Practice*, vol. 1 (1992): 42. Dentists: see p 198.
345. *Journal of Clinical Microbiology*, 30 (1992): 2, 401–406. Also demonstrated on *Panorama* documentary on BBC1 (September 1993).
346. 'Design Improvements', *New England Journal of Medicine*, 319: 5 (1988): 284–288, 308.
347. British Medical Association (April 1990).
348. Numbers infected globally likely to be higher.
349. *Morbidity and Mortality Weekly Report* (22 May 1987): 285–288.
350. 'AIDS: A Doctor's Duty', *British Medical Journal*, 294 (1987): 6. Also suggests a doctor might be struck off the register for refusing to look after someone with AIDS. The risk of getting hepatitis B infection is much greater than the risk of AIDS from a cut or scratch with a needle. *New England Journal of Medicine*, 312 (1985): 56–57.
351. Five million medical rubber gloves imported from Hong Kong to the United States had to be destroyed because they were full of holes. *Daily Telegraph* (8 November 1988).
352. *Canadian Medical Association Journal*, 146 (1992): 2, 227–231.
353. *Lancet*, 2 (1986): 694. A second case was also reported.
354. Simian Immunodeficiency virus in green monkeys and rhesus monkeys. All these viruses belong to the lentivirus group of retroviruses.
355. *Nature*, 333 (18 February 1988): 396.
356. KGB suggested that US made HIV at Fort Detrick, Maryland. *Montreal Gazette* (16 February 1992): 7.
357. Experiments were carried out in the 1920s, transferring monkey testicles and other pieces of tissue into humans. *Lancet*, 338 (1991): 1604. The aim was to help restore deficient hormones.
358. For further discussion see Patrick Dixon, *The Genetic Revolution* (Kingsway, 1993).
359. World Health Organisation 1992.
360. See question on mosquitoes elsewhere. The risk is considered infinitesimal.
361. Dr William Haseltine of Harvard Medical School was reported in the *New York Times* (18 March 1986) as saying that HIV could be transmitted through mosquito bites.

362. 'No evidence for Arthropod Transmission of AIDS', *Parasitology Today*, 2: 11 (1986): 294–295. One dissenting voice is a paper showing that in Africa poor housing and being near water courses made infection more likely, possibly due to insects.

363. *Bulletin of the World Health Association*, 65: 5 (1987): 607–613. There is no association with malaria except some extra cases of AIDS resulting directly from infected blood transfusions used to treat malaria anaemia. *Journal of the American Medical Association*, 259: 4 (1988): 545–549.

364. *Lancet*, 1 (1987): 1094–1098. See also endnote 365.

365. This discussion will continue. Scientists have found that infectious HIV can be regurgitated by the stable fly. If insects are transmitting HIV, it must be very rarely. *AIDS-Forschung*, 7 (1992): 5, 253–256.

366. *Daily Telegraph* (13 September 1992) reporting government figures.

367. *Daily Telegraph* (13 February 1987).

368. I must say that this conflicts with my own experience of serving on the other side of the altar rail in an Anglican church. I think the occasional fragment of a wafer is all I have ever seen.

369. Another vicar, the Rev. Michael Moxon, Vicar of Tewkesbury Abbey, Gloucestershire, England, was reported as telling his parishioners they need not drink the wine if they are afraid of infection by AIDS. *The Times* (5 January 1987).

370. Guidelines on AIDS and communion sent from Archbishops of Canterbury and York to all clergy in their pay slips (March 1987).

371. *Journal of Acquired Immune Deficiency Syndrome*, 5 (1992): 9, 890–903.

372. A hospital chaplain in Essex advised priests to wear rubber gloves and use a spatula when giving communion to people with AIDS! This is totally absurd. *The Times* (5 January 1987). Medically trained people can be just as bad. In County Durham two ambulance personnel collected someone with AIDS in goggles and boiler suits. *Daily Mirror* (22 January 1987). For a scientific discussion see *Journal of Infection*, 16: 1 (1988): 3–23.

373. *British Medical Journal*, 294 (1987): 433.

374. *Lancet*, 341 (1 May 1993): 1155. Failure rate 12.2% per year compared to 19.6% for sponge and 4.2% for diaphragm. Condom failure rates can be anything from 5–15% (see next chapter).

375. *British Journal of Family Planning*, 18 (1992): 36–41.

376. Joseph Lange, *IXth International AIDS Conference News* (June 1993).

377. *Lancet*, 339 (6 June 1992): 1371–1375.

378. National Blood Transfusion Service draft guidelines. Also 'The Patient's Blood Is the Safest Blood', *New England Journal of*

Medicine, 316: 9 (1987): 543–544; 'The Need for Autologous Blood Transfusions', *British Medical Journal*, 294 (1987): 307.

379. Longstanding practice in the United States (Florida): *Journal of the American Medical Association*, 257: 9 (1987): 1211–1214.
380. *Communicable Disease Report* (1991): 1, 13.
381. I have based this figure on the UK government estimate of one in a million risk of HIV infection from a single unit of donated blood.
382. *British Medical Journal*, 305 (29 August 1992): 498–501.
383. This occurred in Glasgow. A leukaemia patient was infected by a pint of blood which tested negative.
384. Many students were giving blood to get an HIV antibody test. *Daily Telegraph* report (8 January 1987).
385. Haemophilia Society figures.
386. Transfusion centres were losing 100 pints a day (15% of their requirements). *The Times* (6 January 1987).
387. *New England Journal of Medicine*, 328 (4 February 1993): 297–302 and *New Scientist* (13 February 1993): 8.
388. *Lancet*, 339 (7 March 1992): 627–628 and *AIDS*, 6 (1992): 2, 223–226.
389. *Morbidity and Mortality Weekly Report*, 36: 19 (1987): 285–288; extra test 389. Two cases of HIV spread between children—probably blood to wound. Extremely rare. *New England Journal of Medicine* 329 (1993); 1835–1841.
390. *Journal of Infectious Diseases*, 165 (1992): 1, 155–158.
391. 'AIDS and First Aid', *Occupational Health Review*, 6 (1987): 12.
392. *Journal of the American Medical Association*, 256: 22 (1986): 3092.
393. For further discussion, see *Lancet*, 340 (22 August 1992): 456–457.
394. *Morbidity and Mortality Weekly Report*, 35: 45 (1986): 699–703; also *Morbidity and Mortality Weekly Report*, 36: 9 (1987): 133–135. TB increase for first time in decades, as more people develop AIDS.
395. *Tubercle*, 67: 4 (1986): 295–302.
396. *Quarterly Journal of Medicine*, 67: 254 (1988): 473–486.
397. *New England Journal of Medicine*, 326 (1992): 703–705.
398. *AIDS Weekly* (2 November 1992).
399. Advisory Committee on Dangerous Pathogens, *Categorisation according to hazard and categories of containment*, 2nd ed (1990).
400. Written communication Royal College of Nursing (November 1992).
401. Advisory Committee on Dangerous Pathogens, *Categorisation according to hazard and categories of containment,* 2nd ed (1990).
402. *AIDS Newsletter*, 7 (1992): 12, 25 quoting PoB3275 from the VIIIth International AIDS Conference.
403. *Reviews of Infectious Diseases*, 10: 1 (1988): 138–150; 151–158.
404. *Journal of Sexually Transmitted Diseases*, 12 (1985): 203–208.

405. *Lancet*, 341 (3 April 1993): 889–890.

406. *British Journal of Psychiatry* special publication no. 9: Silverstone and Barraclough, *Contemporary Psychiatry* (1975): 173–185.

407. Z. Harsanyi and R. Hutton, *Genetic Prophecy* (Granada, 1982). There is some evidence for genetic influence on development of sexual orientation, although this appears to be greatly affected also by childhood experience. In 1952 Kallmann carried out a study showing 100% concordance for orientation in twins raised apart. He later revised his figures, but association remained high. Work repeated in 1968 by Heston and Shields who also found some concordance. *Journal Nerv. Ment. Disorders*; (1952): 115, 283 and *Arch. Gen. Psychiat.*; (1968): 18, 149. The message is that many things about us seem to be influenced by a combination of inherited and environmental factors.

408. Simon Le Vay (Salk Institute, 1991) *Science*, 253 (1991), 1034–1037; and Dr Hamer (US National Cancer Institute, 1993): *Science* 261 (1993), 321–327. For detailed account of genes and their influence, see P. Dixon, *The Genetic Revolution* (Kingsway, 1993).

409. *AIDS-Forschung*, 3 (1988): 7, 392–401; also *Journal of the American Medical Association*, 258 (1987): 14, 1969.

410. *Holistic Medicine*, 2 (1987): 4, 203–215.

411. WHO press release (WHO/54—11 November 1991) for World AIDS Day, 1991 and repeated in 1992.

412. 'Cautions about Condoms in Prevention', *Lancet*, 1 (1987): 323.

413. Family Planning Association Leaflet. 'There are Eight Methods of Birth Control' gives 3–15% pregnant per year but one figure in *Lancet* puts it at 13–15%. *Lancet*, 1 (1987): 323. Studies vary.

414. *European* (20–23 August 1992): 4. Survey by a Dutch consumer group and the world consumer organisation IOCV. The current EC standard is voluntary—ISO 4074.

415. *Self Health* 1987 survey, College of Health. Gross defects. Despite 5 micron sized holes in intact latex (HIV is 0.1 micron) HIV does not seem to pass through except when latex is stretched. 0.1 micron particles leaked in 33% of condoms during simulation intercourse tests. *Sexually Transmitted Diseases* 19 (1992) 230–234. However, free HIV in semen is often low. It may be that transfer to infected cells is greater risk—occurring only through gross defects/tears. *Rubber Chemistry and Technology* 62 (1989) 683; *Journal of Testing and Evaluation* 18 (1990) 352; *Nature* 335 (1988) 19.

416. *Guardian* (21 July 1987). British Standard for imported brands. BSI for Durex is at one hole in 200 condoms.

417. *Consumer Reports* (March 1989): 136; see also notes 410 and 415.

418. See endnote 413.
419. Animated discussion with Family Planning Association. Condom manufacturers take this line for medico–legal reasons, otherwise they could be sued for making false claims. Too small? *The Independent* (15 October 1993).
420. *British Medical Journal* (27 February 1993): 556–557.
421. *Scandinavian Journal of Social Medicine*, 20 (1992): 4, 247–252.
422. *Fertility and Sterilization* (1960): 11, 485–488.
423. *Observer* (23 May 1993): 3. Also *British Medical Journal* (27 February 1993): 556–557.
424. Durex report (1992).
425. Terrence Higgins Trust literature advises: 'A condom should be used as a barrier in heterosexual lovemaking for both vaginal and anal sex. Do not rely on this as a method of birth control, *but use some other form of contraception to avoid pregnancy.*' 'Woman and AIDS', 3.
426. An example: *Lancet*, 1 (2/9 January 1988): 65.
427. *Journal of the American Medical Association* (1987). Report showed only one in twelve became infected. Dangers of premature conclusions. In the brief interval between writing the paper and it being published, the number infected had already risen from one to three out of twelve. *New Scientist* (19 February 1987): 12.
428. *New Scientist* (26 February 1987): 61.
429. 'Women and AIDS.' Terrence Higgins Trust.
430. PO-C11–2833 Milan study presented at the IXth International AIDS Conference (June 1993). Another study by the same team showed anal intercourse with an infected woman exposed a man to greater risk than vaginal intercourse (PO–C11–2854). See also *Archives of Internal Medicine*, 151 (1991): 12, 2411–2416.
431. PO–C11–2828. German study presented at the IXth International AIDS Conference (June 1993).
432. *British Medical Journal*, 304 (1991): 809–813.
433. *The Times* (24 August 1987).
434. *AIDS Newsletter*, 7 (1992): 12, 16.
435. *Sexually Transmitted Diseases*, 18 (1991): 3, 188–191.
436. All condom instructions and most AIDS prevention literature stress the importance of this.
437. Presentation by Gerard Ilaria (New York) at VIIIth International AIDS Conference (July 1992).
438. *Lancet* (1986): 527–529.
439. *South African Medical Journal*, 82 (1992): 2, 107–110.
440. *Family Planning Today* (2nd quarter, 1988): 1. 50% of the students

said they would never use condoms—dulled sensitivity, broke, smelled, were embarrassing to use and meant sex had to be planned. Female condoms (eg Femshield) are experimental but may be less disruptive—inserted by the woman and reusable. See Chapter 5.

441. 42% in UK survey of students. *The Times* (28 August 1987).
442. *British Medical Journal*, 290 (1985): 1176.
443. Leisurewear marketeer Glenn's Style gave away six condoms with every pair of jeans. *Marketing Weekly* (16 December 1988).
444. *Cosmopolitan* (January 1987).
445. *British Medical Journal*, 294 (1987): 1356.
446. See note 440.
447. *Lancet*, 341 (1 May 1993): 1155. See also Chapter 5.
448. *FIRSTAIDS ITV* (20 June 1987).
449. Recent opinion poll.
450. Anxieties over pregnancy risks are lessened by recent reports. *Journal of the American Medical Association*, 261: 9 (1989): 1289–1294. See also Chapter 4 p 98.
451. *Independent* (18 May 1993): 13 and *American Journal of Public Health*, 83 (1993): 4, 574.
452. Voluntary Euthanasia Society opinion poll (1987) showed 30% of family doctors in favour of legalisation—twice the 1985 figure. British Medical Association and House of Lords Committee against.
453. Samaritans had record numbers of calls recently.
454. *AIDSFILE*, 2: 1 (1987): 6–7.
455. The fact that true depression always lifts has made it specially difficult to evaluate anti-depressant drugs, counselling, or anything else.
456. A hospice or palliative care team will usually provide patients, their friends and families, their doctors and nurses with a twenty-four-hour telephone number for help and advice.
457. Regular injections should now be a thing of the past with the new Graseby syringe driver. This is a large matchbox-sized, battery-operated device which holds a syringe containing all the medicines needed for twenty-four hours. The medicine drips in slowly under the skin through a minute needle and thin tube. Unlike big tubes in veins it is comfortable and can remain in place for a long time. These can be set up by a nurse at home or in hospital. Painkillers and sickness medicine are ideally given this way. However, many anti-AIDS drugs have to be given via a different route, into a large vein.
458. He passed away peacefully with champagne on his lips a week later.
459. Medical Education Trust meeting in London (April 1987) came out strongly against euthanasia and advocated more widespread hospice care. In March 1994 the House of Lords rejected new laws.

460. *New England Journal of Medicine*, 318: 15 (1988): 984–988.

461. As experience of doctors grows I hope many tests can be avoided. With any new disease the tendency is always to investigate first and consider options afterwards. After a while common sense prevails and tests are done not to extend understanding of the disease, but only to enable correct treatment to be given. San Francisco now has excellent results in terms of patients' length of survival, with drastically fewer procedures. Hospital stays are greatly shortened (average eight days), and people spend much longer at home (see p. 393).

462. A sample Living Will has been proposed for those with AIDS by the Terrence Higgins Trust. *Guardian* (8 September 1992).

463. This position is also supported by the Catholic Church.

464. Up to thirty-six times more likely to commit suicide than general population. *Journal of the American Medical Association*, 259: 9 (1988): 1333–1337, sixty-six times in Cornell University study 1990.

465. A man: *Independent* (14 March 1987). A man—also shot wife and son; and a woman—also killed husband and children: *The Times* (2 May 1987). Saliva testing—see p 124.

466. There is an antidote but it must be given within a few hours of taking the tablets. There has been some discussion about adding tiny doses of antidote to every tablet sold. It is surprising that such a lethal drug should be so widely available. The reason is that when the correct dose is taken, or higher doses are taken under medical supervision, it is one of the safest painkillers available. It also has virtually no side-effects such as drowsiness or constipation. Figures from Guy's Hospital Poison Centre.

467. Annual representative meeting of the British Medical Association (BMA) rejected World Health Organisation and DSS advice to pass the motion 'that testing for HIV antibody should be at the discretion of the patient's doctor, and should not necessarily require the consent of the patient'. BMA Chairman Dr John Marks has warned that patients could sue for assault (taking blood without consent) and doctors could be brought before the General Medical Council for discipline. It was also agreed that a result would not be passed on to other doctors without consent. BMA and GMC guidelines available in *British Medical Journal*, 295 (1987): 73–74. The Medical Defence Union (MDU) says a doctor will not be prosecuted for informing a family doctor of a positive result without agreement from the patient so long as the family doctor needs the information to prevent the spread of disease or to treat the patient. *Journal of Medical Defence Union*, 2 (1986): 21–22.

468. Fraud: insurance companies are getting scared. They think there have

been several cases where someone has known he is positive, or been almost certain, and has taken out a massive life insurance policy. The family doctor, of course, for reasons discussed earlier is totally unaware of the diagnosis—often even if his patient has full-blown AIDS. The insurance company gets a letter saying the patient is fit and has not been having medical treatment for any condition and issues the policy. Several instances are being investigated. In one case the company was convinced that $630,000 paid to the homosexual lover was for a man who died of AIDS and that it was the result of false information on the original policy. However, because the hospital refused to give any information and the death certificate said 'pneumonia'—as it usually does—nothing could be checked. California and Washington, DC have already made it illegal for insurers to use HIV antibody tests, but most UK insurance companies insist on HIV tests for policies over a certain value. BUPA and Private Patients Plan have paid for private medical care for a few people with AIDS but only where they were certain the policy started before infection was known. *Today* (13 January 1987). In the future, BUPA will not pay for AIDS care where the person has been insured for less than five years, and Private Patients Plan will only pay for initial diagnosis and treatment. *Sunday Telegraph* (5 July 1987). Insurance companies responded in 1988 by increasing premiums for Life cover by up to three times previous rates. While this may have been a cautious but necessary approach in the light of the worst estimates for spread in 1987, no company has reduced premiums since. *Independent on Sunday* (9 May 1993). By 1992, British Life Insurance Companies had already paid out £31.3 million on deaths from AIDS. One policy was for £2 million. *Daily Express* (11 June 1992).

469. *Canadian Medical Association Journal*, 139: 15 (1988): 287–288; also *New England Journal of Medicine*, 319: 15 (1988): 1010–1012. Articles outline the debate in greater detail.

470. Survey showed hospital consultants confused over legal requirements and options. *Lancet*, 1 (1987): 26–28. See endnote 488.

471. A gay doctor writes that he would inform a hospital if admitted for an operation that he could have AIDS, but would expect the surgeon to be fired if he refused to operate. *British Medical Journal*, 294 (1987): 647. See also glossary for description of sex change operations and some issues involved. Ethical code for physicians regarding treatment of people with AIDS: *Journal of the American Medical Association*, 259: 4 (1988): 1360–1361.

472. 'AIDS: A Bill of Rights for the Surgical Team', *British Medical Journal*, 296 (1988): 490.

473. *Canadian Medical Association Journal*, 138 (1988): 6, 490.

474. *AIDS Newsletter*, vol. 8, issue 3 (1993): 1, editorial.

475. *Morbidity and Mortality Weekly Report*, 41 (1992): 43, 823–825 and CDSC 1993.

476. A large United States study concluded that only a third of such accidents were preventable. *New England Journal of Medicine*, 314 (1986): 1127–1132. If minor, each accident may only transmit infection in one out of 200 cases, but the catalogue of accidents is going to become enormous as the number of people needing treatment for AIDS continues to rise rapidly.

477. *Guardian* (5 January 1987). Report on BBC fourteen-point plan to prevent spread of AIDS. A laboratory worker at the Royal Hallamshire Hospital in Sheffield was suspended after refusing to handle blood samples he thought could be infected. *The Times* (24 December 1986).

478. AIDS risk for NHS staff greater outside work. *Health and Safety Journal*, 97 (1987): 33.

479. *Morbidity and Mortality Weekly Report*, 41 (1992): 43, 823–825.

480. *New York Times* (18 May 1993): A1.

481. Ealing Health Authority guidelines ICP23 (November 1986) for operating theatres: 'Ideally the theatre should be allowed to "rest" for at least twelve hours following the operation'—allows fine aerosol mists to settle. 'Student nurses and medical students should be excluded . . . After the operation the theatre should be thoroughly cleaned with hot water and detergent. All surfaces should be wiped with detergent hypochlorate.' Such procedures are unworkable in busy hospitals where HIV infection rates are significant. Similar rules exist for X-ray departments. Some argue that testing does not rule out infection completely. True, but it picks up the majority—after all, testing blood is worthwhile and very few infected donations are missed.

482. *British Medical Journal*, 294 (1987): 44.

483. *British Medical Journal*, 305 (18 July 1992): 106–107.

484. *International Herald Tribune* (11 February 1993): 3.

485. *Journal of Occupational Medicine*, 30: 7 (1988): 578–579; AIDS guidelines for occupational physicians. Employers who breach confidentiality may face charges of invasion of privacy, defamation and intentional infliction of emotional distress with heavy fines. *Occupational Health and Safety*, 57: 7 (1988): 12–19; 31. See p 112.

486. *International Herald Tribune* (2 February 1988): 4.

487. *Today* (4 February 1987).

488. Act of Parliament—Public Health (Control of Disease) Act (1984) and Public Health (Infectious Disease) regulations (1985 and 1988).

489. *The Times* (21 March 1987).

490. *Daily Telegraph* (23 June 1992): 1 and *Guardian* (24 June 1992): 1, 3, 18–19.
491. *The Times* (23 March 1987).
492. *Lancet*, 340 (12 September 1992): 678. Pregnancy risks p 98–99.
493. *Law Society Gazette* (25 March 1987). It is now a crime for a doctor not to inform a spouse in some parts of the United States.
494. *New England Journal of Medicine*, 316: 16 (1987): 1924.
495. 'Partner notification for HIV infection': London Department of Health PL/CO (92) 5 (1992).
496. *Lancet*, 1 (1987): 982–983. Reports twenty-one instances in one London clinic alone.
497. *British Medical Journal*, 306 (9 January 1993): 87.
498. 'Summary of AIDS Law Worldwide', *AIDS-Forschung*, 1: 9 (1986): 505–513.
499. Two lawyers have suggested liability to prosecution under the British Offences Against the Persons Act of 1861 for 'maliciously administering any poison or other destructive and noxious thing'.
500. *Independent* (21 August 1987).
501. *Sunday Express* (11 January 1987).
502. *Sunday Express* (7 June 1987).
503. *AIDS-Forschung*, 2: 11 (1987): 648–651. Munich court judgement.
504. *Nature*, 361 (18 February 1993): 595–596. Also *New Scientist* (20 March 1993): 5.
505. *Independent* (18 February 1993). Also *New Scientist* (20 February 1993): 2 and *Nature*, 361 (18 February 1993): 595–596.
506. *British Journal of Hospital Medicine*; also *The Times* (15 July 1987). Many prostitutes insist on clients using condoms but often a two-tier pricing system exists—if you want it without, you pay more. *Health Education Journal*, 46: 2 (August 1987): 71–73.
507. *International Herald Tribune* (13–14 February 1993): 2. See p 329.
508. *Sunday Times* (21 February 1993).
509. *Guardian* (19 February 1993).
510. *Le Monde* (28 January 1993).
511. Portland Oregan Reuters Report (25 November 1992).
512. 'Identity Cards for People Infected with HIV?', *British Medical Journal*, 294 (1987): 772. See also endnote 513.
513. *Morbidity and Mortality Weekly Report*, 41 (1992): 19, 344–346. Survey of all published and unpublished US data on infected health care workers. In addition to the Florida dentist, by 13 May 1992 CDC had heard of 15,795 test results on patients treated by thirty-two infected care workers. No infected patients were found in 10,270 treated by twenty-three of the thirty-two. Not surprisingly, HIV was

found among the others—you would expect so because HIV is in the general population. Eighty-four were infected. Follow-up is complete on forty-seven: seven had risk factors (eg drug injector), five were previously infected and the remaining thirty-five were prisoners. Risk factors were present in thirty-three, leaving a question-mark over two. Of the other forty-seven of the eighty-four infected patients, a question-mark exists over patients of two dentists: seventeen of one dentist and one from another are having HIV genetic sequences analysed. Results awaited (May 1994).

514. *Guardian* (7 April 1993): 2 and *Daily Telegraph* (7 April 1993): 4.
515. *Lancet*, 341 (20 March 1993): 764. See endnote 513.
516. *Daily Telegraph* (7 October 1993): 1. Three patients infected.
517. *Morbidity and Mortality Weekly Report*, 40 (1991): 23, 377–381.
518. Department of Health AIDS/HIV infected health care workers (interim) (1993).
519. *Lancet*, 341 (29 May 1993): 140. Also, *GMC News Review* (1993): 3.
520. *Journal of American Medical Association*, 276 (1992): 1100–1105. CDC figures USA. UK HIV neg blood transfusion—1 in million.
521. Expert Advisory Group on AIDS. AIDS/HIV Infected Health Care Workers: practical guidance on notifying patients (Department of Health, 1993). Department of Health Executive Letter EL (93) 24 (1993).
522. *Daily Telegraph* (7 July 1992): 4.
523. *The Times* (7 July 1992): 6.
524. 1956 Sexual Offences Act. The Contagious Diseases Act of 1864 allowed police to arrest, forcibly examine and register anyone they thought was a prostitute, designed to ensure healthy prostitutes for servicemen. It led to great brutality and was repealed in 1886, after a twenty-year campaign by the leading feminist Josephine Butler. Today, the Josephine Butler Society does not support legalising brothels to control sexually-transmitted diseases, taking the view that it will only stimulate international trafficking in people and a lawful market for prostitution.
525. *The Times* (7 July 1992): 6.
526. *European* (2–8 April 1992): 5.
527. *Guardian* (16 June 1992): 12.
528. *Nature*, 359 (3 September 1992): 2.
529. *Guardian* (20 August 1993) quoting survey by the UK gay activist group Outrage—campaign to lower age from 21 to 16.
530. 'Because of this, God gave them over to shameful lusts. Even their women exchanged natural relations with women and were inflamed with lust for one another. Men committed indecent acts with men and

received in themselves the due penalty for their perversion' (Romans 1: 26–27). See also endnote 550.

531. *Ottawa Citizen* (3 May 1992): A9.

532. *Daily Telegraph* (3 June 1992): 12.

533. One of these pronouncements came from the Church Society: 'AIDS and the Judgement of God' (July 1987). It states, 'Twice in the AIDS debate, in two separate evangelical publications, it has been written that God does not "zap" individuals. The Bible witness is that he sometimes does.' The report stresses the 'sinful nature of homosexual practices' and that God does judge 'here and now'. The United States Bishops of the United Methodist Church disagree—God does not 'wage germ warfare on the human family'. *International Herald Tribune* (9 May 1988).

534. *Le Monde* (9 February 1993) and *Guardian* (11 February 1993): 8.

535. *Ibid.*

536. The exact words recorded in Greek are, 'Let the sinless one cast the first stone.' Translated in the New International Version of the Bible as: 'If any one of you is without sin, let him be the first to throw a stone at her.' You can read this story in John 8: 1–11.

537. Literally, 'From now, no longer sin' (John 8: 11, New English Bible).

538. 'You have heard that it was said to the people long ago, "Do not commit adultery." But I tell you that anyone who looks at a woman lustfully has already committed adultery with her in his heart' (Matthew 5: 27–28).

539. 'You have heard that it was said to the people long ago, "Do not murder, and anyone who murders will be subject to judgment." But I tell you that anyone who is angry with his brother will be subject to judgment' (Matthew 5: 21–22).

540. 'For the words that the mouth utters come from the overflowing of the heart' (Matthew 12: 34, New English Bible). This is not to say that all wrongdoing is treated the same by God: Scripture shows clearly that some actions and attitudes particularly invoke his anger. We are not looking here at God's reactions in his holy judgement, but at the right of mortal, imperfect humans to stand on a pedestal and condemn others.

541. 'For all have sinned and fall short of the glory of God' (Romans 3: 23).

542. 'Because he himself suffered when he was tempted, he is able to help those who are being tempted' (Hebrews 2: 18).

543. 'But you are a chosen people, a royal priesthood, a holy nation, a people belonging to God, that you may declare the praises of him who called you out of darkness into his wonderful light' (1 Peter 2: 9).

544. 'I urge you to live a life worthy of the calling you have received' (Ephesians 4: 1).

545. 1 Timothy 3: 2–15. The one exception in the list is being 'able to teach'.

546. 'Jesus answered them: "It is not the healthy who need a doctor, but the sick. I have not come to call the righteous, but sinners to repentance"' (Luke 5: 31–32).

547. Luke 23: 43. God's forgiveness when we are truly sorry is absolute.

548. Genesis 12–23.

549. Genesis 2: 24; Matthew 19: 4–6; 1 Corinthians 6: 16.

550. There are those who quote from the Bible (eg, Romans 1: 26–27) to argue that certain sexual sins are particularly abhorrent to God. (See page 209 of this chapter.) The day we start ranking our own or others' sins in some kind of scale of sinfulness is the day we attempt to make God's grace null and void. 'I only lied, cheated, and stole—I didn't commit buggery. I am a reasonably good-natured sort of person—I *deserve* to go to heaven.' The Bible teaches that separation is separation. Even the most humanly perfect person is so imperfect as to be impossibly separated. The only exception is Jesus. You need to read the story again about the woman caught in adultery. There was no such grading in Jesus' mind when he rebuked the crowd. Read the rest of Romans 1: the rest of the list includes gossip and jealousy—but we ignore these. The vital phrase, 'giving them over', is used in verses 24, 26 and 28—not just of sexual sin. The basis of God's anger is explained in verse 21: 'They know God, but do not give him the honour that belongs to him' (Good News Bible). See endnote 567.

551. John 14: 6. Also see Acts 4: 12.

552. 'For it is by grace you have been saved, through faith—and this not from yourselves, it is the gift of God—not by works, so that no one can boast' (Ephesians 2: 8–9).

553. 'Therefore, if anyone is in Christ, he is a new creation; the old has gone, the new has come!' (2 Corinthians 5: 17).

554. John 3: 3.

555. Romans 6: 8.

556. Romans 6: 3–4.

557. Galatians 2: 20, New English Bible.

558. No. They weren't amazed because he'd cut his hair and started wearing a suit. His appearance was exactly the same but something *inside* had changed. The church is so good at sucking people in and pushing identical people out at the other end; same jokes, same dress, same mannerisms. The Christian ghetto rules. The day that happens in my church I want out!

559. Romans 7: 14–25. For discussion of Holy Spirit, see page 238.

560. 1 Corinthians 10: 13; Philippians 4: 13.

561. John 4: 4–30.
562. Luke 19: 45; Matthew 21: 12–13; Mark 11: 15–16.
563. Greek word used is *Ek-ballo*—literally 'to throw out'.
564. Luke 10: 25–37.
565. 'You have heard that it was said, "Love your neighbour and hate your enemy." But I tell you, love your enemies and pray for those who persecute you, that you may be sons of your Father in heaven' (Matthew 5: 43–45).
566. 'He is patient with you, not wanting anyone to perish, but everyone to come to repentance' (2 Peter 3: 9).
567. Acts 4: 12. Separation is the consequence of going our own way and is, I believe, the so-called penalty mentioned in Romans 1: 26–27.
568. 'This will happen when the Lord Jesus is revealed from heaven in blazing fire with his powerful angels. He will punish those who do not know God and do not obey the gospel of our Lord Jesus. They will be punished with everlasting destruction and shut out from the presence of the Lord and from the majesty of his power on the day he comes to be glorified in his holy people and to be marvelled at among all those who have believed' (2 Thessalonians 1: 7–10).
569. Galatians 6: 7.
570. Ephesians 1: 10.
571. 2 Peter 3: 9.
572. Matthew 12: 36.
573. Luke 9: 24, New English Bible.
574. Mark 9: 47, New English Bible.
575. John 1: 12; Romans 8: 14–17.
576. 'But among you there must not be even a hint of sexual immorality, or of any kind of impurity, or of greed, because these are improper for God's holy people' (Ephesians 5: 3–5).
577. 1 Corinthians 7: 32–37.
578. This is a large but incomplete list. The reason I have given it is that many people have never really understood what the Bible says on these subjects.
    (a) Adultery: Exodus 20: 14; Leviticus 20: 10; Job 24: 15; Matthew 5: 27; 19: 9; Romans 7: 3; 1 Corinthians 6: 9; 2 Peter 2: 14.
    (b) Sex outside marriage (general references): Matthew 5: 28; Romans 1: 24; 6: 19; Ephesians 4: 19; 5: 3; Colossians 3: 5; 1 Thessalonians 4: 7; Hebrews 13: 4; 2 Peter 2: 10. *Specific references*: Matthew 5: 32; Acts 15: 29; 1 Corinthians 5: 1; 6: 18; 7: 2; 10: 8; 1 Thessalonians 4: 3.
    (c) Bad attitudes (lust): Proverbs 6: 25; Matthew 5: 28; Galatians 5: 16; Colossians 3: 5; 1 Thessalonians 4: 5; 2 Timothy 2: 22; James 1:

15; 1 Peter 2: 11.

(d) Homosexual practices as a type of sex outside marriage: Genesis 19; Leviticus 18: 22; 20: 13; Judges 19: 22; Romans 1: 27; 1 Corinthians 6: 9; 1 Timothy 1: 10; 2 Peter 2: 4–10; Jude 7.

579. Ephesians 4: 26.

580. Ephesians 5: 18.

581. 1 Corinthians 13.

582. 'If we say that we have no sin, we are only fooling ourselves, and refusing to accept the truth. But if we confess our sins to him, he can be depended on to forgive us and to cleanse us from every wrong' (1 John 1: 8–9, The Living Bible).

583. I suggested diamorphine for breathlessness—safe if properly used.

584. Practice altered today—most places allow viewing of body.

585. Culture I was brought up in. Further discussion in Chapter 8.

586. Imagine the fuss if I had been taking pictures of what happens in a crematorium—of what really happens on the other side of the curtain.

587. Philippians 3: 8–14.

588. Philippians 1: 27.

589. For example, John Wimber's *Power Healing* (Hodder & Stoughton, 1986). A surprisingly balanced book on exercising the gift of healing. Wimber has had an enormous influence on churches as part of the so-called 'charismatic renewal' with its emphasis on God working here and now in supernatural ways. Many rapidly-growing churches have a strong charismatic influence, regardless of their denominational labels.

590. For example, a quote from 'Love and Action' newsletter, September 1993 (Annapolis US): 'Richard has been healed of all pain. . . . He is waiting in faith for confirmation of total healing from AIDS from his doctor.'

591. Matthew 24: 1–31; Revelation 21: 1–4.

592. Matthew 4: 17.

593. John 15: 7.

594. Elizabeth Burnham, *When Your Friend Is Dying* (Kingsway, 1982) is a first-hand account of being on the receiving end.

595. Cadaveric instrumentation is widely practised. The argument is that the patient has died and practising the technique could save a life. The veins usually used for injections empty of blood when the heart stops so are hard to find. Occasionally the only way to inject a drug to try and start the heart again is into a vein deep inside the body. Getting a needle in the right place can be hard. Here is my personal view:

(a) If the patient is dead, then ethically it is not right to experiment without permission of next of kin.

(b) If, as I believe, the patient is usually still dying, then I should act according to what I think the patient would prefer.

(c) The technique is usually practised furtively, in haste, behind closed curtains, with an eye over the shoulder in case relatives arrive. This is not ethical behaviour.

(d) The test is this: Would you ever be able to confess to relatives that you had carried on jabbing, etc, for practice, or would they be too distressed at the thought?

(e) Instrumentation in this way distracts the team from changing gear. It prevents a peaceful death. It robs the patient of a last moment or two of dignity. It delays the introduction of a spouse to the dying patient.

(f) If no relatives or close friends are present outside, I think it permissible for the junior doctor concerned to *ask* any other team member remaining if he or she minds. If permission is granted then one or two brief attempts only and then call it a day. Intubation is easily practised in medical school seven days a week. Subclavian cannulation (inserting a plastic tube into a vein under the shoulder bone to administer drugs during cardiac arrest) is not such a tremendous technique in an arrest. In most cases it will not affect the outcome. I do not think it necessary for every junior in a big hospital to practise this on corpses. Doctors would do *far* better to practise heart massage. A recent study showed that the vast majority of fully qualified hospital doctors could not even massage the heart adequately enough to prevent brain damage (Royal College of Physicians: 'Resuscitation from Cardiopulmonary Arrest.' Training and Organisation. Report July 1987). No wonder so many attempts result in failure: too many doctors being too clever with too many fancy drugs and needles. This is yet another example of appalling lack of common sense in medicine.

We should stand for the rights of the patient, and should show our colleagues that the moments of dying are hallowed ground.

596. Luke 23:40–43.

597. Matthew 19: 30; 20: 16; Mark 9: 35; Luke 13: 30.

598. 'Repentance' literally means in Greek to 'turn back' or 'turn around'.

599. See Chapter 9 for further discussion of supernatural healing.

600. Luke 10: 25–37—the Good Samaritan.

601. Matthew 5: 46.

602. Matthew 5: 44.

603. Luke 10: 25–37.

604. 2 Corinthians 2: 14–16; Galatians 2: 20.

605. 2 Corinthians 2: 15–16. Paul writes that this aroma is the smell of death to those who are perishing, but to those who are being saved it is the fragrance of life.

606. *Pediatrics*, 90 (1992): 3, 482.

607. ACET-linked project in Mbale, Uganda.

608. Total UK spending on AIDS exceeded £200 million in 1993, equivalent to around $300 million. In the same year the entire WHO GPA budget ran on $180 million. UK government figure and WHO press release (15/29 January 1993).

609. WHO press release (June 1993).

610. *Ibid.*

611. World Health Organisation figures (February 1993). See also endnote 613.

612. A doctor in Uganda can earn as little as £25 per month. The annual average UK cost of HIV/AIDS is £5123—or £26 to £261 (HIV), £43 to £2312 (AIDS) per month. *Journal of Public Health Medicine* 15 (1993) 3, 235–242.

613. Many African nations spend £1.50 per person on health per year.

614. UNICEF, *State of the World's Children* (OUP, 1991).

615. *British Medical Journal*, 304 (1992): 388 and Christian Aid figures (1991) 'Banking on the Poor'.

616. Report by the World Bank at the IXth International AIDS Conference in Berlin, June 1993. 'Swaps Against AIDS' is part of the Debt for Development Coalition, funded by USAID. $1 million has already been swapped for programmes in Kenya, Tanzania and Zambia.

617. World Health Organisation figures. Probably a gross underestimate considering the size of the world population. The population of India alone is around 700 million, of which 350 million are adults. How many acts of sexual intercourse take place in that country alone every day? If 70 million couples have sex on average twice a week, then around 20 million couples a day will be having sex. WHO reckons only 100 million for the whole world.

618. If there are countries where it is banned, I am not aware.

619. *New Scientist* (27 February 1993): 12–13.

620. International Planned Parenthood Foundation (IPPF) Medical Bulletin, 26 (1992): 3, 1–3 reporting on Malawi Project which saw condom distribution rise from 3,000 to 600,000 per year.

621. WHO press release (June 1993).

622. *Sexual Behaviour and AIDS in Britain* (HMSO, February 1993).

623. *Sexually Transmitted Diseases*, 19 (1992): 6, 331–334.

624. Research presented by Dr Ekrhardt, New York, at the IXth International AIDS Conference, Berlin, June 1993.

625. Report by Uganda AIDS Control Programme (1993).

626. Research presented by Dr Ekrhardt, New York, at the IXth International AIDS Conference, Berlin, June 1993.

627. Professor John Guillebaud (Margaret Pyke Centre, London) presented

UK findings at a 1992 conference on sexual behaviour. Also *Canadian Medical Association Journal* 149 (1993) 5, 691–696.

628. See *National Symposium on Teenage Sexuality* report (Agape, 20 May 1991). Marc Europe is now Christian Research Association.

629. Marc Europe survey (1991) of 1,729 attenders of 150 church youth clubs across the denominations. See endnote 628.

630. 'Sexual Behaviour and AIDS in Britain', survey of 1,289 men and 1,241 women of all ages; of which less than 1,000 were under twenty years. Figures taken from cumulative sexual initiations of males and females born 1970–76. Average used for each. See figs. 12.3 and 12.4 on p. 123 of the survey. Published by HMSO 1993.

631. This is my understanding of Genesis 1: 26–2: 24 and Song of Songs, a celebration of erotic love. 'There is a frank and open delight in physical attraction, which underlines the fact that God intends man to enjoy physical love within the laws he has given' (*[Lion Bible Handbook*, 1973], p. 376).

632. By 'sexuality' I mean our nature as sexual beings and the feelings we have towards others, that may or may not be expressed sexually.

633. *British Medical Journal*, 305 (11 July 1992): 70–71. Editorial calling for focus of HIV health campaigns to shift to schools.

634. *Morbidity and Mortality Weekly Report*, 41 (1992): 46, 866–868.

635. An estimate from ABI based on demand for the ACET/ABI schools materials. 600,000 colour booklets distributed over 30 months.

636. In the UK such laws include the various education acts requiring sex education to be carried out 'in such a manner as to encourage pupils to have regard to moral considerations and the value of family life' (Education [No. 2] Act 1986, section 46, and also clause 28 of a more recent Act preventing the promotion of homosexual practice in schools).

637. *British Medical Journal*, 305 (8 August 1992): 362–363. Correspondent condemns such an approach as misguided and intolerant of more traditional viewpoints.

638. *The Sun* (29 October 1991) and confirmed to ACET educator during a subsequent visit.

639. 'HIV/AIDS and Sex Education for Young People.' UK All-Party Parliamentary Group on AIDS (occasional paper) 1992, No. 3.

640. WHO presentation by Gary Slutkin at the VIIIth International AIDS Conference—see *AIDS Newsletter*, 7 (1992): 12, 8.

641. In some parts of the UK we have schools workers available, but no home care as yet. Our educators are still involved in caring for those with AIDS in other places, even if on an occasional basis. The personal care factor is always at the heart of what we do.

642. *Journal of School Health*, 62 (1992): 4, 121–5.
643. ACET/Association of British Insurers' figures (1994).
644. ACET UK survey (1991).
645. I met several representatives when advising members of the House of Lords about how they should respond.
646. We need to respect those with sincere convictions, even if we may take a different view. That is how we would all like to be treated ourselves. I have some sympathy with their concerns. My wife and I consider it part of our own parenting role to educate our children about the facts of life, among other things. We also agree that certain teachers can present sex or AIDS in a very mechanistic way, but the government guidelines are clear—"in the context of family life . . . in a moral framework".
647. *Health Education Quarterly*, 17 (1990): 1, 37–51.
648. *Journal of American Academy of Nurse Practitioners*, 3 (1991): 3, 122–8.
649. *Health Education Journal*, 50 (1991): 4, 155–160.
650. *Sexual Behaviour and AIDS in Britain* (HMSO, 1993).
651. *American Journal of Public Health*, 81 (1991): 12, 1596–1601.
652. *AIDS*, 7 (1993): 1, 121–125.
653. *British Medical Journal*, 305 (5 September 1992): 586.
654. Personal communication with ACET educators.
655. *AIDS Care*, 4 (1992): 3, 245–258.
656. *Preventative Medicine*, 20 (1991): 3, 414–430.
657. *Journal of Public Health*, 59 (1989): 6, 246–50.
658. *Journal of School Health*, 59 (1989): 6, 255–263.
659. *Journal of School Health*, 60 (1990): 7, 379–382.
660. *American Journal of Public Health*, 82 (1992): 6, 827–834.
661. Education (no. 2) Act 1986, section 46.
662. *Gynaecology Illustrated* (Churchill Livingstone 1978) p 187.
663. 16 cases per 100,000 per year. Herpes simplex type 2 implicated.
664. *WHO Features*, 152 (December 1990).
665. National Survey of Health and Development (LandMARC, summer 1992). See also *Children in the Middle*, Ann Mitchell (Tavistock, 1985).
666. Population Trends OPCS Household Survey (1992). See also *Birmingham Evening Mail* (19 June 1992).
667. Glasgow, for example. *British Medical Journal*, 305 (October 1992): 3, 801–804.
668. *American Journal of Public Health*, 81 (1991): 5, 617–619. Within nine weeks of distribution, only 61% of needles were returned to one San Francisco project.

669. *American Journal of Public Health*, 81 (1991): 11, 1506–1517.

670. Matthew 7: 1–2.

671. 'Here is a glutton and a drunkard, a friend of tax collectors and sinners' (Matthew 11: 19). 'If this man were a prophet, he would know who is touching him and what kind of woman she is—that she is a sinner' (Luke 7: 39).

672. I cannot justify this statement in statistical terms, but only anecdotally through my own professional contacts. The Christian Medical Fellowship in the UK regularly holds conferences addressing such matters.

673. *AIDS*, 4 (1990): 11, 1153–1155.

674. *Independent* (15 October 1991): 16.

675. Such reports are widely circulating in parts of Asia, but remain unconfirmed.

676. Jackie Pullinger, *Chasing the Dragon* (Hodder & Stoughton).

677. This has been the situation in Spain, where large numbers of ex-drug addicts now live in Christian communities. These are now facing the loss of key leaders and community workers who are ill and dying as a result of previously acquired HIV. (Personal communications.)

678. Small disposable kits for testing blood or others' secretions have been made by Abbott Laboratories in the UK for several years. Excellent results have been obtained using a special device to collect saliva. Many insurance companies and research projects now test for HIV using saliva on a routine basis. Recently I was shown a prototype device to collect saliva into a tube. At the end was a special marker system which was designed to show up positive or negative after around a minute. See also Chapter 5, p 124.

679. Recent reports from Malawi.

680. Personal communication.

681. *Morbidity and Mortality Weekly Report*, 40 (1991): RR–8, 1–9.

682. *Ibid.* The figure of one in five for hepatitis B transmission following accidental exposure is more widely quoted.

683. Personal communications with many expatriate missionary doctors in African countries, confirmed by numerous published reports. The incidence is higher than in the general population, for obvious reasons: HIV infection makes it more likely they will be unwell from a wide variety of other conditions.

684. *British Medical Journal*, 302 (5 January 1991): 51.

685. *New England Journal of Medicine*, 327 (1992): 1461. In four months of using blunt needles there were no accidents of any kind. However, getting hold of sufficiently blunt needles was very difficult and expensive.

686. Three cases of nurses in accident and emergency or midwifery in Africa—studied in the UK. *British Medical Journal*, 305 (19 September 1992): 713.

687. *Ibid.*

688. *The Times* (1 April 1993): 5.

689. *Toronto Star* (17 February 1989).

690. Conservative estimate is $80,000 per patient. *Science USA*, 239 (5 February 1988): 604–610. Some argue that there are no hospital costs: the bed is there anyway; all that happens is that it is filled by someone with AIDS rather than someone with heart disease. Early on when numbers of people with AIDS are small that may be true, but we are already at the stage of planning extra beds which otherwise would not have existed or would have been closed, as a result of AIDS, and the epidemic's effects have hardly begun.

691. Study after study shows that person-to-person education works—especially when peer led, or when educators can relate well to the target audience. *AIDS Newsletter*, 7: 12 (1992): 20. See also Chapter 12.

692. Twelve million dollars in federal funds has established thirteen Regional Education and Training Centres to train health care providers. *Journal of the American Medical Association*, 260: 4 (1988): 2016; also *Morbidity and Mortality Weekly Report* (guidelines for schools), 37: S2 (1988).

693. *Pediatrics*, 82: 2 (1988): 278–280 (American Academy of Pediatrics Committee on School Health).

694. This has always been so for courses on other subjects before AIDS. A Bradford conference for family doctors on AIDS was attended by only ten. *The Times* (24 April 1987).

695. *New York Times* (22 September 1987). Reported fifty-eight homeless in New York hospitals with AIDS. Most needed practical help at home or nursing care. Shortages exist in the community of places and of case-workers to help place people. The situation is far worse today.

696. WHO budget 1993 for AIDS: $175 million (WHO figures—30 April 1993). UK budget 1993 for AIDS: £250 million (*Sunday Times*—9 May 1993). Calculation varies with exchange rates.

697. John 8: 12.

698. John 1: 5.

699. Matthew 5: 16.

700. Matthew 5: 15.

701. Personal communication from a participant.

702. 'Indeed, when Gentiles [unbelievers], who do not have the law, do by nature things required by the law, they are a law for themselves, even

though they do not have the law, since they show that the requirements of the law are written on their hearts, their consciences also bearing witness, and their thoughts now accusing, now even defending them' (Romans 2: 14–15).

703. 1 Corinthians 12: 12–13.
704. John 13: 34–35; 17: 20–21.
705. March for Jesus on 24 June 1994—a global march for millions across every time zone, dozens of nations. Previous marches each year have drawn hundreds of thousands across nations to walk, pray and worship in the open air. Just another pointer to a new spiritual awakening across the globe.
706. Matthew 22: 21; 17: 24–26.
707. Jim Montgomery, *Dawn 2000—7 million churches to go* (Highland Books). Decision by UK denominational leaders to plant 20,000 new churches across the country was made in 1992.
708. Term first introduced by Freudenberger in 1974. *Journal of Social Issues*, 30 (1984): 159–165; *British Medical Journal*, 295 (1987): 284–285.
709. John 11: 35.
710. See 'Withholding treatment', p. 184.
711. 'Healthy People 2000: National Health Promotion and Disease Prevention Objectives', Public Health Reports (1991), 106 (6): 602–603.
712. *British Medical Journal*, 305 (18 July 1992): 135–136.
713. UK government 'Health for the Nation' (1993).
714. Figures obtained from the World Health Organisation and Centre for Disease Control.
715. *Weekly Epidemiological Record*, 27 (2 July 1993).
716. Source: World Health Organisation (May 1994).
717. *Ibid.*
718. *Journal of the American Medical Association* (1992), 268(4): 445–446.

Index

ACET
AIDS Care, Education and Training

ACET is a Christian agency directly involved in the prevention of HIV and in the practical care of those affected by it.

ACET works on behalf of individuals and communities on the basis of their need for HIV/AIDS care, education or training.

ACET, through direct opportunities, partners or associates, trained staff and volunteers, provides:

- Practical care to children, women and men at home with HIV/ AIDS related illnesses, enabling them to live and die in their own homes if that is their wish.
- Youth and schools HIV/AIDS education programmes.
- Training and resources on HIV/AIDS related issues.
- Advocacy, media and policy initiatives on HIV/AIDS issues, including publications and information.

ACET's care, education and prevention initiatives are carried out around the world by ACET Operations Staff and volunteers, ACET Partners or ACET Associates. It has offices in England, Scotland, Ireland, East Africa, Eastern Europe, South East Asia, and has provided resources and training to a number of agencies in several countries.

ACET can provide support, training and materials to churches, groups and individuals who are concerned about HIV/AIDS. ACET does not make financial grants or payments to other projects.

For further information please contact: ACET Central Office
PO Box 3693
London SW15 2BQ
United Kingdom